Until the Cure

Yale University Press   New Haven and London

Until the Cure

Caring for Women with HIV

Edited by Ann Kurth

Foreword by Jonathan Mann, M.D.

Published on the foundation established in memory of William
Chauncey Williams of the Class of 1822, Yale Medical School, and of
William Cook Williams of the Class of 1850, Yale Medical School.

Designed by Deborah Dutton.

Set in Times Roman type by The Composing Room
of Michigan, Inc.

Printed in the United States of America by Vail-Ballou Press,
Binghamton, New York.

Library of Congress Cataloging-in-Publication Data

Until the cure : caring for women with HIV / edited by Ann Kurth ;
    foreword by Jonathan Mann.
        p.   cm. — (A Yale fastback)
    Includes bibliographical references and index.
    ISBN 0-300-05806-3 (cloth : alk. paper). — ISBN 0-300-05835-7
(paper : alk. paper)
    1. AIDS (Disease)   2. Women—Medical care.   I. Kurth, Ann,
    1961– .   II. Series.
    [DNLM: 1. HIV Infections.   2. Women's Health.   3. Women's
Health Services. WD 308 U61 1993]
    RC607.A26U58   1993
    362.1'9697'92—dc20
    DNLM/DLC
    for Library of Congress   93-5550
                                                                   CIP

A catalogue record for this book is available from the British Library.

The paper in this book meets the guidelines for permanence and
durability of the Committee on Production Guidelines for Book
Longevity of the Council on Library Resources.

10   9   8   7   6   5   4   3   2   1

To B. E. K.,
sine qua non

Grateful thanks to Frankie, "Cheryl," Sylvia, "Terry Ann," Grace, Mary, "Patty," Gwen, Michelle, and the other women— named and unnamed—whose words and experiences have enriched this book.

Contents

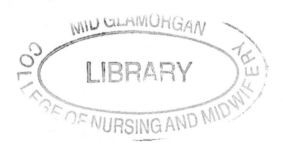

Foreword

AIDS requires us to reconsider our basic assumptions and to question received wisdom in the form of convenient categorizations. One such simplification treats health and human rights as distinct and separate—and often conflicting—concerns; another divides the world into academic thinkers and frontline workers. This book courageously challenges the validity or utility of both oversimplifications.

AIDS is the first pandemic of its kind to occur during the post–World War II era of human rights. Accordingly, health officials have had a dual responsibility in confronting AIDS: they must protect public health and respect human rights. This dual role initially was seen in adversarial terms. Public health policies and programs (such as mandatory testing, isolation, restrictions on movement) were combated as direct threats to individual rights. The public health community gradually realized that concern for such issues as informed consent, confidentiality, and nondiscrimination regarding HIV-infected people and people with AIDS was essential for effective public health work. Finally, and more recently, health experts have discovered that, at a much deeper level, the promotion of human rights and the goals of public health are not only mutually compatible but inextricably linked. For it is now clear that individual, community, and national vulnerability to HIV is directly connected with societal discrimination. Therefore, to the extent that societies can reduce discrimination (based on gender, race, ethnicity, religion, sexual preference, national origin, social class) and promote respect for rights and dignity, they will be increasingly successful in preventing HIV transmission and caring for those who are infected and ill.

This understanding of AIDS, which places the specific problems and concerns of women in the broader context of health, society, and rights, imbues each section of this book. The ethical and legal dimensions of HIV/AIDS and women are not restricted to the chapters by Carol Levine and Michele Zavos but inform many discussions throughout.

The second common oversimplification is acceptance of a dichotomy between thinking and doing. Many books either focus on theory to the exclusion of practical experience or provide a cookbook approach to concrete problems. Wisely and with great sensitivity to differing needs and viewpoints, Ann Kurth has created a book that speaks to varied audiences—from academics to grass-roots activists. The conceptualizers and the practitioners are refused separate-but-equal treatment. The linkages between concepts and action are presented as synergistic and deeply inter-dependent. The conceptual needs to be anchored in and refreshed through contact with concrete and practical problems; local actions must be inspired by a common, larger vision. Nowhere is this interactive richness more clearly evident than in the chapter on working with communities of women at risk, by Helen Gasch and Mindy Fullilove.

Ann Kurth has rendered a great service by editing this superb collection of linked chapters. This book is needed and important: there were more than 8 million women worldwide infected with HIV by January 1993—a number expected to grow to 11 million by January 1996. In the United States, the number of AIDS cases reported among women is rising four times faster than those reported among men. The ever-increasing numbers of women developing AIDS and caring for others who are infected and ill make this book extremely valuable.

By refusing to oversimplify in these two vital areas—health and human rights, and thought and action in confronting HIV/AIDS—Ann Kurth has produced a book that will prepare readers to deal with current problems and to face the complex and uncertain future. In these ways, this book embodies and advances the central elements of the modern paradigm of health itself.

—Jonathan Mann, MD, MPH

Preface

This book was twice inspired. The first and perhaps most obvious reason for undertaking the project was that there existed at the time no single reference for people working on the front lines with women living with HIV disease. What is known as AIDS had been around for more than a decade. Several popular books did address the general subject of HIV and women, but nowhere could the clinician, worker, or woman with HIV disease turn for a comprehensive review of issues faced by women who are infected. The intent of the contributors whose work is gathered here is to create a succinct source of information for those who work with these women. This book is also for HIV-positive women themselves and for their loved ones, for whom living with this disease is a daily reality.

The second inspiration for the book was less direct. Several of the contributors had interviewed HIV-infected women in connection with a small study. Part of the interview involved asking the women what contribution from the health care system would have helped them most in coping with the disease. Several replied, "Nothing but the cure."

On the face of it, there is no arguing with this truth. Everyone wishes for a magic bullet, a medical cure for AIDS. But until there is a cure, women with HIV have needs that the medical, social, and political systems should be addressing more effectively. This book is thus meant to reflect both irony and hope—and the awareness that the needs of women with HIV require creative and consistent response from all providers.

The aim of this book is to help foster this response in providers from the various fields involved in the care of women with HIV: medicine, nursing, sociology, psychology, psychiatry, social work, social activism, women's studies, public health, medical anthropology, ethics, pharmacology, law, and health policy. Several HIV-positive women interviewed for this book give voice throughout the book to concerns and experiences that no provider, however empathetic, can articulate. Their stories appear at the beginning of each chapter. We echo the message these women convey in the hope of building better models of HIV care while waiting for the day when there is less need for these services.

1

Introduction

An Overview of Women and HIV Disease

Ann Kurth

I am the face of the HIV virus. You see me every day, you pass me on the street, you work next to me, yet you don't know my secret. We are invisible. Statistics are not kept, cannot be kept, on those who live with HIV disease. Women are an invisible component of this disease for several reasons: fear of losing custody of children, fear of losing jobs or insurance, and fear of negative judgment.

I am 43 years old, a mother, a lesbian. I learned that I was HIV-positive on March 7, 1989. I had just completed one of my life goals: I had finally graduated from college with a degree in education. I took a job at the University of Arkansas working with disabled students and lived in a small, quaint house with my daughter and my partner. On March 7 my doctor called me at work and gave me the news that I was HIV-positive. . . . My world, my life as I knew it,

> changed completely. Your life feels like a piece of glass that
> shatters to the ground, and the pieces seem impossible to
> pick up. It doesn't go away. But gradually I learned to cope
> with the reality. Today, I am happy to say, my life is very full,
> very content, and filled with joy.
> —Anonymous

A virus spread through sexual intercourse and blood will affect women as well as men. But this biological truism, applied to the human immunodeficiency virus (HIV), has been appreciated slowly, and perception of the impact of HIV disease in women has not kept pace with reality.[1] The first cases of what we now know as acquired immunodeficiency syndrome (AIDS)—but which was then being called gay-related immune disorder—were reported in the United States in 1981.[2] Within months cases in women were reported (Masur et al. 1982; Ellerbrock and Rogers 1990).

By the end of the following year, women constituted about 7 percent of all persons with AIDS (Centers for Disease Control 1983). This proportion had doubled by 1992; in the second decade of the epidemic, cases of AIDS in women comprised 13.5 percent of the total adult and adolescent AIDS caseload reported in the United States (CDC 1993, 9). Globally, one million people are estimated to have been infected with HIV in the first six months of 1992 alone; nearly half of them were thought to be women (Merson 1992).

There are universal concerns faced by women and men living with HIV disease. But the experiences of women who are HIV-positive can be unique in several ways. The clinical presentation can be different from that seen in men, with gynecological symptoms an obvious distinction. The traditional place of many women in society dictates that they experience HIV with a different set of psychosocial needs from those of many men, particularly in the areas of childbearing and child rearing. Some unexamined assumptions continue to underlie discussion about women with

---

[1] Unless otherwise noted, here and throughout this book the term *HIV* refers to human immunodeficiency virus type-1. The second major HIV type, HIV-2, appears to be less widespread and is slower acting than HIV-1, but pathogenic nonetheless. The terminal stages of HIV-2 infection are similar to those seen with HIV-1 (Wilkins 1992). HIV-2 is found mostly in West Africa; only a handful of cases have been identified in North America. On average, women with HIV-2 tend to be about ten years older than women with HIV-1 (Brown 1992).

[2] There is common agreement that what is called AIDS is a late stage of immune system breakdown, caused by long-term infection with HIV and possibly activated by other cofactors. *HIV disease* is a more useful term for this disease process—one that, from HIV infection to the terminal phase of AIDS, may take more than a decade to transpire.

Figure 1.1 Percentage of Total AIDS Cases, Adult/Adolescent Women and Children, 1981–1992

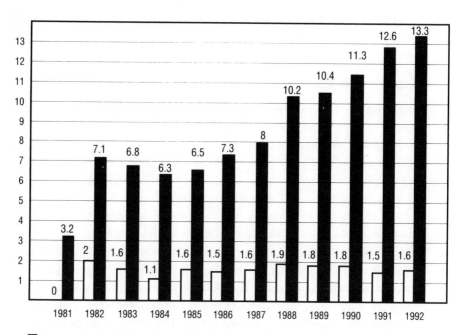

■ Adult and adolescent women as percentage of total
□ Children as percentage of total

Source: Kay Lawton, chief, AIDS Training Section, CDC, May 1993.

HIV; prominent among these is the assertion that the number of pediatric AIDS cases is rising alarmingly because of increased infections in women. Although the total numbers of female and pediatric AIDS cases continue to climb, the rates are different and diverging. Pediatric AIDS cases have remained steady at an average of 1.5 percent of the total adult/adolescent/pediatric AIDS caseload reported since 1981, even though the percentage of AIDS cases in women has increased each year (see figure 1.1). All females with AIDS made up 14.1 percent of cases reported in 1992 (CDC 1993).

Some HIV-positive women do go on to bear children, but transmission from mother to baby is not inevitable, occurring in about one in four cases. As more women learn of their HIV status, it is hoped that they will receive care for their own disease, but not only in the context of potential transmission to their children.

The goal of this book is to provide information regarding such care. Because readers have different backgrounds and interests, the book is organized by topical areas. Chapters 2 through 8 concern the provision of clinical care. Ethical, legal, and epidemiological analyses follow in chapters 9 through 11. The last third of the book, chapters 12 through 15, is devoted to the psychosocial context in which support to HIV-positive women and their families is delivered. The final chapter outlines the need for campaigns to get effective prevention messages to women and men who are not yet infected.

Research on Women

AIDS is estimated to be the fifth leading cause of death for all women aged fifteen to forty-four in the United States (Chu, Buehler, and Berkelman 1990). Most women and men with HIV disease live in the so-called developing countries. Although at least 60 percent of all HIV-infected people are thought to live in Africa (Wilkins 1992), less than 4 percent of biomedical journal articles on HIV have discussed the problem of AIDS there (Elford and Summers 1991).

Despite its growing importance as a cause of premature morbidity (illness) and mortality, HIV disease in women has been similarly understudied. As the authors of one editorial in a leading American medical journal mused, perhaps the attention to AIDS in women and children is lagging because "women and children are a politically weak group in this country" (Heagarty and Abrams 1992). The percentage of scientific articles containing references to women and HIV/AIDS in a widely used biomedical database between 1985 and 1991 averaged 4.4 percent, though during the same year the percentage of people with AIDS who were female averaged 11 percent in the United States and even higher worldwide.[3]

Science is not generally conducted in the absence of funding. Has the area of women and HIV received sufficient allocation of research monies? Two-thirds of the federal monies earmarked for research on AIDS in women and children has been used for research on children[4] (see figure 1.2). This unequal allocation persists even though infected women outnumber infected children by almost 6:1. The comparative neglect of research on women may begin to be rectified as several large studies get under way (see Anastos and Vermund, chapter 11).

The issue of AIDS is emotionally affecting, as is any life-threatening illness. Yet too often a distinction has been made between "innocent victims" (such as children) versus, by implication, the non-innocent. Some insurance carriers have specified coverage for HIV costs only for people who acquired the disease through blood transfusion or hemophilia treatment (Arno 1992). The first question many

[3] MedLine, the bibliographical database of the National Library of Medicine, contains about 75 percent of all citations published in English in the biomedical literature (more than 3,200 journals as of December 1991).

[4] As of February 18, 1992; data provided by D. Adderly, National Institutes of Health.

Figure 1.2 Women and Pediatric AIDS Cases vs. Funding, 1990–June 1992

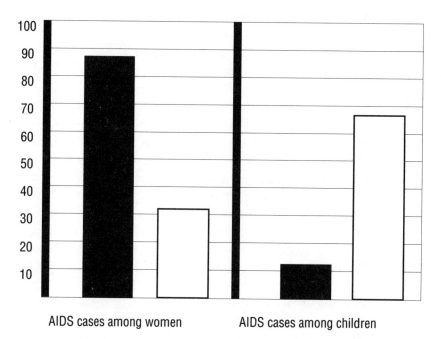

■ Percentage of AIDS cases
☐ Percentage of funding

Source: CDC

people still ask upon hearing that someone has HIV disease is, How did she get it? The projection of a value-laden judgment onto what is a biological entity prevents HIV from being seen as just another disease. Many people living with this illness bear the additional burden of societal and personal stigma, extremes of fascination or of shunning, pity or shame. What women and other people with HIV need is the support required by anyone facing a serious challenge.

Transmission

In the United States most transmission occurs through injection-drug use (IDU) by women themselves or through sexual contact with an injection-drug user. Particularly in women, HIV disease can be described as a disease of poverty. The majority of HIV-positive women in the United States are black (52.9 percent) or Hispanic (20.9 percent); and 25.2 percent are white (CDC 1993). These percentages are almost four times higher than would be expected by the proportion of African-

American and Latina women in the general population. But a recent poll of 1,157 women of color found that 84 percent of African-American women and 83 percent of Latinas said they had little or no chance of getting AIDS (CCCM 1992). Seroprevalence rates for HIV in black women have been documented to be five to fifteen times greater than for white women dwelling in the same state (Gwinn, Pappaioanou, George et al. 1991). Some of the possible explanations for this disparity are explored by Gasch and Fullilove in chapter 13.

Heterosexual contact is one of the fastest growing transmission categories in the United States. In fact, 6.5 percent of the total AIDS caseload can be traced to heterosexual contact (CDC 1993), and that percentage is expected to double by 1995 (Allen and Setlow 1991). Heterosexual transmission accounted for 35.8 percent of all female adult/adolescent AIDS cases reported through 1992 and fully 39 percent of all AIDS cases in U.S. women in 1992 alone (CDC 1993). Women now constitute almost two-thirds of all heterosexual transmission cases. Ninety percent of HIV infections occurring in 1992 throughout the world are estimated to have been transmitted through heterosexual intercourse (United Nations 1992). Transmission has been documented, though infrequently, among lesbians who have no other identified risk factors (Chu et al. 1990). It has been pointed out that the surveillance reports kept by the Centers for Disease Control and Prevention (CDC) do not include a category for female-to-female transmission, which may affect reporting accuracy (Cole and Cooper 1991). Such cases fall into the "no identified risk" category, the percentage of which is more than double that of men—7.4 percent versus 3.6 percent as of December 1993 (CDC 1992).

In most cases, AIDS strikes women who are fifteen to forty-four years old (Minkoff 1991), and it is thought that 100,000 or more American women in this age group are HIV-positive. Nearly one-quarter of these women were twenty to twenty-nine when their AIDS was diagnosed (CDC 1993). Because there is a latency period of ten or more years between infection and overt symptoms, these women were probably infected as teenagers. The CDC has reported 946 cases of AIDS in people aged thirteen to nineteen in 1993. These numbers, while small, are disturbing. Through 1992, more than 19 percent of AIDS cases among thirteen- to twenty-four-year-olds and AIDS deaths among fifteen- to twenty-four-year-olds were female (CDC 1993).

Older women also have many of the same risk factors as their younger counterparts; one retrospective chart review of hospitalized patients found that 25 percent of the HIV-infected patients sixty and older were female (Scura and Whipple 1990).

These figures indicate that much more HIV disease in women is on the way, and several trends have already outlined the impending wave, as is detailed in chapters 11 and 12. From January 1987 to April 1991, diagnosed AIDS cases in women increased by 900 percent (CDC 1991a). The ratio of male-to-female seropositivity has approached parity in some populations. In Africa the sex ratio is already 1:1 or higher among females (Berkley et al. 1990); among applicants to the U.S. Job Corps, young women aged 16 and 17 had a significantly higher level of HIV infection than did young men of the same age—2.3 per 1,000 versus 1.5 per 1,000 (St. Louis et al. 1991). Seroprevalence among young women and men in the U.S. Army is almost equal at 1:1.09 (Burke et al. 1990). As Ickovics and Rodin point out (1992), the gender gap is closing, particularly among adolescents. These trends will have an inevitable effect on the sex-curve distribution of HIV cases: by the end of the twentieth century there will be as many women as men with AIDS worldwide (NIAID/NIH and CDC 1991a).

As with some other sexually transmitted diseases (STDs), the efficacy of HIV transmission between men and women appears to vary, at least in the short term. This may be the result of a dose-response effect: there is a higher inoculum of HIV in a sperm deposit than in vaginal fluid (Williams 1992). HIV has, however, been found in vaginal secretions and is known to be harbored in dendritic cells (Langhoff, Terwilliger, Poznansky et al. 1991), which line the vagina and anus and thus may serve as a reservoir for viral secretion. The National Academy of Sciences reports that other factors that may affect transmission include frequency of exposure, host susceptibility, infectiousness of the HIV-positive person and virulence of HIV isolates, and the presence of other STDs or cofactors (Institute of Medicine 1988, 45). Infectivity may be related to the transmitting person's disease state, with higher rates of transmission during early infection and during the more advanced stages of HIV disease.

Researchers have established that during vaginal intercourse the risk of infectivity from a man to a woman is greater than from a woman to a man[5] (Padian 1987, 1991; Institute of Medicine 1988). Estimates are derived only from aggregate averages, however. Each episode of unprotected sexual contact involving the exchange of fluids carries with it a risk of potential transmission, regardless of whether that exchange occurs between heterosexual or same-sex partners.

Some behaviors may carry more inherent risk than others. Anal intercourse, for example, is more likely to lead to lacerations than is vaginal intercourse (Modan et al. 1992). In this light it is important to note that several studies have documented that anal intercourse is a behavior occurring with some frequency among heterosexuals. Wyatt and coworkers (1988) found that 43 percent of white women and 21 percent of African-American women contacted in a telephone survey reported at least some experience with anal intercourse, with about 6 percent reporting anal sex on a regular basis. Among the women's cohort followed at Project AWARE in San Francisco, 48 percent initially reported having anal sex (Cohen and Wofsy 1989).

[5] In places like Africa, where rates of genital ulcer disease are higher, heterosexual transmission may be more equally bidirectional.

Jaffe and coworkers (1988) found 25 percent of 148 adolescent girls surveyed reported having had anal sex, with only 11 percent always using condoms.

The exact quantification of HIV transmission risk by oral sex remains undetermined (Gorna 1992). A small number of HIV cases have been traced to fellatio, though the risk appears to be much lower than that of unprotected anal or vaginal sex (Lifson et al. 1991); few cases have been liked definitively to cunnilingus, though at least one case report exists (see Keeling 1993).

Survival Rates

Early studies showed that the group of people diagnosed with AIDS who died the fastest were women, especially low-income urban blacks and Latinas (Rothenberg et al. 1987; Verdegem, Sattler, and Boylen 1988). As Anastos and Vermund document in chapter 11, however, more recent data seem to indicate that this survival gap has diminished, with no significant differences seen between cohorts of HIV-infected women and men in the same clinical setting (Ellerbrock et al. 1991; Anastos 1992). Diminishment of the survival gap has also been documented by several studies presented at the Eighth International Conference on AIDS in July 1992 (Dorrucci et al. 1992; Melnick et al. 1992; Szabo et al. 1992).

This equity appears to be related to treatment access, however. Stein and coworkers (1991) found that males were more likely than females to be offered AZT, as were whites and those with insurance. In another study of 5,000 men and women in Atlanta, median survival after diagnosis was less for women (13 months) than for men (18 months; $p<0.05$), even when differences in the two groups' immune systems (as measured by CD4+ counts) were controlled. The authors postulate that this difference may be due to AZT use. During followup only 71 percent of women, but 91 percent of men, with CD4+ counts below 50 were using AZT ($p<0.002$). This difference was most pronounced for African-American women (Creagh et al. 1992). The finding echoes other studies that found poorer prognosis for women and for those less likely to be taking AZT (Lemp et al. 1992).

Several theories have been postulated to account for the sex-based survival differences. Access to care is one; many HIV-positive women are economically disenfranchised, which may lead to a late entry into the health care system. And, as Creagh and coworkers show (1992), attending a clinic does not by itself ensure that clients within the same system are undergoing similar regimens. Management strategies may not have been as well developed for women as for men; many women's primary contact with the health care system is with an obstetrician or gynecologist, who may not have been attuned to suspect HIV disease in female patients. Finally, the caretaker role played by many women may have kept them from seeking care promptly—or getting any care at all—for themselves. What has become increasingly clear, though, is that access to early care improves survival for women and men.

Another issue of contention has been the definition of AIDS developed for surveillance purposes by the Centers for Disease Control. The original definition was based on initially identified clinical presentations—that is, those symptoms seen in what was almost exclusively a gay white male population.[6] Advocates argued that gynecologic presentations such as pelvic inflammatory disease or recurrent, intractable candida vaginitis (monilia, or yeast infection) may not be suspected as HIV-related, thus possibly delaying aggressive therapy and leading to an undercounting of cases in women. As the following excerpt illustrates, it also meant that women may not have received such benefits as Social Security Disability Income and Medicaid, dying before ever having received a formal AIDS diagnosis (see chapter 10 for a detailed discussion of this issue).

> Let me describe M. C., who had the following medical history between 1981, when she believes she was infected, and June 1990, five years after she initially applied for [Social Security disability] benefits, when she was found eligible: eight hospitalizations for PID [pelvic inflammatory disease]; five for carcinoma of the cervix and ovaries; five bouts of bacterial pneumonia; recurrent UTIs [urinary tract infections]; chronic yeast infections. Her records also classify her as HIV-infected and asymptomatic (no medical person had even suggested an HIV test for her until 1988). No one administered a test to determine her CD4+ count. M. C. is dying now—she is lucky she saw any benefits before she died. (McGovern 1992)

Though developed for tracking purposes, the CDC definition has been used around the world to define populations for epidemiological, clinical, and even benefit-determination purposes. The original definition was amended in 1985 and 1987 to include more presentations, such as wasting syndrome and HIV encephalopathy, making a total of twenty-three diseases that constitute AIDS when they occur in the presence of HIV-seropositivity. The authors of one study conducted a retrospective review of death certificates of women aged fifteen to forty-four that listed HIV/AIDS as the underlying cause of death; they found that only 35 percent of the certificates listed opportunistic infections covered in the 1987 case definition (Chu, Buehler, and Berkelman 1990).

Following much discussion, a new case definition was enacted in January 1993. Under the new definition, individuals with HIV and a CD4+ T-lymphocyte count of 200 cells/mm^3 or fewer (severe immunosuppression) automatically qualify

---

[6] These include opportunistic infections, generally seen when CD4+ T-lymphocyte cell counts are below 200 cells/mm^3; certain neoplasms, such as Kaposi's sarcoma (rarely seen in women); and neurological illnesses (e.g., dementia).

as having AIDS, regardless of other symptoms. Pulmonary tuberculosis, invasive cervical cancer, and recurrent pneumonia (occurring within the previous twelve months)—were also added to the new case definition (see table 2.1). These are conditions that tend to affect or are particular to women. It is thought that the definition change may increase 1993 cases by 75 percent (CDC 1993). Authors who calculated the projected impact of this case definition in New York state (exclusive of New York City) found that it might increase the reported number of AIDS cases in women by as much as 83 percent, nearly twice the expected increase in men (Smith et al. 1992). It is unclear whether there will be increased funding available to provide services to the additional persons identified as having AIDS.

HIV Disease in Women

Data on the natural history of HIV disease in women are still limited. In addition to having many of the opportunistic infections seen in men, women have sex-specific symptoms that are often gynecological in nature (see chapters 3 and 11). For example, persistent, treatment-resistant vulvovaginal candidiasis is nearly a clinical marker of impending AIDS in HIV-positive women, often presenting a number of months before oral thrush shows up. Candida esophagitis, mucotaneous herpes simplex virus, wasting syndrome, and Pneumocystis carinii pneumonia (PCP) seem to be common AIDS-defining events. There also appears to be a link between human papilloma virus (HPV), cervical cancer, and HIV; it is suspected that immunosuppression may play a role in the progression of HPV-mediated cervical cytologic abnormalities. Multiple studies have shown a strong association between advanced cervical neoplasia and declining immune function (Vermund and Kelley 1990; Klein et al. 1992; Anastos et al. 1992).

A Papanicolaou smear is the most common test used to collect cervical cells for analysis. Test results are reported using two systems, both of which describe cellular changes related to benign infections (atypia), dysplasia (abnormal/precancerous cells), or cervical cancers (carcinoma or cervical intraepithelial neoplasia [CIN]). As Denenberg outlines in chapter 3, women with HIV should receive a pelvic exam and a Pap smear every six months (Minkoff and DeHovitz 1991). A Pap smear alone may be insufficient in some cases, however. A study of thirty-two HIV-positive women found a 3 percent rate of cervical intraepithelial neoplasia detected by Pap smear, but colposcopy revealed an actual CIN rate of 42 percent in these women (Auer 1992). Colposcopy should be done if the woman's Pap smear results are difficult to interpret or indicate evidence of cervical cancer (Minkoff and DeHovitz 1991); some practitioners feel that anoscopy should be done as well. Recurrence of CIN is significantly higher in HIV-infected women than in uninfected women (Fruchter, Maiman, and Serur 1992). Other genital-tract infections—like herpes simplex virus, PID, and genital cytomegalovirus—have been reported to occur at higher frequency and with greater resistance to treatment among women with HIV (see Hoegsberg et al. 1990).

The question of whether pregnancy advances disease progression in women with relatively intact immune systems remains open. In chapter 5 the authors survey current options regarding the obstetrical and related medical needs of women. The authors also provide an overview of pediatric HIV and protocols for the management of HIV-positive women during pregnancy.

Studies presented at the Eighth International Conference on AIDS regarding the natural history of HIV disease in men and women appeared to reach a premature conclusion that significant differences in the opportunistic infections experienced did not exist; for example, in four studies PCP was the most common AIDS-defining illness for both sexes (Creagh et al. 1992; Szabo et al. 1992; and Melnick et al. 1992). On a panel of six presenters, however, only one represented a study that had bothered to collect gynecological data from its cohort. Thus, a claim for parity in disease presentation might appear to be a questionable assumption until more comprehensive data are collected. Those data, in the case of women, should encompass any disorders of the reproductive tract, including menstrual changes, infections, and neoplasms, as well as any other manifestations that may reveal a gender difference in rates of occurrence, such as bacterial pneumonia and possibly wasting syndrome.

Clinical Care

Although women's gynecological needs are obviously great, it is important that practitioners and policymakers not make the mistake of viewing women merely as reproductive tracts. In the absence of gender-specific data for prophylactic and treatment strategies, women with HIV will need at least the same management men need. This includes antiretroviral therapies, medications for the prevention of PCP, and other monitoring, as well as access to comprehensive primary care. As noted previously, evidence for gender difference in the use of standard antiretroviral and PCP prophylaxis regimens has been found. Several studies show that white males have the highest and black females the lowest rates of receiving PCP prevention and AZT even when immune status is the same. What determines this difference? Socioeconomic access (ability to pay, access to private versus public clinics, physicians, and care providers)? Differing cultural acceptability of medical regimens? Unless more attention is focused on improving access to care for women and men across the continuum, this disturbingly inequitable trend may continue. In chapter 2 Young provides protocols for HIV management in the primary care setting.

Other needs for women with HIV include psychological and psychiatric services. There is no consensus on the type and prevalence of neurological abnormalities associated with HIV-2 infection (World Health Organization 1990), but there are clear disorders related to HIV-1 itself and as sequelae to HIV-related infections and malignancies. It is known that the brain is affected by HIV directly (AIDS dementia), and indirectly (opportunistic infections and neoplasms). Sanders reviews these concerns in chapter 6.

Access to Pharmaceutical and Other Research

The history of clinical research in HIV disease has been unusual in many respects. Even more than with other illnesses, the scientist/clinician and the patient/advocate have crossed paths. Their meeting has produced fascinating, frustrating, and fruitful exchange. People living with HIV and their advocates have demanded changes in the way research is usually done and the rapidity with which results are translated into useful treatments. They have pushed to streamline Food and Drug Administration procedures for drug approval and have expanded access to drugs still under investigation ("parallel track"), broadening the involvement of women and minorities in clinical trials and changing the design of the trials themselves (see, e.g., Gonsalves and Harrington 1992).

Everyone living with HIV disease needs access to experimental therapies for what is essentially a new and life-threatening syndrome. Certain biological and social factors may affect women's experience with therapies that are considered standard of care. For example, women have more adipose tissue, which may lead to different distribution of a drug in their bodies. The issue of women's involvement in clinical trials conducted by the federal government, community-based centers, and pharmaceutical companies is discussed by Korvick and Long in chapters 7 and 8.

Just as there have been few data on the gender-specific natural history of HIV, so too have clinical therapies been studied less thoroughly in women than they have been in men. This has been true of research beyond HIV as well. Only in September 1990 was an Office of Research on Women's Health established at the National Institutes of Health; its purpose is to address the inequities in women's health and to ensure that women are included in clinical research (Pinn 1992). In March 1993 the NIH announced a $625 million study of older women's health. Health and Human Services Secretary Donna Shalala stated that this initiative needed to be followed up by "ensuring the place of women's health in the mainstream of biomedical research."[7] In chapter 9 Levine provides historical background on the exclusion of women from clinical research trials. Korvick and Long further examine the question of the involvement of women—or reasons for their prior underenrollment—in research trials of new therapies. Women must be included in such trials at least proportionately, a fact that the FDA has now formally recognized. More recent enrollment figures—14 percent of AIDS Clinical Trials Group enrollees were fe-

---

[7] Associated Press interview, *New York Times*, March 31, 1993.

male as of early 1993—indicate that the tide may be turning. In December 1992 a coalition of AIDS advocates petitioned the Food and Drug Administration to change its 1977 guidelines recommending that women of childbearing potential be excluded from clinical trials. In March 1993 the FDA announced its intention to do so.

Prevention and Policy

Much of the medical and policy literature of the 1980s (studies of prostitutes and perinatal transmission) focused on women as vectors of disease rather than as human beings who function in relationships. Seroprevalence research on sex workers has consistently shown their HIV-positivity to be most associated with injection drug use, not with sex work; despite this finding and the fact that women are more at risk biologically from sexual encounters than are males, only in the 1990s did prevention campaigns begin to target prostitutes' clients.

Strategies to prevent the spread of sexually transmitted diseases in the United States prior to the advent of HIV have a long history, not all of it illustrious. During World War II, for example, up to 60,000 female sex workers were put in concentration camps as a "prevention" measure. The Navy also removed doorknobs from ships as it was thought that these contributed to the spread of gonorrhea (Brandt 1986).[8]

Today some of these policies seem ineffectual at best and a travesty at worst. Ironically, however, some of the same mistakes may be repeated if the context that places women at risk is not well understood. The usual message of many prevention interventions—"Wear a condom"—is the one mechanical contribution that depends on male cooperation for safer sex. A recent study conducted among three groups of heterosexuals at an urban STD clinic found that men who received a "condom skills" course as their intervention had the lowest rate of new STD infections in subsequent visits to the clinic. The researchers also documented that none of the interventions studied reduced the rate of new infections among women. As the primary investigator noted, women "seem to feel they have very little control or power over their men. Many women said they would rather have unprotected sex with an unfaithful partner than risk hurting their relationships" (D. Cohen 1992).

The other common recommendation—that sexually active people use latex barriers along with such spermicidal/virucidal agents as nonoxynol-9—also may have an unintended effect. As many as 47 percent of women in one study experi-

---

[8] A more recent, sinister rumor of "STD control" comes from Mynamar (formerly Burma). In April 1992 it was alleged that twenty-five HIV-positive Burmese women who had been abducted and forced to work in brothels in Thailand were, upon their forced repatriation, executed with cyanide injection by the military government of Mynamar (International Gay and Lesbian Human Rights Commission 1992).

enced vulvar and vaginal irritation, burning, and ulceration with high rates of nonoxynol-9 use, a situation that may actually increase rather than minimize the risk of HIV transmission in some women. This study also found that the contraceptive sponge with nonoxynol-9 was not efficacious in preventing HIV transmission among a cohort of Kenyan sex workers (Kreiss et al. 1992). Real-use studies have found far fewer side effects (Elias and Heise 1993). Important considerations regarding birth control and safer sex methods are reviewed in chapter 4.

Several authors have called for further research and development of methods that can be controlled by women (Stein 1990; Gollub, Rosenberg, and Michael 1992; Guinan 1992). These may include new barrier methods and, for women who wish to conceive but at reduced risk of acquiring HIV, vaginally applied agents that will kill HIV but not sperm. The lack of evidence that vaginally applied spermicide alone can prevent HIV transmission, coupled with the fact that cervical caps and diaphragms still leave vaginal mucosa exposed to STD organisms (Stone and Peterson 1992) make the creation of completely safe female-controlled methods a challenge. Nevertheless, response to this call has been less than swift. For example, efficacy and acceptance data from several dozen studies on the female condom had been presented at international meetings for a number of years, but the Food and Drug Administration gave approval for its sale in the United States only in May 1993. The silicon-coated polyurethane device has been available in Switzerland, Austria, Britain, and France and is being marketed in other countries (Leary 1992).

When discussing prevention efforts, it is important to acknowledge the most common portrait of women with HIV disease: a young woman of color and low socioeconomic status. But it is equally critical to recognize that HIV affects women of all races, ages, classes, and sexual behaviors. Until the heterogeneity of women at risk is recognized, many women may see HIV prevention campaigns as irrelevant. Given the seriousness of the HIV epidemic, it is time to examine both the message and the medium of HIV prevention for women, as Wagner and Cohen do in chapter 16.

Men must be included in messages about safer sex, and the sexual taboos and constraints for both women and men must be openly discussed. In the United States through the late 1980s, as Wofsy has pointed out (1987), condom advertisements and safer-sex guidelines appeared in virtually all magazines targeted at female audiences but in almost none aimed at males. Magazines such as *Ms.* (May 1989; January–February 1991) and *Essence* (April 1990) have discussed women and HIV. This is not to say that all popular women's magazines have been models of enlightenment. *Cosmopolitan* chose to print articles about the "myth" of heterosexual HIV, remarking that "by featuring women as typical potential victims, the AIDS-prevention advertising was designed to scare the hell out of everybody" (March 1992). In December 1992 William Haseltine, a Harvard AIDS researcher, testified before the U.S. Congress that HIV could infect as many as one billion people by the year 2025, and 85 percent of them would be infected through heterosexual inter-course, specifically vaginal sex (Chemical and Engineering News 1993).

Reproductive rights

Much funding and policy emphasis for HIV in women has focused on prenatal antibody testing. It could be argued that this has precluded a focus on the clinical and psychosocial needs of women with HIV.

The impact of drug and alcohol addiction has been a monumental contribution to the breakdown of many familial and community networks in the United States (see chapters 13 and 14). Drug use by women has become an increasingly strident policy issue, with more punitive than rehabilitative initiatives being launched. Many women who are addicted see pregnancy as a time of hopefulness, and they are motivated to stop their substance use entirely (Williams 1990). Few treatment programs will take a pregnant addict, however. As Zavos points out in chapter 10, some addicted women have already been criminally charged in relation to their children.

Small studies are beginning to document the possible teratogenic and other effects of male substance use upon progeny. This idea was called a new concept as late as 1980 (Soyka and Joffe 1980, 64). Research conducted at Temple University suggests that cocaine can attach to sperm, enter the egg, and possibly inflict on the developing embryo such defects as learning disabilities and memory problems (Yazigi et al. 1992). Another research group found a pronounced connection be-tween tobacco smoking, low vitamin C intake among males, and increased DNA damage in sperm cells, which may predispose offspring to genetic anomalies, birth defects, and cancers. Decreased vitamin C levels were generally caused by an unbalanced diet and by smoking cigarettes (study by Motchnik et al., reported in Brody 1992). It is hard to imagine, however, that a campaign to promote prenatal smoking cessation and vitamin ingestion among males will be developed soon, much less that fathers will face criminal charges for their drug use in relation to their offspring.

Women with HIV who get pregnant decide to carry to term or abort for many of the same reasons that motivate HIV-negative women, as Hutchison and Shannon detail in chapter 4. Those who choose to continue their pregnancies understand that there is a risk of transmission but generally hope that their child will remain uninfected—a hope that bears out about 75 percent of the time. This phenomenon has been described elsewhere as "parallel thinking" (Kurth and Hutchison 1990) and has been documented in other contexts in the cognitive-psychology literature (Cicourel 1983). For some women, pregnancy may be a way to subsume feelings of grief about their own illness, and providers may help address the woman's own adaptation to the diagnosis of HIV.

Although commentators like Mitchell and Levine have affirmed the particular value of childbearing in the African-American and Hispanic communities, it may be that the desire for parenting cuts across socioeconomic classes and cultural and ethnic groups. This is evidenced by the desire of HIV-discordant hemophilic couples (many of whom are white and middle-class) to become parents in the face of possible HIV infection (see Kraus et al. 1991).

Providers must examine their own emotions regarding the issue of drug use and HIV in the context of pregnancy in order to provide nonjudgmental professional care. Earlier detection of the infant's true HIV status (made difficult because maternal antibodies can persist in the child's bloodstream for up to fifteen months) and improved prophylactic regimens for mother and baby have led to calls for more prenatal screening of women. It must still be recognized that the risks and benefits of testing and treatment ultimately rest with the woman, who must be supported in whatever decision she makes.

Multiple Roles of Women in Society

Women with HIV are many things: parents, partners, sexual beings. Around the world, as Carovano and Schietinger point out in chapter 12, women are living with this disease and caring for those who die of it. Yet it is not always clear on whom women rely to support them through this process. As noted by the Society for Women and AIDS in Africa (SWAA), "The greatest challenge for HIV-infected women and women with AIDS appears to relate to dealing with the stigma, abandonment, rejection, loss of job or source of income, lack of support services to cope with sick children/spouse and absence of a viable future plan. . . . [These women are often isolated from] the rest of the family, thereby limiting the family support system that women would otherwise rely upon during illness and distress. . . . [T]he plight of women living with HIV/AIDS has yet to receive adequate attention, as most action still centers around prevention" (SWAA 1991).

Because women are more often the primary caretakers of children, with the attendant financial, emotional and physical responsibilities, many women with HIV state that their greatest concern is who will take care of their children in the future. Ideally, providers can discuss family law and life planning with women before times of crisis like hospitalization (see chapter 10). HIV in families has again raised the specter of orphanages, as kinship and other foster care systems may become unable to meet the needs of the growing numbers of children orphaned by AIDS. Simpson and Williams describe the experience of kinship foster parents in chapter 14 and make recommendations for supporting families living with HIV.

The context in which many women experience HIV is centered around their children and family—often their extended family. Helping women cope with the disease thus means more than simply providing medical care, as Sunderland and

Holman describe in chapter 15. More important to some women than getting AZT right away may be finding housing so that they and their family members can stay together. The New York City Task Force on Women and AIDS noted in its 1992 policy document that "in their pivotal role as mothers, sisters, daughters, aunts, mothers-in-law, and grandmothers, women are traditionally called upon to minister to ill family members as well as care for those who are not ill . . . . Older women, in their roles as mothers and grandmothers, are faced with the unforeseen circumstances of caring for chronically ill children and their dependent grandchildren. . . . Younger women, often infected themselves, are confronted by the physical and emotional needs of chronically ill partners and dependent children while coping with bouts of debilitating illness." To help preserve family integrity, housing and other social service agencies need to work together.

Health care systems also can improve the way they meet the needs of HIV-positive women. These women often require transportation, day care, or on-site child care. Appointments for mother and children should be linked if at all possible (see Diaz et al. 1990). In chapter 15 Sunderland and Holman describe one such system in Brooklyn, New York, and in chapter 13 Gasch and Fullilove describe the "family-centered, community-based, comprehensive care model" in a discussion of the need for community building in areas ravaged by HIV and other epidemics. Clinical, social, and psychological providers must work together in caring for women and families affected by HIV: "The appropriate clinical response to this situation is to create therapeutic environments that address the hierarchy of human needs, from food, shelter, clothing, and medical care to psychological and interpersonal issues such as trust, autonomy, self-esteem and intimacy" (Benson and Maier 1990).

The entire area of human sexual and addiction behaviors is still relatively uncharted territory. Extensive population-based sexual surveys have been released recently in Britain and France (ACSF Investigators 1992; Johnson et al. 1992). In the United States, where there is the highest number of reported AIDS cases in the world, funding for such research is restricted by congressional decree and political expedience. Across many cultures learned and unspoken norms are prescribed, if not adhered to, regarding the number, combination, and types of partners and sexual acts that are sanctioned or condemned. Many of these norms leave women powerless to assert their sexual autonomy and safety, much less their desires. Yet these same societal norms may also constrain men from changing their sexual behaviors, for a different set of reasons.

It is not clear how health-improving changes in sexual behavior are to be achieved without a more fundamental understanding of the whys and hows of current sexual activity. In the absence of this understanding, health educators are often left to function on a number of assumptions in the provision of their work. It may be wise to examine these assumptions as we proceed with such work; the specter of HIV disease dictates as much. Most HIV/STD prevention messages tell people how to have safer sex. Rarely are people asked why they have sex and how they learned to have it. It may be fruitful to help women and men learn to have sex that is communicative as well as technically safe. Such an approach, however, requires open dialogue not just between individual sex partners but at the level of cultural archetypes.

The impact of HIV on women—who are family caretakers, sexual and emotional partners, professionals, clinicians, researchers, and people living with the infection—is increasing. HIV forces a reexamination of many issues related to sex, gender, social and economic roles, and health care access. For this reason HIV may represent an opportunity amid sadness and loss. Women and men around the world can learn that sexual expression can be mutually pleasurable and free from coercion and danger; that taking care of upcoming generations is not just a woman's ordained duty but a function of the human family. Until a medical cure is found, people working in health care, political, and social systems must ensure that women—and all others affected by HIV disease—get the care they need.

2

A Primer of Health Care

Mary Young

I am an African-American woman who knows she must be heard in order to pave the way for the women who come behind her.

I lived in poverty the younger part of my life; my mother was a practicing alcoholic and my father lived in someone else's home, not knowing anything of his family or their well-being. I was raised by my grandparents to know only how to conceive a baby at the age of 13. . . . As a teen and a mother, I sold drugs of any kind, not expecting to become my own best customer. [Drugs] drew me into a world of prostitution and stealing, [and I abandoned] my child. After my marriage failed, I went back into a life of prostitution and drugs only to lose custody of my second child.

I relocated to Washington, D.C., ended up in a detoxification center, and began to want to live differently.

So I went on to get my life together with another man, who truly loved and wanted me, and was pregnant again. This time it was different. I was happy and very hopeful.

I went to the hospital and was asked to take the AIDS test. The results came back positive, and then the doctors told me I should abort my baby because it would stand a fifty-fifty chance of living with full-blown AIDS and dying in three to five years, or dying within weeks after birth. . . . I went on a mission of suicide for my baby and myself. I went back into the life I knew best—prostitution with no safe sex—in the hopes that someone would help me kill myself because the alcohol and drugs were not doing it.

When the baby was born she was not breathing. I felt a very deep hurt inside of me that my baby was not going to live but I was. I began to cry and pray that God would help both of us, and then my baby started to cry. Moments later the Child Protective Services came into the room and told me I had just lost custody of my newborn on the grounds of child abuse on an unborn infant.

Finally I was ordered by a judge to complete a long-term drug-treatment program. After eighteen months, my little girl tested negative for antibody. That gave me a lot of hope, knowing my baby was okay and I could be too if I just took care of myself.

—Frankie E. Mason

Although a great deal is known about the management of HIV disease in children and men, relatively little has been published regarding the care and treatment of HIV-infected women. Nevertheless, a consensus is emerging, one that is outlined here, with an understanding that HIV treatment is constantly changing. Comprehensive management, particularly in the later stages of the illness, requires interdisciplinary care and often subspecialty medical consultation. It is important for nonspecialist providers—family- and general-practice physicians, internists, nurse-practitioners, and others—to realize that women and men with HIV disease can benefit from a comprehensive primary-care approach.

Who should take the time to understand this approach to care? When a disease is in flux, as is the case with HIV, the affected person is her or his own best advocate. Women infected with HIV should become well informed regarding standards of care and promising new developments. And those health care providers to whom women have traditionally turned—gynecologists, family practitioners, obstetricians, midwives, nurse-practitioners, and internists—need to understand risk behavior, testing protocols, signs and symptoms, and, when feasible, the management of HIV, particularly early in the progression of the disease. As the number of those infected with HIV grows, care will need to be drawn from the resources of the health delivery system, from public health clinics to private offices to tertiary care centers. The goal of comprehensive care is to help women navigate this complex system smoothly and efficiently.

The underlying philosophy of primary care lends itself to this goal, viewing health care providers as clinicians who interact with clients as human and social beings. Primary care aims to manage and supervise all the medical concerns of the individual and, sometimes, the family. Continuity of care, health maintenance, primary prevention, and client education are its cornerstones (adapted from Goroll et al. 1987).

What Is HIV?

AIDS is the end stage of a long disease process caused by a virus known as human immunodeficiency virus (HIV). It takes as long as ten years from HIV exposure to AIDS diagnosis in about half of those individuals infected. The early stage of HIV infection may be "silent"—the person looks and feels healthy, and routine laboratory work and physical exams are normal. But the hallmark of HIV disease is the steady and inexorable loss of immune function. In the middle stage of infection, nonspecific signs and symptoms may develop. As immune dysfunction becomes more severe, those infected become susceptible to unusual or opportunistic pathogens and cancers. People are considered to have AIDS when they experience one of a number of opportunistic infections, malignancies, or brain disorders, or a drop in certain immune cells (CD4+ T-lymphocyte cells) to 200 cells/mm^3 or fewer, with or without other symptoms.

Infection occurs when HIV, a retrovirus belonging to the Lentivirinae family, gains access to an uninfected host following significant exposure to infectious material, most commonly blood, semen, or vaginal secretions. The virus enters through interruptions in the epithelial surface of the rectum, vagina, mouth, or skin as a result of unprotected sexual intercourse or the sharing of needles or works during injection-drug use. The virus then attaches through high-affinity binding to cells expressing a glycoprotein receptor called CD4. These cells include T-helper lymphocytes (T_4 or CD4+ cells), B-lymphocytes, monocytes-macrophages, dendritic cells, Langerhans cells, and such nonimmune system cells as glial cells and astrocytes. HIV replicates by using specific enzymes, including reverse transcriptase, which converts viral RNA to DNA, allowing for integration into the host cell. The virus can lie seemingly dormant (unexpressed) for years (Greene 1991), though there is now evidence that it is sequestered in high quantities in the lymph tissue, creating an extensive period of "prepotency" (see *Nature* 1993a). Reverse transcriptase enzyme is the target of such nucleoside analogues as Retrovir (AZT), Videx (ddI), and Hivid (ddC), the antiretrovirals licensed for treatment of HIV infection.

Studies have demonstrated that monitoring the CD4+ T-helper lymphocytes can lead to accurate predictions regarding a person's risk for opportunistic infections (Polk 1987). The CD4+ cell count, used as a surrogate marker of clinical status, is now a mainstay of clinical trials for new therapies. It is the most important test after the HIV antibody test itself in managing the care of a person infected with HIV. The studies that defined the role of the CD4+ cell count were carried out primarily in gay men. Until more gender-specific studies are completed, the guidelines established in the studies on men are being followed in the treatment of women.

A CD4+ cell count of 600–1,200 cells/mm^3 is considered normal. A CD4+ cell count of less than 200 cells/mm^3 indicates compromise of the immune system and the risk of opportunistic infections or malignancies. Although it is not normal, a CD4+ count of 200–500 cells/mm^3 does not appear to be associated with opportunistic infections, but patients may complain of such nonspecific symptoms as fatigue, unexplained weight loss, fever, or diarrhea. Oral and vaginal thrush may occur, and skin conditions like seborrheic dermatitis may manifest. Recent studies have also demonstrated that a CD4+ cell count below 50 cells/mm^3 represents the most severe immunocompromise, with risk for multiple infections and subsequent death.

Because CD4+ cell counts can fluctuate from reading to reading and from laboratory to laboratory, multiple readings are needed to establish trends over time. A second test, the %CD4+ (available as part of the lymphocyte subset), may be more precise, and it is helpful in interpreting fluctuating absolute counts. Studies and guidelines in treating HIV were established using the absolute count, however. A %CD4+ greater than 35 is considered normal, and a %CD4+ of 20 roughly corresponds to an absolute count of 200 cells/mm^3.

Who Is at Risk for HIV?

Early in the epidemic workers spoke of "risk groups"—gay men, injection-drug users, and prostitutes. It later became apparent that the risk was not in who one was but in what one did. Workers then began to speak of "risk behaviors"—unprotected sexual intercourse of any kind and the sharing of needles and works. For women especially, it is these behaviors that place them at risk.

Protocol 2.1 Sex and Substance Use History-Taking

- Do you have or have you had sex with men, with women, or with both?
- Have you undergone any gender surgery?
- Do you use barrier methods when you have sex (e.g., condoms, dental dams)?
- Have you or your sex partner ever had a sexually transmitted disease?
- Have you or your sex partner ever injected drugs?
- Do you use recreational drugs like alcohol, cocaine, marijuana, or amphetamines?
- Have you ever had hepatitis B?
- Did you receive blood, blood products, skin grafts, artificial insemination, or an organ transplant between 1978 and 1985?

Source: Adapted from Nadler 1992.

In the early years of the disease most HIV-infected women identified sharing needles or works as their risk behavior. But an increasing number of women reported having heterosexual contact with injection-drug users or bisexuals. In 1988, 18 percent of AIDS cases in the United States occurred among women whose only risk was heterosexual exposure. By 1990 this had increased to 33 percent (CDC 1990a). Women with HIV tend to be from urban areas, though the incidence in more rural settings is also on the rise; they also tend to be women of reproductive age, women of color, and mothers or caretakers of partners and children.

In testing for HIV, a sexual and substance-use history should be taken to help the woman identify possible exposures—non-barrier-protected sex with someone who may have been infected; needle use; a history of other sexually transmitted diseases; and blood transfusion between 1977 and 1985, before testing of the blood supply for HIV was routine—particularly if she is considering pregnancy or already is pregnant (see protocol 2.1). Because for many women heterosexual contact is the only known risk factor, all women—especially those who live in high seroprevalence areas—should be routinely offered testing.[1]

The mainstay of HIV testing is the ELISA (enzyme-linked immunosorbent assay), which measures a protein (antibody) that is made in response to the virus. The sensitivity and specificity of the test approach 99.5 and 99.8 percent, respectively. But false positives can occur, so the Western blot is always done to confirm the result. Although it is also an antibody test, the Western blot measures antibodies to certain structural components of the HIV and is considered more specific than the

[1] In one study of 76 HIV-positive women, for example, 36 percent had no identified risk; 57 percent reported sexual contact with a man at known risk for HIV infection (see Allen and Marte 1992).

ELISA. Only when both the ELISA and the Western blot are positive is an individual said to be infected. Antibody to HIV is normally detected two to twenty-four weeks after exposure to the virus (Chaisson and Volberding 1990). During this "window period" an infected person may still test negative. Therefore, a woman with a high-risk exposure whose test result is negative should be retested in three to six months. Alternatively, nonantibody tests may be helpful, but they require research facilities and are much costlier. Such tests involve detection of the virus by culture, detection of HIV DNA by a gene-amplification technique called polymerase chain reaction, and detection of a specific viral antigen called p24.

Because of the emotional, personal, and societal impact of a positive test result, HIV testing must be voluntary, confidential, and offered with counseling and referrals. Confidentiality is critical, and access to anonymous testing should be available.

A negative HIV test represents an opportunity for counselors to reinforce risk-reduction behaviors. A positive test result is always difficult to convey, but it should be presented with accurate information, immediate HIV staging, referrals, and a clear message of hope. A positive result that is given insensitively can affect a woman's relationship with the health care system for months, delaying the initiation of therapy and causing an abiding distrust of the medical system.

The delicate task of informing the patient of a positive test result must be done within the social framework of each patient's support system, family responsibilities, insurance and economic status, history of substance abuse (including alcohol), and coping mechanisms and resources. Education on the difference between HIV and AIDS, the implications of CD4+ cell counts, and the availability of treatments must be provided within the patient's cultural framework, with some understanding of that individual's definition of health and philosophy of a healthy lifestyle. Hope is the key at this stage of intervention.

How HIV Affects Women

An understanding of how HIV manifests in women—the specific infections to which women are susceptible and the gynecological presentation—is critical to establishing early intervention strategies and therapies. Although no large multicenter cohort studies of women are available, several groups have investigated differences in presentation in smaller numbers of men and women.

In studies such as those by Carpenter et al. (1989, 1991), candida esophagitis, wasting, and mucocutaneous herpes simplex virus were found to be the most common AIDS-defining events. In contrast, the Community Programs Clinical Research in AIDS (CPCRA) study reported Pneumocystis carinii pneumonia (PCP) as the most common event, followed by wasting syndrome, then candida esophagitis (Rodriguez et al. 1991). Studies that have compared men with women have found PCP to be the most common AIDS-defining event, occurring equally in men and women (Fleming et al. 1991; Grant et al. 1991; Thompson et al. 1991).

These and more recent reports, though helpful, are limited by cohort size and retrospective techniques. But the incidence of PCP is significant enough to warrant similar prophylaxis recommendations for men and women. Women appear to be at increased risk for development of candida esophagitis, but whether this reflects a predisposition in women or a lack of awareness on the part of practitioners earlier in the disease process is unclear.

Another way to study HIV in women is to examine their presenting symptoms. For example, Mayer et al. (1991) reported on a group of 117 symptomatic women whose initial presentations included recurrent vaginal candidiasis (N=43), persistent generalized lymphadenopathy (17), bacterial pneumonia (15), acute retroviral syndrome (8), constitutional symptoms (8), oral thrush (6), thrombocytopenia (6), leukoplakia (4), shingles (2), PCP (2), HIV encephalopathy (1), and cytomegalovirus retinitis (1). The women later presented with vaginal candidiasis (89), oral thrush (36), genital warts (32), bacterial vaginosis (28), bacterial pneumonia (26), candida esophagitis (24), and trichomonas vaginitis (18).

This study and others have shown that women may present with recurrent severe bacterial infections, such as non-Pneumocystis pneumonia (now part of the CDC case definition of AIDS), and that gynecological disorders may serve as early markers of HIV infection. Although candida is common in immunologically competent women, severe recurrent vaginal candida should prompt a discussion of risk behavior for HIV and voluntary testing. Pelvic inflammatory disease (PID) has been seen with increased incidence in HIV-positive women (Safrin et al. 1990), often with a more frequent need for surgical intervention (Hoegsberg et al. 1989).

Staging and Early Treatment

Treatment of HIV disease has progressed rapidly with the introduction of anti-retroviral agents and prophylactic regimens to prevent the most common AIDS-defining illnesses. An understanding of the natural history of HIV has helped define stages of the illness, from the asymptomatic to the end stage. With earlier recognition and diagnosis, more women than before can be expected to present at the less symptomatic stage. Many of the women who are diagnosed early may be most appropriately treated in the primary-care setting.

The initial workup following diagnosis should include staging of HIV disease and screening for associated illnesses (AMA Physician Guidelines 1990). Practitioners may use the CDC's 1993 revised HIV disease classification system to determine the patient's status along the disease continuum (see figure 2.1).

Aside from the absolute and %CD4+ cell counts, initial laboratory tests include baseline complete blood counts (CBCs), chemistries, and urinalysis. Addi-

Figure 2.1 CDC Disease Staging

CD4+CATEGORIES	CLINICAL CATEGORIES		
	A Asymptomatic or PLG	B Symptomatic	C AIDS-indicator conditions
1 > 500/mm^3	A1	B1	C1
2 200-499/mm^3	A2	B2	C2
3 < 200/mm^3	A3	B3	C3

Source: CDC 1992

tional early tests are screenings for syphilis with rapid plasma reagent (RPR), for hepatitis B with the hepatitis B surface antigen and hepatitis core antibody, and for tuberculosis with placement of a purified protein derivative (PPD) and appropriate anergy controls. A baseline chest X-ray when the patient is asymptomatic is helpful, because early signs of PCP may be subtle. Some practitioners include a screening toxoplasmosis titer at this time.

It is important that the initial workup include a gynecological evaluation, including Pap smear. Current CDC guidelines advise annual Pap smears, but some practitioners recommend the test every six months in women with CD4+ counts of less than 200 cells/mm^3. Concurrent infection with human papilloma virus (HPV) warrants colposcopy and biopsy, and many sites utilize colposcopy every six months as standard of care for women with concurrent HIV and HPV. Sexually transmitted diseases should be treated aggressively. In women with low CD4+ cell counts, in-hospital treatment of PID is warranted (Minkoff 1991; see also Thompson and Swift 1992 for management protocol).

Many women presenting with HIV infection have additional medical problems— asthma, hypertension, diabetes, arthritis, anemia, allergies, obesity, alcohol and drug abuse—that complicate the course of HIV infection and its treatment. Anemia, for example, which is common in women of childbearing age, may be seriously exacerbated by AZT therapy. Drug and alcohol problems may keep the client from participating fully in health management. Preventive health assessments, such as baseline mammography for clients age forty and older, must be administered regularly. A comprehensive problem list should be compiled for all clients, with the goal of stabilizing acute and chronic medical problems.

At the initial visit, referrals to support groups, counselors, substance-abuse programs, and entitlement programs should be made and the importance of notifying partners stressed (see protocol 2.2). Risk reduction is an ongoing counseling objective. Protocol 2.2 summarizes key points for the initial visit. The practitioner should be prepared to cover many of the same topics on subsequent visits.

The second visit should be scheduled as soon as the CD4+ cell count is available. Women often approach this session with more focused questions, and time should be spent discussing the response of family and friends to the diagnosis. Continuing education regarding HIV and AIDS should be undertaken with culturally appropriate and literacy-appropriate materials. With the results of the CD4+ cell count, a therapy plan can be formulated. Because the count can fluctuate, two determinations taken over time will give a more accurate assessment of the HIV stage. In general, women with CD4+ counts of 500 or greater should be reassured that they are in the asymptomatic stage of illness. No specific therapy is recommended, but another count should be done in six months. A count of 200–500 should initiate discussion of antiretroviral therapy (generally AZT or ddI). A count of 200 or less should initiate discussion of antiretroviral therapy and PCP prophylaxis. With CD4+ counts in mind, followup gynecological care should be scheduled.

During the early visits, pneumococcal vaccine should be given unless the patient has already been immunized. Influenza vaccine should be given annually. For those at risk of contracting hepatitis B but with no history of exposure, vaccination should be offered (see protocol 2.3). For children, immunizations should be updated following accepted guidelines. In general, live vaccines should be avoided.

At all stages of HIV disease, consideration should be given to the availability of clinical treatment trials through the federally sponsored Aids Clinical Trial Group, the CPCRA initiative, and drug-company-sponsored private trials (see chapters 7 and 8). Practitioners should be aware of resources within their community and should direct women to these important programs whenever possible.[2] Women who care for children or partners require special consideration, and practitioners should make efforts to keep such women in treatment trials and ongoing care. Issues to be

---

[2] NIH/NIAID maintains an information line on ongoing clinical treatment trials. The telephone number is (800) TRIALS–A.

Protocol 2.2 Initial HIV Workup

Medical History

- History of bacterial, viral, parasitic, and fungal infections, and other STDs
- Sexual and drug-use history
- Travel in developing countries or where endemic fungal infections are found
- Pets in household
- Immunization history

Social History

- Family system (biological or family of choice)
- Occupational history, socioeconomic needs (insurance, disability benefits, housing, etc.)

Physical Exam

q visit	• Weight (assess baseline nutritional status, then q visit); height or body surface area; BP; temp
q visit	• Psychiatric (affect, history, medications, or suicidality)
q visit	• Skin (lesions, etc.), nails (fungus, clubbing)
q visit	• Oral cavity and tongue
q 3 mos.	• Eye exam (ideally with mydriatics; fundoscopic: assess retina)
q 3 mos.	• Lymph nodes, ears, and nose (visualize turbinates, palpate facial sinuses)
q 3 mos.	• Heart and lungs
q 3 mos.	• Abdomen (liver and spleen)
q 3 mos.	• Extremities (muscle mass, myositis, etc.)
q 3 mos.	• Neurological (mental status exam; cranial nerves; reflexes; gait; fine motor skills)
Annually	• Breast exam
Annually	• Genital and perirectal area

Pelvic Exam

q 6 mos	• Pap, GC, chlamydia, HPV, wet mount
	• Refer for colposcopy if concurrent HPV or abnormal Pap results

Labs

- CBC with differential and platelets
- Lymphocyte panel (CD4+ and %CD4+)
- Chemistry panel, including liver functions (e.g., ALT, AST, alkaline phosphate, bilirubin)
- RPR/serological syphilis
- Toxoplasma antibody
- Hepatitis B panel (HBsAg, Anti-HBc, Anti-HBs)

(continued)

Protocol 2.2 (*Continued*)

- PPD with anergy
- Urinalysis
- Baseline chest X-ray (PA and lateral)

Disease Staging (based on above data)

Counseling

- Referrals for support groups, substance abuse tx, entitlement programs
- Risk reduction and partner notification

Sources: Adapted from Valenti 1992; Thompson and Smith 1992.

addressed in ongoing care include risk reduction, family planning, living wills and medical power of attorney, and custody determinations for children. Living with HIV is stressful, and ongoing discussion of substance abuse and coping mechanisms must be established.

Antiretroviral Therapy

As of June 1992 three antiretroviral agents have been approved by the Food and Drug Administration for treatment of HIV disease: AZT (Retrovir or zidovudine); ddI (Videx); and ddC (Hivid), approved for use in combination with AZT. Each works by inhibiting the enzyme reverse transcriptase. Of the agents, AZT is the most studied; ddI may be used only by those who failed with or were intolerant of AZT. The new agent D4T, or stavudine, is available on a trial basis.

In early trials, AZT delayed deterioration of the immune system and decreased the frequency of opportunistic infections, with no significant differences between outcomes for men and women. For women with two consecutive CD4+ cell counts of less than 500 cells/mm^3, AZT is recommended at 500 mg daily, usually divided into three or five doses. Few serious side effects are seen with these levels of AZT, though some patients experience nausea, headache, vomiting, myalgia, and insomnia during the initial weeks of therapy. A temporary dose reduction to 300 mg daily is recommended to resolve these problems. CBC with differential and platelets needs to be monitored during therapy at two weeks, at one month, and, if the value is stable, every three months thereafter (see protocol 2.4). A macrocytosis that is not responsive to therapy with vitamin B$_{12}$ or folic acid often occurs. Patients may also develop normocytic anemia, neutropenia (drug should be withheld for neutrophil counts of less than 500), and thrombocytopenia. Patients should also be monitored

Protocol 2.3 Vaccinations for Adults with HIV

- Polyvalent pneumococcal vaccine   _____ × 1
- dTetanus vaccine   _____ q 10 years
- Influenza virus vaccine   _____ q November
- Hepatitis B vaccine _____ baseline _____ 1 mo. _____ 6 mos.
- Consider *Haemophilus influenza* type B conjugate vaccine

Source: Adapted from Bronx-Lebanon Hospital Center 1992; Falloon 1992.

for such allergic responses as fever or rash; myopathy has been seen with long-term usage of AZT.

Gynecological abnormalities with AZT use have not been described, though animal studies have demonstrated vaginal tumors in female mice on high and prolonged doses. The significance of this for women is not known. There are no compelling data to suggest that AZT behaves differently in women than in men, but clinicians caring for women should report any unusual experiences with the drug to the FDA.

The second antiretroviral, ddI (Videx) was released for use in 1991. Like AZT, it is a reverse transcriptase enzyme inhibitor. Studies on long-term effects are under way, as are comparison trials with AZT as combination therapy. At present the drug is reserved for use in patients who are intolerant of AZT—those who are suffering such intractable side effects as nausea, fatigue, refractory anemia, or neutropenia— and for those who "fail" AZT—developing recurrent opportunistic infections or rapidly losing CD4+ cells while on therapy. Mechanisms for failure may include the development of resistance by HIV to these agents, a process that takes, on average, eighteen months in patients on AZT. The clinical significance of this resistance has not been proved, but the problem has encouraged the development of new agents and trials of therapies that combine such antiretroviral agents as AZT or ddI to delay or prevent the emergence of resistance.

The current recommended dosage of ddI is based on patient weight, with a standard dose of 200 mg twice daily, administered as chewable tablets. Potential side effects include nausea, diarrhea, neuropathy, and pancreatitis. Patients with a history of pancreatitis or with markedly elevated triglyceride levels should probably avoid this agent. Because this agent was introduced later that AZT, more women were involved in the initial trials. No specific gender differences have been reported. Because relatively small numbers of women have been exposed to ddI, clinicians should be alert to unusual side effects and report them to the FDA.

The third antiretroviral, ddC (Hivid), had been shown to be less effective than AZT as monotherapy. In June 1992, ddC in combination with AZT was approved

Protocol 2.4 CD4+ Counts and Therapy Guidelines

CD4+ count	Action
• >600/mm³	No recommended intervention; repeat CD4+ count q 6 mos.
• 500–600/mm³	Possible antiretroviral (case-by-case); repeat CD4+ count q 3 months
• 300–500/mm³	Antiretroviral as indicated; repeat CD4+ and labs q 3–6 mos.
%CD4+ >22	Evaluate for toxicity and disease progression q 3–6 mos.
• 200–300/mm³	Antiretroviral agent(s) and possible PCP prophylaxis
%CD4+ >20–22	Repeat CD4+ q 3 mos.
• <200/mm³	Antiretroviral agent(s)
%CD4+ <20	PCP prophylaxis Rifabutin prophylaxis for MAC (FDA approval for CD4+ <100) Monitor for development of serious infections, including clinical evaluation and laboratory tests q 1–3 mos.
Patient Education	Don't pin all emotions on a single lab result; get T-cells tested at roughly same time of day each visit

Toxicity Management of Antiretroviral Therapy

Anemia	Neutropenia
Hg 9.5–10.5 gm/dL: Monitor CBC q 2 wks	ANC 1,000–1,500/mm³: Monitor CBC and diff. q 2 weeks
Hg 8.0–9.4 gm/dL: Monitor CBC q wk	ANC 750–999/mm³: Monitor CBC and diff q wk
Hg 6.5–7.9 gm/dL: Stop drug; monitor CBC 1–2 × week; transfuse if symptomatic; when Hg improves (8–9.4 or better), restart zidovudine at lower dose (300 mg qd)	ANC 500–749/mm³: Stop drug; monitor CBC and diff. 1–2 × week. Observe for symptoms of infection. When ANC improves (≥750–999), restart zidovudine at lower dose (300 mg qd)

Note: ANC (absolute neutrophil count) calculated as percentage segs plus bands multiplied by total WBC.

Sources: Adapted from Falloon 1992; Santangelo and Schnack 1992; Thompson and Smith 1992.

for the treatment of advanced HIV infection (CD4+ count of less than 300 cells/mm³) in patients who have demonstrated significant clinical or immunologic deterioration. This recommendation was based on data from two small studies that were not designed to measure clinical efficacy or effect on clinical progression. More controlled trials are under way. At present, most clinicians are using this combination in those who have failed a course of AZT followed by a course of ddI or who are intolerant of these agents. Other agents and combinations are being studied in treatment protocols.

Opportunistic Infections and Prophylaxis

A major advance in the treatment of HIV disease has come with the early recognition and treatment of Pneumocystis carinii pneumonia. Early in the epidemic PCP frequently resulted in death, but today it can often be managed in an outpatient setting. Equally important has been the recognition—derived from the experience of patients who have undergone organ transplants—that small doses of the same antimicrobials used to treat PCP can prevent the development of the infection. This use of antibiotics to prevent or delay disease manifestation is known as prophylaxis. Recommendations regarding prophylaxis and treatment change periodically, and new agents are under investigation.

PCP remains a significant risk, and the NIH advises that when CD4+ cell counts fall below 200 cells/mm³, prophylactic regimens should be initiated. The current drug of choice is trimethoprim/sulfamethoxazole (Bactrim, Septra); one double-strength tablet is taken once daily or three times weekly. Potential side effects include fever, rash (including Stevens-Johnson syndrome), leukopenia, anemia, thrombocytopenia, azotemia, nausea, and hepatitis.

For patients who are allergic to sulfa-containing drugs or intolerant of trimethoprim/sulfamethoxazole, pentamidine 300 mg may be given as a nebulization (aerosolized treatment) once monthly. Some patients experience bronchoconstriction with this agent and should be pretreated with an inhalant bronchodilator. Other side effects include cough and occasionally pancreatitis.

Dapsone, an agent used to treat leprosy, has been used alone or in combination with pyrimethamine for prophylaxis, but studies comparing efficacy are not yet completed. A new investigational agent used to treat active PCP, 566C80, is also being studied as a prophylactic agent.

Disease caused by Mycobacterium tuberculosis has become a concern as increasing incidence and the appearance of new strains that are resistant to multiple drugs have sparked a parallel epidemic, especially in cities like New York and Miami, which have high rates of HIV. People with HIV-related immunosuppression are at much greater risk for manifestation and rapid progression of active tuberculosis disease than are non-HIV-infected people. But tuberculosis in HIV-infected individuals is preventable and treatable, and all efforts should be made to diagnosis the condition early. Once the diagnosis of HIV infection has been established and a CD4+ cell count determined, women should be screened for TB exposure (see protocol 2.5). A 5TU intradermal PPD and anergy battery should be given. If the PPD is positive (at least 5 mm of induration) a chest X-ray should be performed and isoniazid prophylaxis initiated. An abnormal X-ray warrants aggressive workup for active tuberculosis. When the X-ray result is normal, the test should be repeated annually.

A negative PPD may be caused by anergy; therefore, controls should be placed

Protocol 2.5 Tuberculosis Screening and Treatment Algorithm

- All persons with HIV should receive PPD skin test with anergy panel: place 5TU PPD by Mantoux method with two or more DTH antigens (candida, mumps, or tetanus toxoid).

- Any induration measured at 48–72 hours is considered evidence of DTH response; failure to elicit response (0 mm induration) indicates anergy.

- Persons with a positive PPD reaction (≥ 5 mm induration by CDC; some sites use ≥ 2 mm) are considered infected with MTb and should be evaluated for isoniazid (INH) prophylaxis after active tuberculosis has been ruled out.

- If active disease suspected, CXR and collect sputum smear for acid fast bacillus.
  a. If AFB is positive, start on INH and rifampin with respiratory isolation.
  b. Await culture reports (6–8 wks); if positive MTb growth, begin full course of tx (minimum of 12 months with 3–4 agents).
  c. Followup for exposed contacts (household members, coworkers, etc.)

- HIV-positive persons who are PPD-negative but are anergic and at risk of MTb (estimated risk ≥ 10 percent) should be considered for prophylactic INH (10–15 mg/kg/day in a single dose $\times$ 12 months, regardless of age).

Sources: Adapted from CDC 1991a; O'Grady and Frasier 1992; Thompson and Swift 1992.

(see CDC 1991b and protocol 2.5). If these are positive the PPD is repeated yearly. If the anergy panel is negative, a chest X-ray is obtained; if the X-ray is abnormal, a workup for TB is initiated. If the X-ray is normal in the anergic patient but she has history of exposure to TB or has spent time in communities with a high prevalence of the disease, prophylaxis with isoniazid 300 mg daily for twelve months should be strongly considered (CDC 1989a).

As the CD4+ cell count falls, the risk of opportunistic infections increases. Clinical trials are under way to assess the utility of other prophylactic regimens— like rifabutin or the newer macrolides, such as clarithromycin, azithromycin—to prevent Mycobacterium avium complex (MAC). Rifabutin is now FDA-approved for the prevention of MAC. Fluconazole is being evaluated as a prophylactic agent for such fungal infections as cryptococcosis. There are no definitive recommendations regarding other prophylactic regimens, but many of these may be forthcoming.

Health care providers who work with women with HIV disease face the challenges of treating disenfranchised clients and watching previously healthy and generally young people die. They must summon the energy to learn about a disease that seems to be constantly changing and for which most of the potential therapies are still under investigation. It is not surprising that many providers feel unequal to the task.

It can be argued that HIV illness legitimately belongs within the spectrum of primary care. It is a life-threatening, chronic condition with a long asymptomatic phase during which clients benefit from monitoring and treatment. Primary-care providers, knowingly or not, are seeing women at risk for HIV disease and are treating conditions that are often caused or exacerbated by HIV. Their familiarity with the process, signs and symptoms, and treatment strategies of the disease will improve care for the woman living with HIV.

3

Gynecological Considerations in the Primary-Care Setting

Risa Denenberg

I was diagnosed in November 1990; I had lots of symptoms before then, but I was an IV-drug user so you learn to take care of the problems by getting high. I should have been diagnosed when my son was, since we got high together sometimes. He died while I was in the hospital and would have been thirty-two this Saturday.

I needed the drugs to help shut my mind down, and when that happened, that was glorious. . . . I got through withdrawal while I was in the hospital. Now I feel fantastic— don't like to see needles even for a blood test! Of course, my children and family were in back of me, even through my drug thing. . . . I've been married for a year now to a man I met at the Baker House shelter where I was sent after I got out of the hospital. I have ups and downs, but they're child's play compared to what I've been through. This may sound weird, but if it weren't for this virus, I might still be acting stupid. Together, we make each day count now.

People make life too complicated. They look at simple stuff and say, "That's not rational." I look for the simple thing every time. People always ask me the same question— "Why are you always in a good mood?" It's easier than being sad! I did a photo shoot recently for an AZT ad, and the photographer asked me to look serious. "Well," I said, "that'll be a problem!"
—Grace Simons

Biological differences between women and men are important to health care management. For example, women have a greater distribution of body fat and a unique and complex cyclic hormonal system. They are subject to such organ-specific diseases and conditions as pelvic infections, cervical cancer, and vaginal thrush. They also suffer a higher incidence of certain diseases than men do, including simple urinary tract infections, breast cancer, and human papilloma virus (HPV) infections. Women also experience more complications of such common disorders as gonorrhea and chlamydia. Many of these concerns fall into the general category of gynecology.

Recognition of the early manifestations of immunocompromise in the genital tracts of women is crucial to forestalling progressive undiagnosed HIV infection. Likewise, medical strategies for treating gynecological infections and cancers must consider the woman's current immune status to be effective (Allen 1990).

Providing Gynecological Services in Primary-Care Settings

Too often women do not receive comprehensive gynecological care in the primary-care setting (Marte 1989). This disservice to all women poses additional hardships for those with HIV infection. All primary-care providers are trained in routine gynecology, so why is this area of care so often ignored? In some cases, there may be provider reluctance to compile a comprehensive menstrual, sexual, and reproductive history. After all, the gynecological history brings to the surface difficult and unpredictable topics: early sexual abuse, current domestic violence, sexually transmitted infections, concerns about fertility, menstrual problems, pelvic pain, and sexual dysfunction. The care provider may feel inadequate to the task, and a woman with such problems would be better served by a specialist. A male care provider may feel burdened by the need to have a female observer present during examinations. And the task of educating the client on such topics as safer sex, frequency of gynecological care, douching or use of tampons, family planning, and self-breast examination may seem overwhelming. Yet health maintenance, disease prevention, and client education make up the very fiber of primary care.

In some primary-care settings it may not be feasible for all providers to perform gynecological evaluations on HIV-positive clients. Sessions staffed by a gynecologist, nurse-practitioner, certified nurse-midwife, physician's assistant, or other trained primary-care provider can be established. When women receive gynecological care in a familiar setting, continuity with the regular medical provider is enhanced (Denenberg 1992). It may also be optimal to provide simultaneous pediatric care in the same location.

The only expensive equipment required for providing gynecological care is a good microscope for wet-prep slides to diagnose vaginitis. Other required supplies include disposable speculums of all sizes, materials for Pap smears, cultures for gonorrhea and chlamydia, viral cultures for herpes simplex virus, medications for the treatment of simple genital warts (trichloroacetic acid is preferred), sanitary pads, patient examination gowns and drape sheets, saline and potassium hydroxide (KOH) solutions for wet preps, microscope slides, and cover slips. Examination tables should be equipped with stirrups, and the exam room should include a private area for undressing.

As do many simple medical procedures, gynecological examinations pose the risk of blood exposure to the examiner. Universal precautions include wearing gloves and disinfecting spills according to standard guidelines and institutional policies (CDC 1988a, 1991c).

Staff in-service training and excellent referral sources are critical to the establishment of successful gynecological services for HIV-positive clients. In-service training should ideally involve all levels of personnel: physicians and other medical providers, nursing staff, social workers, and others involved in patient care. It is essential that a sensitive, skilled gynecologist be available for prompt referral.

Gynecological screenings of HIV-positive women often uncover much pathology. In some studies, as many as 45 percent of HIV-positive women had abnormal Pap smears that called for colposcopy (Sillman and Sedlis 1987; Provencher et al. 1988; Schrager et al. 1988; Feingold et al. 1990; Maiman et al. 1991; Anastos et al. 1992). Immunocompromised women with moderate to severe pelvic infections may be at greater risk of developing tubo-ovarian abscesses than are other women, and they need ready access to hospitalization (Minkoff 1991). Women may request services—like tubal ligations—that are beyond the scope of care provided in the primary-care setting, so referral sources for prenatal and obstetric care and for abortion services are essential.

Risa Denenberg

Protocol 3.1 Gynecological Screening

- Pelvic exam q 6 mos., including
  a. Papanicolaou smear
  b. STD screen (GC, chlamydia, HPV)
  c. Wet mount (r/o candida, BV, trich)
     Pap results
        If inflammation: treat, followed by repeat PAP smear
        If atypia of undetermined significance: refer for colposcopy
        If dysplasia/CIN: refer for colposcopy and endocervical curettage/biopsy of
           any lesions

- Counseling at time of initial pelvic exam:
  HPV, cervical cancer, STDs, candida, contraception and pregnancy, safer sex

- RPR q 6 mos.
  or for suspicious lesion or history of exposure

- Medications available on prn schedule:
  acyclovir, topical $+/-$ oral ketoconazole $+/-$ fluconazole (monitor LFTs)

Source: Adapted from Marte 1989.

Gynecological Screening

HIV-positive women are ten times more likely than uninfected women to have abnormal cervical cytology. Abnormal findings include inflammatory changes, vaginal pathogens (monilia, trichomonas, and bacteria), cellular atypia, and cervical intraepithelial neoplasias (CIN) of all grades. The severity of the abnormality is believed to correlate with the degree of immunosuppression (Feingold et al. 1990; Maiman et al. 1990; Anastos et al. 1992). The entire lower genital tract may be affected and at risk of developing squamous cell cancers. In immunocompromised women this type of disease tends to persist, recur, and extend, even with conventional treatment. Further, in one study of thirty-two women, Pap smears did not uncover cytological abnormalities that were evident from colposcopically directed biopsies obtained at the same time (Maiman et al. 1990).

The vast majority of squamous cell abnormalities in the genital tract are associated with HPV, specifically with strains 16, 18, 31, and 33 (Becker, Stone, and Alexander 1987). Immunocompromise accelerates the progress from viral infection to neoplasias both in renal transplant patients on immunosuppressive therapy and in HIV-positive women with lowered CD4+ counts. Several recommendations therefore seem prudent. Cytological screening for HIV-positive women—particularly those with AIDS and depressed CD4+ counts—needs to occur frequently. Most clinicians feel that Pap smear screening should be performed every six months. At the time of screening it is equally important to culture the cervix for gonorrhea and chlamydia and to diagnose and treat vaginitis (see protocol 3.1).

Routine on-site colposcopic evaluation of HIV-positive women probably is not feasible in most institutions, so liberal referrals for such evaluation must be provided. All Pap smears with atypias, CINs of all grades, and carcinoma-in-situ (CIS) should be referred for colposcopic evaluation within six weeks. It is important to use a cytology laboratory that is consistently accurate and employs the Bethesda system for reporting (Lundberg 1989; National Cancer Institute 1989).

Treating Infections

Gynecological infections—genital ulcers, vaginitis, simple urinary tract infections, postpartum endometritis, or pelvic inflammatory disease—may be an early sign of HIV illness. These infections may be recurrent and difficult to treat, warranting close attention and followup because they may indicate underlying immuno-compromise (Minkoff and DeHovitz 1991).

Sexually transmitted diseases and genital lesions are likely to facilitate the transmission of viruses (Pepin et al. 1989; Moss and Kreiss 1991). These STDs and lesions include genital ulcer diseases (GUD): syphilitic chancres, genital herpes, chancroid, and, rarely, lymphogranuloma venereum and granuloma inguinale (donovanoses). Other lesions that may accompany HIV infection include genital warts and molluscum. Chronic vaginitis may predispose women to HIV transmission and to other STDs (Schmid 1990).

In managing women with gynecological infections, caregivers should take the client's sexual history, ask about symptoms, perform a speculum and bimanual examination, and obtain laboratory specimens. They also must consider the client's overall health and degree of immunocompromise. Clients with lowered CD4+ cell counts are often pancytopenic, which increases their susceptibility to infection and complicates their response to treatment. Further, their white blood count (WBC) may not rise in response to systemic infection, thus rendering an important test less useful. Erythrocyte sedimentation rates (ESR) are often elevated in chronic illness and therefore become less useful in the diagnostic workup for such acute infections as pelvic inflammatory disease (PID). It has been observed that immunocompromised women with acute PID often are less symptomatic than their immunocompetent counterparts, even with marked disease (Marte and Allen 1991).

Several nonprescription agents are available for treatment of vaginal yeast, but the cost of such drugs can be prohibitive. HIV-positive women should be trained to recognize the signs and symptoms of this vaginitis—which include an itchy, cottage cheeselike discharge—and should be cautioned to expect them when placed on other antibiotics. Self-treatment weekly or every other day can prevent outbreaks, but for more severe recurrences or when standard therapy fails, such systemic agents as ketoconazole or fluconazole are useful.

In general, full-course therapy is recommended over any abbreviated courses for vaginitis, urinary tract infection, and PID. For example, it is preferred that metronidazole be used for a full seven days in treatment of trichomonas and that antifungal creams or suppositories be administered for a full week in the treatment of vaginal thrush, rather than single-dose or three-day treatments. It also seems prudent to have the client return for a followup visit so the effectiveness of treatment can be ascertained, even for minor cases of vaginitis or urinary tract infection. Consideration of the stage of HIV illness is useful in planning followup. All STDs must be treated according to CDC guidelines, and the cures must be tested for effectiveness (Aral and Holmes 1991). Treatment of sexual partners should be arranged when appropriate. Counseling regarding safer sex must be reinforced frequently to help prevent new infections and to preserve overall health and freedom from new infections.

Particularly troublesome are recurring and hard-to-treat infections. Immunocompromise predisposes many clients to repeated outbreaks of genital herpes, which may become resistant to acyclovir. Genital warts may rapidly turn into a florid infection that will not respond to such ordinary measures as local application of trichloroacetic acid. Vaginal thrush may recur or fail to clear with suppositories or vaginal creams (Sobel 1990; Dupont 1990). It is important that aggressive therapy and supportive measures be available. Clients may require constant high-dose treatment with acyclovir for persistent herpes lesions, and cryotherapy, interferon injections, laser therapy, and 5-fluorouracil creams (5-FU) often need to be employed to treat difficult warts (Allen 1990; Lebowohl and Contard 1990; Minkoff and DeHovitz 1991). Systemic antifungals and rigorous prophylactic measures may be required for recurrent vaginal thrush. The client's comfort may depend on the clinician's familiarity with the safe use of such home remedies as sitz baths, soothing lotions and creams, and with nutritional considerations and judicious use of pain medications. Persistence, sensitivity, and consideration on the part of the clinician are likely to be rewarded with improvement, or at least improved comfort, for these clients. Table 3.1 reviews differential symptoms and management of vaginitis.

Few regimes are available for prophylaxis of common fungal infections in women. Although oral agents such as clotrimazole (Mycelex troches) have been effective in preventing oral candida, no recommendations are available regarding vaginal prophylaxis. Patients should be advised to decrease their dietary sugar, and many clinicians recommend daily ingestion of acidophilis-containing yogurts (Hilton 1992). Use of vaginal suppositories of nystatin or clotrimazole on a weekly, three-times weekly, or daily schedule is also a good preventive measure. Trials are needed to assess which agents and dosages will provide the safest prophylactic

Table 3.1 Vaginitis

Condition	Symptoms	Wet Prep	TX	Prevention/Comfort Measures
Bacterial vaginosis	Odorous, frothy discharge	pH > 4.5 clue cells + whiff	Metronidazole 500 mg BID × 7 d; avoid alcohol Alt: Augmentin 500 mg TID × 7 d	Treat female partners with goldenseal sitz bath (1 TB goldenseal powder in warm water)
Trichomonas	Copious, itchy discharge	Motile trichomonads	Metronidazole 250 mg TID × 7 d; avoid alcohol	Treat all partners with garlic suppositories (wrapped in gauze QD @ HS × 2–3 wks) if metronidazole contraindicated
Yeast (candida, vaginal thrush)	Itchy, clumpy discharge with irritation	pH < 4.0 hyphae and spores on KOH slide	Antifungal creams or supp. HS × 7 d, repeated as needed; add ketoconazole 200 mg QD × 5–14 d as needed	Daily intake of lactobacillus-containing yogurt or acidophilus capsule and decrease dietary sugar; for inflamed labia: mycolog or lotrisone Rxs or A + D, Desiten or zinc oxide ointment
Atrophic vaginitis	Irritation, burning, or discharge; atrophic appearance to mucosa	pH > 6.0; no vaginal pathogens	Estrogen creams per vagina 2 × weekly; appropriate workup for systemic HRT	Daily perineal massage with calendula cream, vitamin E oil, or wheat germ oil; 3 × daily Kegel exercises to increase circulation
Herpes HSV infection	Painful, blisterlike sores anywhere in genital area; swollen inguinal nodes	—	Apply BID Acyclovir 200 mg 5 × d @ initial outbreak; 400 mg BID for maintenance	Therapeutic vitamins and lysine 500 mg QD; zinc oxide ointment to new sores; goldenseal sitz bath

Source: Denenberg 1992.

Risa Denenberg

Table 3.2 Use of Exogenous Hormones in HIV Infection

Oral Contraceptives

Pros	Cons
Contraceptive efficiency	Unknown drug interactions
Menstrual regulation	Possibly increased vaginitis
Decreased PMS	Increased gingivitis
Scant menstrual blood loss	Increased respiratory infections
Reduced menstrual-related anemia	Bothersome side effects in some
Treatment for dysfunctional uterine bleeding	Contraindicated in smokers and those with asthma, liver disease
	Possibly reduced immune function

Hormone Replacement in Menopause

Pros	Cons
Controls bothersome symptoms (hot flashes, dysuria, vaginitis)	Unknown drug interactions
May improve mood, appetite, sleep	Uncertain impact on immune response
Improves urethral syndrome	
Helps distinguish symptoms of menopause from symptoms of opportunistic infections	
Prevents osteoporosis	

Source: Denenberg 1992.

approach; a clinical trial evaluating the use of intermittent fluconazole in the prevention of mucotaneous candidal infections may soon provide guidance in this area.

Menstruation and Menopause

HIV-positive women frequently complain of changes in their menstrual cycles: irregular, heavier, or scantier periods, and increased premenstrual symptoms (breast pain, cramping, fluid retention, anxiety, and depression). It is not known whether these changes are caused by HIV itself or by medications, particularly AZT, or both. Other variables that may affect the menstrual cycle include use of street drugs (particularly heroin), and weight loss.

Current standards of care neither approve nor forbid hormone therapy during menopause or for birth control or menstrual regulation. But too often, in an effort to "do no harm," health care practitioners withhold hormones from women (see table 3.2). This policy may be subtly reinforced by the idea that all immune-suppressed patients will progress to AIDS in the near future, so the long-term benefits of such therapy will not be useful to them. There may also be subconscious opinions that women with HIV infection become "asexual" or that they should not have sex and therefore do not have the same concerns others have about menstruation, menopause, and sexuality. These biases deny women appropriate care.

There are almost no data available regarding the use of exogenous hormones in clients who are transsexuals (male to female). Hormones are used both before and after surgery to develop and maintain desired secondary sex characteristics. Providing appropriate clinical supervision may enable clients to lower a high use of estrogen. The possible negative consequences of high rates of exogenous hormone use include an increased risk of breast cancer and other cancers. Reinforcement of needle-cleaning instructions may be warranted, as silicon injection—sometimes with shared needles—can be a practice in the transsexual community.

Menstrual problems can affect a woman's health adversely during HIV illness. Blood loss from heavy periods can predispose a woman to anemia or exacerbate the problem. Irregular or absent periods may signal significant systemic illness.

Amenorrhea should be investigated in all women (Speroff, Glass, and Kase 1989). The diagnosis can usually be accomplished in the primary-care setting, but consultation with a gynecologist or an endocrine specialist may be necessary. Sexually active women should undergo a pregnancy test. If the result is negative, the woman should be scheduled for a pelvic examination to rule out a pelvic mass. If a mass is noted, a sonogram can be scheduled for confirmation. Tests measuring the levels of thyroid-stimulating hormone and prolactin should be ordered to determine if the problem lies outside the reproductive tract. If these values are normal and pregnancy is ruled out, the woman can be given a progesterone challenge—usually 10 mg of provera daily for five days—to induce bleeding. If withdrawal bleeding occurs following this challenge, it is established that the woman is producing estrogen but is not ovulating. Anovulatory women may be at increased risk of developing endometrial or breast cancer owing to constant unopposed estrogen.

If no withdrawal bleeding occurs with the progesterone challenge, the woman is experiencing either ovarian failure to produce estrogen or hypothalamic failure to produce follicle stimulating hormone (FSH) or luteinizing hormone (LH). This is the time in the workup to order LH and FSH levels. Hypothalamic failure, which will demonstrate low levels of FSH and LH, is usually related to stress or weight loss and often will resolve without treatment. High levels of FSH prove that the ovaries are being properly stimulated but are not producing estrogen. Ovarian failure can be caused by premature menopause, autoimmune disease, or a destructive disease of the ovaries. Diagnoses and proper treatment should be established.

Menopause, the natural ending of the menstrual cycle, does not generally require treatment. But premature menopause seems to be more common in immune-suppressed women than it is in others. Hormone replacement is indicated for severe symptoms of menopause, which include hot flashes, atrophic vaginitis, urethritis, vaginal dryness and itching, and discomfort during urination. Replacement hormones may also prevent osteoporosis and damage to the cardiac system. The main concern about hormone replacement is that it increases the risk of endometrial and breast cancer. Current regimens combine estrogen with progesterone to reduce the risk of cancer.

In women with HIV, symptoms of ovarian failure, such as hot flashes, may be worse at night than during the day. They may be easily confused with night sweats brought on by such infections as tuberculosis or Mycobacterium avium complex (MAC). Atrophic vaginitis and urethritis may be mistakenly and repeatedly treated as vaginal thrush and may cause openings and sores on the genitals. These symptoms may interfere with normal sleep, appetite, and sexual functioning.

Reproductive and Sexual Health

HIV-positive women do not differ significantly from any other women in how they make decisions regarding pregnancy and abortion. It seems clear that efforts to interfere in personal and family decision making not only are invasions of a woman's privacy, but they also tend to impose distance between the health care system and HIV-positive women. When health care providers are seen as supportive of women's rights and abilities to make informed decisions, the provider-client relationship is generally preserved.

A common response to the discovery of HIV infection—among both women and men—is to shun sexual relations for a period of time. This often is a symptom of depression and altered self-esteem. HIV-positive clients need support and encouragement to attain healthy and safe relationships where affection and sexuality are experienced. But they may need to go through the stages of grieving for the loss of their healthy and whole self-image and in anticipation of their own death. The stage of HIV illness must be taken into account in assisting clients through this grieving process. It may be helpful to counsel the client individually and with her partner. The hopeful message that sexual dysfunction (often accompanied by such symptoms as sleeplessness and poor appetite) is most likely temporary sets the stage for teaching about safer sex practices. A positive attitude about sexuality includes acceptance and encouragement of its safe expression.

Furthermore, women often need support and assistance in learning how to disclose their HIV status to sexual partners, how to incorporate the use of condoms into the sexual relationship, and how to experience pleasure during sex.

An important challenge for clinicians is working with "discordant" couples—those in which only one individual is HIV-positive—who desire a child. By offering support and referrals for alternative insemination, infertility workups, and adoption agencies, clinicians can help a couple avoid unsafe sex while achieving their goal of having children.

Client Education

Health care workers should view every encounter with an HIV-positive woman as an opportunity to provide useful and appropriate information and education. This sharing of information can take place during the provider visit and nursing interview. Health educators are valuable team members. Social workers are often viewed by clients as knowledgeable about the complexities of HIV illness and the medical system and willing to address clients' concerns. Use of an interdisciplinary team approach will increase the likelihood that clients' need for information can be met.

Specific areas of client teaching that encompass gynecological, reproductive, and sexual health include:

• the need for frequent gynecological examinations and Pap smears;

• the relation between immunocompromise and gynecological problems;

• early reporting of such symptoms as irregular bleeding, vaginal discharge, pelvic pain, sores, missed periods;

• the need for monitoring, treatment, and prophylaxis for vaginal infections, particularly thrush;

• strategies for implementing safer sex with male and female partners;

• advice regarding douching, use of tampons, and sexual activity[1];

• home remedies for cutaneous rashes, chronic herpes infection, recurrent vaginitis, and other problems affecting the genital area;

• contraceptive advice and information;

• and accurate information regarding pregnancy, perinatal transmission of HIV, and HIV testing of children at risk.

Summary

The woman with HIV illness confronts a multiplicity of needs: psychological, social, financial, nutritional, sexual, and medical. Primary-care settings strive to meet these needs by undertaking the complex tasks of early detection, prevention, and management of illness. Routine early referral for potential problems may improve the likelihood that HIV-positive women will maintain their jobs, homes, families, and psychological well-being or receive medical benefits or treatment for drug addiction in a timely way. This early-referral approach is often most available and effective in the primary-care setting.

Primary-care facilities cannot afford to lose the resources available for treating HIV-positive clients, who often end up in the primary-care setting with or without

---

[1] Women with recurring pelvic infections probably should never douche; women must not insert anything into the vagina following a cervical biopsy, cryotherapy, or other similar treatment.

their own or their clinician's knowledge. When primary-care facilities have identified the proportion of their clientele at risk for HIV infection—and incorporate policies, training, and protocols for treating such clients—it will become easier to maintain appropriate funding.

The challenge of delivering comprehensive primary care to the women with HIV must be borne by a multidisciplinary team of doctors, nurses, physicians assistants, nurse-practitioners, nurse-midwives, social workers, health educators, and nutritionists. The task ahead may be among the most important work that health care practitioners will undertake in this decade.

4

Reproductive Health and Counseling

Margaret Hutchison and Maureen Shannon

I felt like I was totally destroyed, like I was going to die, and that's all I understood. I was afraid because I had a lot of kids and I didn't want to leave my children alone. . . . I didn't want them to go to foster care, and I didn't know what my family would do. I was mentally torn apart.

Everybody that has HIV should look for a person that's working in that field who always thinks . . . positively. . . . You have to have somebody that you can actually touch. The phone is great, but somebody . . . that can put their arms around you to make you feel like a person, you know, [so] that you don't feel dirty. Because it's a horrible thing to feel dirty.

I think it took me about a year to realize that I wasn't going to just drop dead next month, you know, so I started trying to get my mind together for that aspect. My biggest

> fear was that I would die before my oldest child became 18,
> and I didn't want that to happen. I wanted to wait for her to
> become 18.
> —"Terry Ann"

Decisions on whether to become pregnant or to continue a pregnancy involve complex personal issues for all women, particularly in this time of besieged reproductive freedom. The decision-making process is confounded by HIV-positivity, which superimposes the reality of a chronic infectious disease that will considerably diminish the quality and length of most women's lives.

Contraceptive compliance and reproductive decision making are shaped by a multitude of factors—variables that are as important to women with HIV as to those who are uninfected. But for an HIV-positive women, selection of a contraceptive method is influenced by the method's efficacy in preventing both pregnancy and transmission of disease. In this chapter we focus on these concerns in order to assist the care provider who works with HIV-positive women in the context of their reproductive lives.

Family Planning

Ideally, a contraceptive method for an HIV-positive woman will thwart both the horizontal transmission of sexually transmitted diseases (STDs) and the vertical transmission of HIV by preventing pregnancy. Family planning counseling is inadequate when it focuses on contraceptive methods that are highly effective in preventing the transmission of STDs (especially HIV) but are less successful in preventing pregnancy. Evaluating a woman's needs on the basis of her sexual practices and her relationship with her partner or partners is essential in determining whether a particular method will be appropriate and successful.

Table 4.1 presents the failure rates, benefits, and possible side effects associated with the methods discussed in this chapter; for a comprehensive presentation of family planning methods see Hatcher et al. (1992).

Barrier Methods

Barrier methods of contraception include condoms (male and female), diaphragms, cervical caps, and vaginal sponges. An additional benefit of these methods, especially when they are used in conjunction with a spermicide like nonoxynol-9, is protection against several of the pathogens that cause STDs. There is wide support for the use of one or more of the methods for HIV-positive women and women at risk of HIV exposure.

Table 4.1 Contraceptive Methods and Use in HIV-Positive Women

Contraceptive Method	Failure Rate (percentage)	STD Protection	Risks and Side Effects	Indications for HIV-Positive Women
Abstinence	0%	Maximum.	None except possible pregnancy or STD if sexual assault occurs.	No contraindications.
Contraceptive sponge Parous Nulliparous	9–28% 6–18%	Documented decreased risk of gonorrhea and chlamydia; risk of other pathogens and nonoxynol-9 irritation; no evidence of HIV prevention.	Increased risk of pregnancy (for parous women especially), vaginal candidiasis, and microabrasions/lacerations; possible increased risk of toxic shock syndrome.	Limit use as a long-term contraceptive because of associated risks. Should be used only if no other option is available at time of coitus. Avoid use during menses and remove within recommended time period. Use with latex condom to enhance STD and pregnancy prevention.
Diaphragm	6–18%	Documented decreased risk of pelvic inflammatory disease, gonorrhea, chlamydia, and cervical neoplasia. Use with nonoxynol-9.	Latex allergy and increased risk of urinary tract infections, TSS, microabrasions, and pregnancy.	Use with caution because of possible side effects (avoid during menses) and risk of pregnancy if used improperly. Use with latex condom and nonoxynol-9 spermicide to enhance STD and pregnancy prevention.

Table 4.1 (*Continued*)

Contraceptive Method	Failure Rate (percentage)	STD Protection	Risks and Side Effects	Indications for HIV-Positive Women
Cervical cap	6–18%	Theoretically similar to diaphragm (decreased risk if nonoxynol-9 used).	Latex allergy, difficult removal, increased risk of microabrasions and possible increased risk of pregnancy and abnormal Pap and TSS.	Limited use because of side effects and risks. Use with latex condom and nonoxynol-9 to enhance STD and pregnancy prevention.
Latex condom (male)	2–12%	Documented decreased risk of gonorrhea, chlamydia, herpes, hepatitis B, HPV, HIV; nonoxynol-9-containing latex condom further decreases risk of STDs.	Latex allergy, increased pregnancy rate.	Recommended for STD prevention. Use with nonoxynol-9 to enhance prevention of pregnancy and STDs.
Polyurethane condom (female)	12–26%	Laboratory evidence of impermeability to HIV, hepatitis B.	Latex allergy, increased pregnancy rate.	Protects against other STDs (e.g., HPV). Use with nonoxynol-9 to enhance effectiveness.
Spermicides containing nonoxynol-9	3–21%	Documented decreased risk of HIV, gonorrhea, chlamydia, herpes.	Mucus-membrane irritation, microabrasions, pregnancy.	Recommended for STD and pregnancy prevention. To enhance STD and pregnancy prevention, use with barrier method.
Intrauterine device (IUD): Progestasert Copper T 380 A	2% 0.8%	None.	Increased risk of PID, intermenstrual spotting, and bleeding.	Contraindicated because of increased risk of PID and theoretically greater risk of HIV transmission.

Method	Failure rate		Comments
Oral contraceptives (OCs) Combination, low-dose	0.1%	Documented lower risk of PID (though PID risk caused by chlamydia may be unchanged).	Possibly greater immunosuppression and cervical neoplasia. Cervical ectropion with greater risk of STD (CT), no HIV protection, intermenstrual spotting, interaction with medications.	Use with close followup because of side effects until more data are available, especially women in advanced stages of immunosuppression. Concomitant use of latex condoms and nonoxynol-9 essential to lower STD exposure.
Oral contraceptives (OCs) Progestin-only	1.1%	None documented.	Increased menstrual cycle changes, including intermenstrual bleeding, increased pregnancy rate compared with combined OCs.	Use with close followup until more data are available. Concomitant use of latex condoms and nonoxynol-9 is essential to lower STD exposure.
Subdermal implants	0.4%	None documented.	Increased menstrual cycle changes, including intermenstrual bleeding during first few months after insertion.	Use with close followup until more data are available. Concomitant use of latex condoms and nonoxynol-9 essential to lower STD exposure.
Tubal ligation	0.4%	None.	Increased risk of ectopic pregnancies and abnormal menstrual patterns.	Recommended in women definitely desiring cessation of childbearing. Use latex condoms and nonoxynol-9 to lower STD exposure.

Failure rate: Percentage of women experiencing unplanned pregnancy during first year of method use (Trussel et al. 1990).

Source: Shannon 1992.

Margaret Hutchison and Maureen Shannon

Male Condoms A compilation of data from numerous investigations demonstrates that latex condoms, especially those containing spermicides, provide substantial protection against several STDs, including gonorrhea, chlamydia, human papilloma virus, herpes virus, hepatitis B, and HIV (CDC 1988a; Judson et al. 1989; Minuk et al. 1987). Natural-membrane condoms are not recommended as a means of preventing STDs, however, because they have been documented to leak HIV during laboratory simulations of penile thrusting (Van de Perre, Jacobs, and Sprecher-Goldberger 1987).

Consistency of condom use among HIV-positive women and their partners is difficult to assess. Studies of condom use among women engaging in risk behaviors showed that accessibility to condom supplies does not correlate with increased compliance. Major deterrents to consistent condom use among women include the inability to negotiate condom use effectively with a partner, lack of perceived risk of STDs or pregnancy, crisis-oriented problem solving and behavior, and poor access to health care. The health care services provided to HIV-positive and at-risk women should include community-based STD prevention and family-planning programs that advocate a nonjudgmental approach in order to encourage patient compliance *(Contraceptive Technology Update* 1992).

Female Condoms There are two types of female polyurethane condoms currently available or in development. Their advantages are similar to those of the male condom, with the additional advantages of protection during cunnilingus and control of the method by the woman. Disadvantages may include expense (especially with frequent coitus), problems with partner negotiation, and lack of data regarding efficacy rates for pregnancy prevention (Connell 1989; Hatcher et al. 1993). The female condom may be most useful for HIV-positive women who anticipate infrequent coital activity.

Cervical Barrier Methods The diaphragm, the cervical cap, and the contraceptive sponge are among the barrier methods of contraception approved for use in the United States. When used with a spermicide these methods can reduce the acquisition and transmission of STDs. Additional advantages include reversibility, relative inexpensiveness, and control of the method by the woman.

These methods have not been documented to effectively prevent HIV transmission, however, and should be used with caution by HIV-positive women. Use of such methods has been associated with the development of microabrasions and lacerations (Hatcher et al. 1993), and breaks in the mucosa of HIV-positive women could provide a mechanism for transmission of HIV and other STDs. Although these methods provide a barrier over the cervix, most of the woman's vaginal vault is unprotected (except for the chemical protection of a spermicide), and the vaginal mucosal surfaces and their secretions could also afford an opportunity for the transmission and acquisition of STDs (Hatcher et al. 1993).

Some cases of toxic shock syndrome have been reported with the use of the contraceptive sponge and the diaphragm (Faich et al. 1986; Hatcher et al. 1993). Although no similar data exist regarding the cervical cap, there is some concern because the mechanism of action is similar to that of the sponge and diaphragm. Use of the cervical cap has been associated with increased incidence of rapid develop-ment of abnormal Pap smear results (Bernstein 1986); however, other investigators have not found such a correlation (Gollub and Sivin 1989; Richwald et al. 1989). The theoretical risk must be considered when an HIV-positive woman wishes to use the cervical cap, though, because HIV-positive women are already at an increased risk for the development of cervical intraepithelial neoplasias (CIN) as their immu-nosuppression advances (Maiman et al. 1990).

Because of these potential complications, cervical barrier methods should be considered by HIV-positive women only when no other contraceptive option is available. To enhance prevention of pregnancy and STDS, these methods should be combined with use of a latex condom by the woman's partner.

Vaginal Spermicides

Spermicides are chemical surfactants that attach to sperm and immobilize or destroy them (Connell 1989; Hatcher et al. 1992). They also are effective in the prevention of STDs: nonoxynol-9 has demonstrated an inhibitory effect against gonorrhea, chlamydia, syphilis, trichomonas, herpes simplex virus types 1 and 2, and HIV (Austin et al. 1984; Hicks et al. 1985; Malkovsky, Newell and Dalgleish 1988; Louv et al. 1988; Niruthisard et al. 1991).

Anecdotally, however, some women using nonoxynol-9 report irritation and a burning sensation after sex and during urination, urethral and vulvar irritation, and rash. This has led to concern over a possible association between the use of sper-micides and the development of vaginal abrasions and lacerations, a complication that may foster the transmission of all STDs. But because microabrasions have been reported in women following vaginal intercourse without spermicide use (Novell et al. 1984), it is unclear whether nonoxynol-9 contributes to the development of vaginal and cervical abrasions. Until this finding is studied further, the use of spermicides as a means of preventing STDs in sexually active HIV-positive women is recommended (CDC 1989; Connell 1989; Hatcher et al. 1992). Women who experience vaginal or other irritation with nonoxynol-9 may use spermicidal prepa-rations with a similar anti-HIV effect but slightly different chemical composition—such as silicon or SK-70. Combining spermicide with a barrier method, especially a latex condom, will maximize its contraceptive and STD-preventive effects.

Margaret Hutchison and Maureen Shannon

Hormonal Contraceptive Methods

Several methods of hormonal contraception are currently available in the United States, including combination oral contraceptive pills (OCs), progestin-only contraceptive pills, progestin-secreting subdermal implants (such as Norplant), progestin injections (Depoprovera), and progestin-secreting intrauterine devices. Gonadal steroids exert some influence on the regulation of both humoral and cell-mediated immunity. Studies of immune function in women using combination OCs have reported conflicting data regarding the hormones' effects on immunosuppression (Allen 1990; Baker et al. 1985). Currently, there is no documented evidence that OC use by HIV-positive women contributes to the progression of their immune disease (Contraceptive Technology Update 1992; Minkoff and Dehovitz 1991).

Because of the association between estrogen levels and the development of cervical ectopy with OC use, there is a theoretical concern about increased risk of HIV transmission. Cervical ectopy leads to increased cervical secretions, which contain lymphocytes and monocytes with CD4+ receptor sites to which HIV attaches (Meirik and Farley 1990). Since cervical secretions of HIV-positive women contain the virus (Vogt et al. 1986; Wofsy et al. 1986; Archibald et al. 1987), an increase in secretions could increase the risk of transmission to an infected woman's sexual partner. OC-induced ectopy also leads to eversion of the columnar epithelium, which can increase the risk of transmission to women (see chapter 11).

Plummer and colleagues (1991) reported a statistically significant increase of HIV transmission among Nairobi prostitutes using combination OCs when compared with controls. This finding was independent of other variables, including genital ulcer disease, but it has not been replicated in other populations (Carael et al. 1988; Allen et al. 1991). Its significance may in fact illustrate the importance of using STD protection (latex condoms and spermicides, for example) in conjunction with effective methods of pregnancy prevention.

There is no consensus on whether OCs increase the risk of cervical neoplasia. Despite their numerous methodologic difficulties, some studies suggest an increased risk in women using OCs for five or more years (Vessey et al. 1983; Negrini 1990; Brinton 1991). The possibility of an increased risk of cervical neoplasia in HIV-positive long-term OC users has not been investigated. Some studies have demonstrated an increased incidence of CIN in HIV-positive women, however, especially as immunosuppression progresses (Maiman et al. 1988; Spurrett, Jones, and Stewart 1988; Maiman et al. 1990). Given the need for more data, the potential risks for the development of cervical neoplasia must be measured against the potential benefits of avoiding pregnancy in HIV-positive women.

There has been some interest in the use of subdermal hormonal implants in HIV-positive women. The possible adverse effects are unknown, but implants combined with STD protection may be a viable and attractive option for HIV-positive women who desire sustained contraceptive benefit without the permanence of a tubal ligation.

Concern about hormonal contraceptive use by HIV-positive women is appropriate given the paucity of information available regarding the methods and their possible interactions with the pathologic conditions of this infection and the pharmacologic agents used to treat it. But until further studies clarify these complex interactions, the elimination of a highly effective method of contraception for HIV-infected women—especially those who are in the early stages of infection and relatively immunocompetent—seems unwarranted.

Intrauterine Devices

The contraceptive benefit of an intrauterine device (IUD) is presumed to be a result of several factors, including a local inflammatory response of the woman's endometrium that prevents successful implantation. This response has been cited as a cause of concern regarding use of IUDs by HIV-positive women: such a response and the resulting increase in the number of lymphocytes and monocytes could both provide additional receptor cites for HIV and expose an HIV-positive woman's sexual partner to HIV-infected genital secretions. In addition, the tail of an IUD can cause penile trauma, breaking the skin and providing a port of entry for HIV (Allen 1990; Contraceptive Technology Update 1992). In addition, the increased spotting and bleeding observed in IUD users could increase exposure to HIV-infected secretions (Contraceptive Technology Update 1992), as well as contribute to the development of anemia.

The increased risk of pelvic inflammatory disease (PID) associated with IUD use is another concern. Current contraceptive guidelines cite impaired immune response and behaviors associated with an increased risk of STDs and PID as strong relative contraindications for the use of an IUD (Allen 1990; Hatcher et al. 1992). These risks, along with those discussed previously, make IUD use by HIV-positive women inadvisable.

Voluntary Surgical Contraception

Voluntary surgical contraception is the interruption of tubal patency for both women (tubal ligation or occlusion) and men (vasectomy). Although the reversal of these procedures is possible, they should be considered a permanent cessation in childbearing. There are no studies of voluntary female sterilization and complications in HIV-positive women. Since tubal ligation does not afford any protection against STDs, a woman and her partner must be educated about the need to use latex condoms each time they have sex.

Margaret Hutchison and Maureen Shannon

Therapeutic Abortion

The earlier in gestation a therapeutic abortion (TAB) is performed, the more likely it is that the woman will avoid such complications as infection, bleeding, cervical or uterine injury, or death (Hatcher et al. 1992). The safety of TAB procedures in HIV-positive women has not been studied. Extrapolation of findings from studies of HIV-positive women who were pregnant or being treated for gynecological diseases (such as CIN) has indicated an increased risk of morbidity as immune functioning deteriorated (Maiman et al. 1990). Because late-gestation terminations are linked to increased incidence of complications in the general population, it seems prudent to make TABs available to women who want them, regardless of their HIV status, as soon as possible to reduce morbidity.

Artificial Insemination

There are several reports in the literature of HIV transmission via artificial insemination (Stewart et al. 1985; Rekhart 1988; Chaisson, Stoneburner, and Joseph 1990; CDC 1990b). Both the Centers for Disease Control and Prevention and the American Fertility Society have developed guidelines for screening prospective donors that include testing at time of donation, freezing and quarantine of semen, and retesting of the donor six months later and before use of the semen (CDC 1988b; Peterson, Alexander, and Moghissi 1988). Because no method has been shown to eliminate HIV from semen consistently, the CDC in 1990 also advised against donation by known HIV-positive men. Although the overall incidence of HIV transmission by donor semen is low, documentation that such transmission occurs should be considered by all involved in the process.

Pregnancy

When an HIV-positive woman wants to become pregnant, she and her partner must receive counseling about the timing of coitus to limit HIV exposure and transmission—no intercourse during menses, and only selectively during ovulation. Fertility-awareness methods of family planning may need to be considered. If artificial insemination is pursued, the risks must be discussed.

Safer Sex Techniques and Counseling

Much has been written about behaviors associated with increased risk of acquiring STDs. Activities that pose the greatest risk of HIV transmission are receptive anal intercourse (Koop 1986; Padian et al. 1987), unprotected vaginal intercourse (Koop 1986; Fischl et al. 1987; Padian et al. 1987, 1991), and exposure to blood during coital activity (Holmberg et al. 1989; Allen et al. 1991). HIV transmission also appears to be enhanced by the presence of other STDs, especially those associated with genital ulceration (syphilis, herpes, chancroid) and cervicitis (Carael et al. 1988; Holmes and Kreiss 1988; Holmberg et al. 1989; Allen et al. 1991; Holmes 1991; Marx et al. 1991; Plummer et al. 1991; O'Farrell, Windsor, and Becker 1991).

The incorporation of safer practices into an HIV-positive woman's sexual activity is integral to her health care. Reduced exposure to STDs and their attendant complications is an obvious advantage for the woman and her partner. The acquisition of other STDs by an HIV-positive woman can result in serious health consequences, including neurosyphilis, PID from exposure to gonorrhea or chlamydia, CIN from human papilloma virus infection, and recurrent herpes virus infections. The successful treatment of such diseases is often difficult and protracted in HIV-infected women (Hoegsberg et al. 1990; Maiman et al. 1990), especially in those at more advanced stages of immunocompromise. Because viral replication in HIV-positive individuals can be stimulated by infections, a reduction in exposure to and acquisition of such infections is an important goal (see table 4.2). In addition, preventing the transmission of HIV between an HIV-positive woman and her partner not only reduces the partner's risk of infection, it also prevents reexposure and an increased viral load in the woman whose partner is also HIV-positive.

In addition to reviewing risk and prevention strategies, clinicians must assess the HIV-infected woman's sexual preference, number of partners, types of sexual behavior, contraceptive method, her partner's involvement in STD prevention, and her ability to negotiate safer sex with her partner or partners. Although a questionnaire can be used to obtain this information, a followup interview is essential to clarify responses, educate the woman about her specific needs, and provide safer-sex guidelines.

A woman's knowledge of how to prevent the transmission of STDs is beneficial only if she can put it into practice. Her decision on whether to do so may be affected by cultural and family influences, religious beliefs, drug use by the woman or her partner, economic instability, and domestic violence, as well as by her awareness of her vulnerability to STD exposure.

Studies indicate that knowledge of HIV transmission and prevention does not consistently provoke changes in sexual behavior, even among people living in areas of high HIV seroprevalence (Kegeles, Adler, and Irwin 1988; Jemmott and Jemmott III 1991). But a perceived susceptibility to HIV may be a key factor in a person's decision to decrease risk-taking behaviors and increase preventive measures (Kegeles, Adler, and Irwin 1988; Solomon and DeJong 1989). Therefore, assessing an HIV-positive woman's perceived risk of exposure to STDs is an essential component of the counseling process.

When possible, the woman's partner should be included in the counseling

Margaret Hutchison and Maureen Shannon

Table 4.2 Risk Behaviors and Prevention of HIV Transmission

	Safest	Low Risk	Possibly Unsafe	High Risk
Behaviors	Abstinence Self-masturbation Monogamy (both partners uninfected and not engaged in risk activities) Hugging, massaging, touching, mutual masturbation* Dry kissing Drug abstinence	Wet kissing Vaginal intercourse with latex condom Anal intercourse with condom and spermicide	Cunnilingus Fellatio	Unprotected receptive anal intercourse Unprotected vaginal intercourse Unprotected anal penetration with hand Oral-anal contact Multiple sexual partners if unprotected sex Sharing sex toys or douches Sharing needles for any purpose
Prevention Strategies	Avoid increased risk behaviors	Avoid exposure to possibly infected body fluids. Consistently use latex condoms and spermicide with vaginal intercourse. Avoid anal intercourse, but if anal sex occurs, use latex condoms and spermicide.	Use dental dam or female condom with cunnilingus. Use latex condom with fellatio.	Avoid exposure to possibly infected body fluids. Consistently use condom and spermicide with vaginal intercourse. Avoid anal penetration (penile or hand); if anal penetration occurs, use condom with anal intercourse, latex glove with hand. Avoid anal-oral contact. Do not share sex toys or douching equipment. Do not share needles, but if sharing needles, clean them with bleach before and after use.

*If no breaks in skin.

Source: Adapted from Cohen 1990; De Ferrari 1989.

sessions. This allows an assessment of their perceptions regarding the effectiveness and acceptability of safer sex techniques, as well as an opportunity to reinforce those techniques with thorough instructions. Emphasizing the importance of avoiding other STDs and infections to prevent unnecessary illness may encourage the use of safer-sex methods. In cultures in which the man is regarded as the head of the household, stressing his responsibility to protect the family and maintain its well-being may enhance his compliance with such methods (Schilling et al. 1989; Maldonado 1990).

Psychosocial factors can have a major impact on an HIV-infected woman's compliance with therapeutic interventions, including safer sex practices. She may experience denial, guilt, anger, depression, and anxiety in facing this disease and its effects on her life and family. These elements of the grieving process (Kübler-Ross 1969) may delay her integration of safer sex practices, especially if she and her partner are experiencing denial.

In addition, a woman who is psychologically or economically dependent on her partner may have little or no say about sexual practices in the relationship. Her suggestion regarding condom use may seem to imply mistrust or infidelity. Furthermore, a partner may oppose methods to prevent STDs because of his desire for a child. Such dynamics can jeopardize a woman's economic stability and emotional support system and possibly subject her to physical abuse from her partner (Karan 1989; Anastos and Palleja 1991). Disclosure of HIV serostatus to explain why safer sex practices are desired may further jeopardize her relationship and therefore may not be perceived as a viable option.

A chemically dependent woman's need to obtain a drug may supersede her desire or ability to use safer sex practices. The effects of the drug may alter her sense of vulnerability to STDs, resulting in decreased condom use. Her physical and psychological craving may override a rational approach to negotiating safer sex with partners who will provide her with drugs or money for drugs (Marx et al. 1991). A recent study by Schilling and colleagues (1991) documented the successful incorporation of condom use by black women and Latinas enrolled in a methadone-maintenance program after they participated in five group sessions designed to increase their knowledge of AIDS risks, their acceptance of condom use, and their ability to negotiate safer sex. This approach to education and building negotiating skills among high-risk women may be necessary to effect behavioral changes that will reduce the risk of STD exposure.

Antibody Testing

Most HIV testing of women takes place in family planning, gynecology, STD, and prenatal clinics. Practitioners involved in testing should consider both the purpose of testing (whom the information will benefit) and how testing should be offered.

The applicability of universally or selectively offered screening depends on local seroprevalence rates and specific characteristics of the at-risk population (Landesman et al. 1987; Barbacci, Repke, and Chaisson 1991; Institute of Medicine 1991). Most high-seroprevalence areas offer testing to all women who come in for care; in areas with low incidence of HIV, testing is often discussed only with women who acknowledge risk behaviors. Informed consent and pre- and post-test counseling are essential components of both screening methodologies.

Practitioners and facilities should be apprised of these testing philosophy issues as well as of the particular needs and limitations of their setting. Preserving the confidentiality of test results and offering support and referral are necessary parts of care. The many issues involved in the testing of women are presented in the 1991 Institute of Medicine publication. For HIV-testing protocols in the antepartum setting, the reader is referred to Holman et al. (1989) and Tuomala (1990). Protocols for nonpregnant populations have been published by Carr and Gee (1986) and McMahon (1988).

Counseling About Reproductive Options

The issue of reproductive choice is a most difficult and ethically charged aspect of the HIV testing and counseling of women. Numerous studies representing diverse cohorts of women—drug users, low-income women, women in the military, and partners of hemophilic men—show that knowledge of HIV-positivity has little or no effect on contraceptive behavior (Fischl 1987; Price et al. 1989; Selwyn et al. 1989; Brown and Rundell 1990; Dattel et al. 1991). Similarly, two studies of low-income women found no significant differences in rates of pregnancy termination between women with known HIV-positivity and matched seronegative controls (Sunderland et al. 1988; Selwyn et al. 1989). Other studies have examined the reproductive behaviors of HIV-positive women (Barbacci et al. 1989; Kaplan et al. 1989; Wiznia et al. 1989; Brown and Rundell 1990; Jason et al. 1990; Johnstone et al. 1990); a summary of available data found that in most cohorts 50 percent or more took their pregnancies to term (Sunderland 1990).

Decision-Making For HIV-positive women, serostatus has been documented as only one of many factors that influence reproductive decision making. Other factors are individual, community-based, or religion-based morality or ethics regarding abortion; a desire to parent; the influence of partner, family, and friends; religious faith/optimism; risk evaluation (acceptable versus unacceptable odds); access to care; prior experience with HIV; maternal health concerns; cultural norms; parenting concerns; psychological adaptation to HIV; and non-HIV-related psychological issues (Sunderland et al. 1988; Selwyn et al. 1989; Sunderland 1990; Hutchison and

Kurth 1991). Many women speak of the importance of motherhood in their lives, and children may be a source of strength or a reason to live. For some addicted women, a pregnancy provides the impetus to become drug-free and holds the promise of normal family life (Cancellieri et al. 1988; Mitchell 1988). The value of motherhood may also be shaped by culture. For example, some Latin communities hold mothers in especially high esteem (Worth and Rodriguez 1987), and children in black and Latin cultures have a role in the preservation of cultural identity (Mays and Cochran 1988).

How women perceive the risk of perinatal transmission of HIV also influences decision making. The conceptualization of risk may vary with life context. In one study, some Kenyan women with HIV sought to better their chances for healthy offspring by having more children (Temmerman et al. 1990; see also chapter 12). In the United States the risks associated with daily living—including the risks of perinatal, infant, and child mortality—vary greatly by socioeconomic class and life circumstance. It is important to note, however, that risk calculation in the face of a reproductive decision may be a difficult task for women of *all* socioeconomic backgrounds (see Faden 1987).

Psychological variables are clearly involved in many reproductive decisions. It may be difficult for women with preexisting psychiatric morbidity (such as addiction) to adapt to an HIV diagnosis and to make reproductive choices (Cancellieri et al. 1988), and decision making by women with and without psychiatric problems is confounded by the process of adaptation to HIV (Kurth and Hutchison 1990). Women with HIV may pass through stages similar to those described by Kübler-Ross (1969) or struggle with the ambiguity of asymptomatic seropositivity. For pregnant women, the psychology of adaptation to AIDS and HIV is superimposed on the psychology of pregnancy, with as yet undetermined effects (see Varney 1987; James 1988).

The impact of HIV-related grief on pregnancy decision-making has been only minimally explored. The only study of the effects of grief on reproductive behavior that could be found in the general pregnancy literature shows that sexual intimacy and pregnancy fulfill needs related to the recent death of a parent (Swigar, Bowers, and Fleck 1976).

The data thus far described were collected predominantly from low-income cohorts, groups that are representative of the majority of HIV-positive women. But studies of women in the military (Brown and Rundell 1990) and of partners of hemophilic men (Jason, Evatt, and the Hemophilia–AIDS Collaborative Study Group 1990) document both planned pregnancies and decisions against therapeutic abortion in the context of known HIV-positivity among women who are generally well-educated, employed, and without known risk behaviors other than sex with their male partners. Rationales for the decision to bear children are only briefly discussed in these studies, with quotes from hemophilics' female partners who either know of their HIV-positivity or have unknown positivity but known risk. Their reasons echo those of the low-income women with HIV. They express "denial that the offspring really could become infected" and show a "willingness to 'take their chances'" along with an "unwillingness to consider the possible consequences" (Jason, Evatt, and the Hemophilia–AIDS Collaborative Study Group 1990, 487).

There may be a danger in emphasizing socioeconomic elements of reproductive decision making—that is, the assumption that poor women have special reasons for having babies while women of higher socioeconomic or educational status choose "rationally." This perception of women with HIV who choose to reproduce is arguably parentalistic and divisive, ignoring factors already identified in the reproductive decision-making literature that have little or nothing to do with socioeconomic status. Even more egregiously, it is blind to the continued childbearing of women who do not fit the usual profile of the woman with HIV. More research is clearly needed to understand the reproductive behaviors of *all* women.

There has been heated ethical debate about the appropriateness of various modalities for the reproductive counseling of women with HIV. For more on this issue the reader is referred to chapter 9 and to the literature by Bayer (1990), Nolan (1990), Arras (1990), and Faden, Geller, and Powers (1992). For both ethical and pragmatic reasons, many care providers working with HIV-positive women espouse the genetic nondirective counseling model. The role of the genetic counselor is to "translate scientific possibilities into personal calculations" (Rapp 1987, 1) in the course of helping women to decide what is right for them and their families.

What does this model mean for the care provider faced with reproductive counseling of the HIV-positive woman? It provides a useful framework if the care provider accepts the basic premise that a reproductive decision for a woman with HIV is hers alone to make. For some, this precept is not acceptable; others may embrace it theoretically but balk at the disturbing realities of some women's choices. To be effective, counselors must be comfortable with the moral terrain of HIV and reproduction as well as with sexuality and drug abuse.

Counseling involves providing up-to-date information about HIV and its impact on infected women and discussing such topics as perinatal transmission, pediatric disease and assessment, and the effects of pregnancy on maternal HIV disease and on prenatal care; care of the child with HIV and plans in the event of worsening disease; and psychosocial support systems. These topics must be discussed in language appropriate for each woman. According to Rapp (1987, 7), the counselor engages in a "tug-of-war of words" as she or he seeks to find the parlance that has most meaning to the client, taking into consideration the woman's educational level, primary language, and idiomatic or regional speech patterns.

Cultural and social or peer-group belief systems also can influence the efficacy of communication. Williams (1990) found that a majority of a group of women at risk for HIV through their own or a partner's injection-drug use believed that maternal-fetal transmission of HIV occurred during every pregnancy. Their belief was based in part on the assumption that drugs in a pregnant woman's bloodstream will enter the child. Cultural differences in perceptions of disease and health may confound the counseling interaction as well. For example, a study of the health beliefs and practices of low-income African-American women in Los Angeles County found that "AIDS had been integrated into the traditional conceptualization of illness, health practices, and healing" (Flaskerud and Rush 1989, 210).

Ideally, a health system responds to the cultural diversity of its clientele by providing culturally matched counselors and providers. In reality, it must often suffice for staff members to become sensitive to cultural differences (including class, race, and social group) and to remain open in each counseling session to navigating a course to better understanding (see chapter 13).

The client's perception of the counselor may complicate the communication process. In some Latin cultures, for example, deference to authority may cause women to withhold their feelings throughout a counseling session (Medina 1987). And wariness of a message delivered by the medical establishment may also have cultural roots, as exemplified by the black community's historic and well-founded distrust of public health interventions (Levine and Dubler 1990).

Finally, grief can also influence the counseling session. A counselor must strive to identify grief stages and tailor interventions accordingly. The following summarized case study (Hutchison and Kurth 1990) illustrates some of these principles:

> Amy is a 37-year-old mother of seven children who has been in and out of drug treatment for fifteen years. She has been pregnant twice since learning of her HIV-positivity. The first pregnancy occurred five months after her diagnosis, while she was waiting to learn if a previous child had acquired perinatal HIV. She felt immobilized by guilt and by her anxiety about HIV's possible effects on her infant and the fetus she was carrying, and she finally decided to abort the pregnancy. The second pregnancy she chose to keep: she felt well-informed about the risk she was assuming, her life was stable, and she was optimistic about living with HIV.

This case illustrates various stages of Amy's adaptation. During her first pregnancy she said, "The only thing that registered in my mind was that I had AIDS and that I was going to die, which means that my child was going to die" (Hutchison and Kurth 1990, 47). She was overwhelmed by information she had received; she became emotionally unstable and unable to care adequately for her children. Counselors focused not on the specifics of perinatal HIV but rather on helping Amy recognize her emotions and the impact that another potentially HIV-positive child would have on her life.

Margaret Hutchison and Maureen Shannon

During the second pregnancy Amy had shifted her perspective to view her future positively. There is a fine line—one that may be blurred by cultural variations—between this thinking and denial; it was the counselor's task at this point to help Amy once again see what was best for her life. This meant trying to break through denial by reflecting her own words back to her, reminding her of past responses to difficult situations, and helping her to look at possible future scenarios. During such grief stages as denial, anger, or shock, women may be difficult to reach with interventions. In all interactions, however, a counselor's genuineness will facilitate both the goal of engaging the woman in care and the usefulness of counseling to the woman as she makes her decision.

Reproductive counseling for women with HIV calls on the provider's every resource. All the methods discussed above are time-intensive, ideally involving multiple counseling sessions. But the constraints of most care systems rarely allow for this luxury, leading the providers to cut corners in assessments and care. This may mean inadequate time to develop trust, find a common language, or uncover the appropriate intervention strategy. Unfortunately, the same intervention that helps one woman make the right decision for her life may propel another into a state of immobility that prevents her from making any decisions or accessing appropriate care. The task of individualizing counseling is sometimes overwhelming; whereas some women are helped by such scare tactics as visiting a child with AIDS, others may become unreachable by any intervention the health care provider may attempt.

The system further frustrates clients with its intractability, with the provider's individual lack of control over what other service providers or systems might do or say, and with the lack of resources for women with multiple medical and social problems. A provider may feel powerless given these systemic problems or what she or he perceives as poor choices by the women counseled. Providers who seek to help women take control of their lives may feel disheartened when their agenda is not met and when they realize that they are "very much constrained by the social and cultural experiences of pregnant women: messages given are not necessarily messages received" (Rapp 1987, 16).

For many women, HIV is just one of countless problems, and taking away the option of reproduction may take away all that gives meaning to their lives. Counselors have little to offer to replace the role of reproduction. This is not to suggest that removal of all social ills would spell the end of reproduction by women with HIV, or that it should; but choice becomes more real when it involves more than two options.

A caveat to the discussion of counseling for women with HIV is Faden's finding in her 1987 study of women's attitudes toward the abortion of defective fetuses: attitudes changed dramatically when probability of defect rose from 95 to 100 percent. She argues that "counselors should be sensitized to the fact that although 95-percent accuracy in diagnosis is very acceptable to many professionals, to parents, the psychological difference between any chance and certainty may be tremendous, and may make the difference between deciding to abort the fetus or to bear the child" (p. 290).

Conclusion

For health care workers and women in the United States, the sociopolitical climate is the inescapable backdrop to any discussion of reproductive counseling and family planning. In a time when women's access to abortion is under attack and there is increasing focus on the fetus as patient, it is hardly surprising that a large part of the public-policy response to women and HIV has revolved around the issue of perinatal transmission. This emphasis on women as childbearers can have both an overt and an insidious effect on those who care for women with or at risk for HIV, one that demands constant questioning of our own premises and those of federal, state, and institutional policies.

Interventions based on unfounded assumptions about how women think or act are doomed to fail. Decision making and behavior changes associated with sexuality and reproduction are complex undertakings that are seldom based on the facts offered by care providers. Gaps in our understanding of women with HIV, including the effects of grief on reproductive decision making and the biologic effects of OC use on HIV-positive women, must be filled. Our approaches must be formulated from the perspectives of those to whom we seek to provide care.

Finally, energies must be put into implementing culturally sensitive programs that empower women to use medical information about HIV for prevention and care. Such interventions demand more time and creativity than traditional public health strategies, but they represent an investment that is long overdue and for which there is no alternative.

5

Obstetrical Management

Janet L. Mitchell, Ilene Fennoy, John Tucker,

Patricia O. Loftman, and Sterling B. Williams

I've just started going to support groups, and I think
they're just the best. You get those night terrors when you
first find out, then you realize you have three choices: move
on, go back, or lose it entirely. I found out that I was positive
at work. A physician called and said, "You've got AIDS." I felt
like one of those test dummies in the drinking and driving
commercials . . . crash. The biggest thing is you need
support. For a long time I held this in, never dreamed there
was support like this out there for me.

I tell people who work with HIV to show some
compassion for the women you see. Women do tend to care
for others instead of themselves, so when they do come in
for care they're really sick. I've had my share of traumas,
and it's taken its toll, but I won't give up. I've always looked

at things realistically but could never say these things. But now I've already made my will out. There's days when I don't get out of bed, and other days when I can run a mile.

Someone at my support group said that people who give up hope die fast; I believe that's true. I don't want to be on a machine, and I feel when it's time to go it's time to go. I've attained all my dreams in life. If I died now, I'd be happy. All you can think about when you're first diagnosed is anger and sadness. Then you've got to make a choice. I chose to stick around for my kids. And I've made arrangements for my mom and sister to take them, which I would have had to do anyway. I just had to do it sooner.

—"Patty Youngheart"

Nearly 85 percent of all reported cases of AIDS in women occur in those of reproductive age, fifteen to forty-four (CDC 1993). Most infected women in this age group are not yet aware of their infection, and perinatally acquired HIV continues to account for about 1.5 percent of all AIDS cases. For this reason the Centers for Disease Control and Prevention (1985) published recommendations on preventing perinatal transmission of HIV; those recommendations were then endorsed by the American College of Obstetrics and Gynecology (ACOG, 1987). The CDC advised that all women of reproductive age be offered HIV counseling with voluntary testing in accordance with state statutes, and many states and private institutions initiated plans to achieve this. Several states mandated that prenatal or family planning programs receiving state funding comply with the recommendations.

Although the intent of the recommendations may have been to provide infected women with information that might affect their reproductive choices, the immediate result was the identification of many women who were already pregnant. Rapid developments in therapeutics—antiretrovirals and prophylaxis for opportunistic infections—have created additional incentive for counseling and testing. Because of these recommendations and the resultant policies, increasing numbers of HIV-infected women are being identified.

HIV is distinguished in the field of health care delivery because education and counseling about intimate matters are the foundations on which care is given. Providers have been forced to initiate discussions about sexual practices and possible illegal behaviors, as the predominant risk behaviors for many women involve the use of mood-altering substances. Infected women are predominantly women of color, poor, and from cultures alien to most providers, creating additional awkwardness.

Pregnancy makes these issues all the more complex, leading many care givers to refer women to specialists. But advancements in treatment and the availability of antiretrovirals have changed HIV infection from a rapidly progressive terminal illness to something resembling a chronic disease, and optimal care for patients with chronic diseases and their families requires coordination by a primary-care provider. Thus the growing numbers of HIV-infected women require that obstetricians, nurse-midwives, and other primary-care providers for pregnant women be knowledgeable about all aspects of care for this population.

HIV and the Parturient's Health Status

There are no data to suggest that pregnancy accelerates the progression of HIV disease. Initial concerns were based on the fact that pregnancy alters the immune status of women so that the fetus, an allograft, is not rejected. Pregnancy often obscures diagnosis and thereby delays appropriate treatment for medical or surgical conditions, however, because of unawareness on the part of the provider or concern for the fetus. A similar delay in diagnosis and treatment can occur in HIV-positive women because of the theoretical risk and the unknown long-term effects of many of the drugs used to treat primary infections and other complications. These issues have been addressed in the literature and in the recommendations of the obstetricians who serve as consultants to the AIDS Clinical Trials Group (ACTG). Specific concerns are discussed later in this chapter.

The effect of HIV on obstetrical outcomes is less clear. Part of the problem is the methodology of many of the studies. Drawing from research on other medical complications of pregnancy, more severely ill women tend to have poorer outcomes than less ill women. Overlooked in initial studies were the background rates of problems associated with pregnancies in substance-using women. One study that attempted to consider these two potentially confounding factors discovered that the obstetrical outcomes of HIV-infected women were not different from those of uninfected women. The greatest determinant for poor outcome was continued use of cocaine throughout pregnancy. The majority of the infected women were asymptomatic, and the authors cautioned that sicker women may have different outcomes (Selwyn et al. 1989a).

Clinical Issues of HIV in Pregnancy

No discussion of the clinical issues of HIV in pregnancy can be undertaken without some understanding of the population that is at highest risk for infection. That population is most likely to be using a mood-altering substance, often by injection, and is apt to be made up of African-Americans or Latinas. More important, the women are likely to be poor and to receive their health care at public facilities

(Mitchell 1988). These factors are important clinically because they are associated with late presentation for care. Because of previous experiences with negotiating systems, prejudicial attitudes of staff, and other survival priorities in their lives, many HIV-infected women will enter the health care system only when they are acutely ill or at the time of delivery. Consequently, medical services for this group are more likely to offer intervention than prevention.

An additional complicating factor is the emphasis placed on pregnancy as a time for identifying HIV-infected women. Because of the recommendations of the CDC and ACOG, many women are informed of their HIV serostatus during pregnancy, often to the surprise of the women and their providers. This creates an uncomfortable situation for the woman and the provider: the woman may need time to come to terms with the knowledge and miss appointments and withdraw from support, and the provider may need to reexamine her or his own fears and perceptions about this infection, often sending an unconscious but negative message to the woman. This too may lead the patient to withdraw from care. The following guidelines have proved successful in providing continuity of care for HIV-infected women with or without a history of substance abuse.

Agency Preparation

Policies and procedures such as those outlined in protocol 5.1 should be established and documented because many obstetrical services will not see large numbers of HIV-infected women. Ongoing staff education and in-servicing are fundamental, given the rapid changes in HIV knowledge and the constant need to address the myths and pressures staff may encounter from family members and friends. It is unrealistic to expect all staff to manage these pressures without support.

Continual reinforcement of universal precautions for handling blood and body fluids is also important (CDC 1988). Many staff members will strictly adhere to these precautions when they know someone is HIV-infected. But staff members may be less cautious with women they perceive to be not at risk, in effect putting themselves and their colleagues in greater jeopardy. Newborn-screening seroprevalence studies of women of childbearing age note that most HIV-infected women are unidentified at the time of delivery.

Because of uncertainty about which fluids are covered by the CDC recommendations, staff members often institute procedures that are interpreted as somewhat punitive by the patient and those who support her. In addition to blood and visibly bloody fluids, the body fluids covered by the recommendations are vaginal secretions; semen; cerebrospinal, synovial, pleural, peritoneal, pericardial, and amniotic fluids. Not included in the recommendations are urine, feces, saliva, breast milk, vomitus, sputum, nasal secretions, tears, and sweat.

Liaison with medical or infectious-disease specialists is critical, even if obstet-

Mitchell, Fennoy, Tucker, Loftman, and Williams

Protocol 5.1 Agency Preparation

- Regular, ongoing in-services for all agency staff.
- Monitoring of adherence to Universal Precautions.
- Liaison with medicine and/or infectious disease to promote continuity of medical care after delivery.
- Liaison with pediatrics to ensure optimal followup for the infant and for the woman's other children.
- Knowledge of other AIDS activities, especially those that relate to legal matters, drug treatment and other mental and psychosocial matters.

Source: Authors.

rical providers are knowledgeable about HIV. Identifying providers in medicine who are interested in the care of women prior to delivery makes for a smoother transition for the patient after delivery.

The same holds true for pediatrics. At present there is no widely available test to identify babies that are HIV-infected at birth, so many departments of pediatrics monitor all infants born to HIV-infected mothers for a year or two. This also ensures that the pediatricians assigned to the infants will be knowledgeable about HIV infection.

Because HIV also affects the patient in ways that go beyond the traditional bounds of medicine, knowledge of other activities and agencies involved with AIDS is imperative. Issues that are particularly difficult for providers in maternal and child health are those concerning death and dying. The life expectancy of HIV-infected individuals is longer than it was five years ago, but child custody, extent of lifesaving measures, and wills need to be discussed with all patients.

Antepartum Management

Many women still initially perceive their HIV status as a death sentence. They need time to work through various issues of living with the disease. Ironically, pregnancy often allows HIV-positive women to accept the reality of their situation while ceasing risky sexual behavior. During pregnancy, concern for the infant becomes a high priority.

Women who receive their positive results during pregnancy may need to deal with the guilt and anxiety surrounding the pregnancy before they can inform their sexual partner. For drug-using women this may also be a time of relapse. Coming to terms with positive results may take weeks and translate into missed appointments and noncompliance with other aspects of care. The ongoing involvement of the staff is necessary. It is critical that a team approach be used when women are told of their

Protocol 5.2 General Antepartum Care

- Address and support the needs and concerns of newly diagnosed and known HIV-infected women about the outcomes of the pregnancy for the woman and her unborn child.
- Involve the partner and significant others in her life as the woman permits.
- Refer women who actively use drugs or alcohol to treatment.
- Begin to discuss attitudes toward safer sexual practices and family planning.
- Begin exploration of the issues of death and dying—of the woman and/or her child.

Source: Authors.

positive status and that various scenarios be discussed so that the woman can perceive that her response is "normal."

As is well known to providers of obstetrical care, pregnancy denotes involvement with family—biological, extended, or family of choice. This may complicate care for the woman who is HIV-infected if she prefers to keep her status a secret, especially from the father. Most states do not have partner notification regulations for HIV, but providers encourage women to inform their sexual partners and, in this instance, the father of the baby. In addition, discussions about safer sexual practices and contraception have more impact if they are discussed with both parties. Regardless of ethnicity, class, or economic status, sexual behaviors are greatly influenced by the attitudes of the woman's partner.

Women traditionally perceive the obstetrician-gynecologist as their primary-care provider. Women experiencing other diseases during pregnancy are usually managed by the primary obstetrician in conjunction with a medical specialist or by an obstetrician with training in high-risk obstetrics. HIV-infected women should be managed similarly. If the care provider is an obstetrician, maintaining a link to a specialist in infectious diseases is important for care of the woman after delivery or if she is hospitalized during pregnancy for an HIV-related illness. A relationship with a pediatric specialist is equally important for the continuing care of the infant. It is imperative that women who are chemically dependent be in treatment. Fortunately, pregnancy motivates many women—even those using cocaine or crack—to seek both medical and drug treatment. The key to success is that the program be appropriate for the needs of the woman. But because most drug treatment programs offer no on-site prenatal services and minimal primary medical care, the obstetrician and infectious disease specialists will continue to be responsible for the care of these women. Recommendations for antepartum care are summarized in protocol 5.2.

When a pregnant woman is diagnosed as HIV-infected or when an HIV-infected woman becomes pregnant, a baseline CD4+ (T-cell) count should be obtained as soon as possible. Although the majority of women will be asymptomatic at diagnosis, some will have CD4+ counts of 500 cells/mm³ or less. Most obstetricians and infectious disease specialists with expertise in caring for HIV-infected women agree that if a confirmed CD4+ count is 200 cells/mm³ or less, the woman should be offered the prevailing standard of care for HIV-infected persons (Minkoff and Moreno 1990; Sperling et al. 1992). This includes treatment with zidovudine (AZT) and a prophylaxis for Pneumocystis carinii pneumonia (PCP) (Fischl et al. 1987; NIAID 1990; CDC 1989b).

Experience with zidovudine in pregnancy is limited (Brown and Watts 1990). The National Institutes of Health has conducted phase I trials (Schuman et al. 1990) and currently is conducting a phase III protocol to assess the usefulness of zidovudine in reducing perinatal transmission (ACTG 076). The mother begins taking the drug after fourteen weeks of gestation.

The use of zidovudine is based on a more traditional approach to the treatment of diseases during pregnancy. If a pregnant woman has a life-threatening disease, the decision to treat is historically weighed against the risk of withholding treatment until after the pregnancy has ended. If the risk of progression or death is thought to be high, treatment is instituted, and the significance of HIV infection as a cause of death among women has been documented (Koonin et al. 1989; Chu, Buehler, and Berkelman 1990). The safety of most drugs used in pregnancy is established through experience, not through clinical trials.

In discussing therapies with pregnant women, the usual maternal response is concern for the fetus. It is important that the woman understand that the risks to the fetus from these therapies are theoretical; however, the risks to the mother of delayed treatment are well documented. A toll-free telephone number to collect data on exposure to zidovudine during pregnancy has been established.[1] Every woman taking AZT during pregnancy, no matter how limited her exposure, should be reported.

The benefit of using zidovudine during pregnancy by women with CD4+ counts between 200 and 500 cells/mm³ is debatable. In the expanded criteria, the benefit was in delaying the onset of HIV-related illness (NIAID 1990). But the risk-benefit ratio is not as clear in this group of women. Delaying use of the drug until after pregnancy may not have an untoward effect on the progression of HIV infection. Many obstetricians feel that in this range the decision to take or not to take zidovudine should be left to the woman. Repeating the CD4+ count every trimester may be beneficial. If there is substantial change, one might elect to recommend treatment. A confirmed count of less than 200 cells/mm³ would reclassify the woman into the treatment category.

The two drugs most commonly used for treatment of PCP—trimethoprim-sulfamethoxazole and pentamidine isethionate—are now recommended for pro-

---

[1] Phone (800) 772–9292 for the Burroughs Wellcome Zidovudine in Pregnancy Registry.

phylaxis. Trimethoprim is a folate antagonist, and sulfamethoxazole is a sulfa antifungal. Sulfamethoxazole carries the theoretical risk of causing kernicterus in the infant, but a review of the literature did not substantiate this risk (Minkoff and Feinkind 1989). Neither drug has demonstrated an increase in fetal anomalies. Experience with using pentamidine during pregnancy is also limited. The aerosol form of pentamidine is recommended for prophylaxis, but the choice of a PCP prophylaxis is institution-specific. If trimethoprim-sulfamethoxazole and aerosol pentamidine are both available, a locally applied medication that has little system absorption would seem best.

The CDC recommends that neither aerosol pentamidine nor trimethoprim-sulfamethoxazole be used during pregnancy; this is standard policy for any drug whose use in pregnancy is limited (CDC 1989). But CDC's own data show that the highest mortality in pregnancy of HIV-infected women is related to PCP (Koonin et al. 1989).

Other drugs, such as dapsone, also have also been recommended as prophylaxis. Until more data are available on these compounds, it is best to use pentamidine or trimethoprim-sulfamethoxazole during pregnancy.

Opportunistic Infections

Many of the drugs used to treat an HIV-infected woman may potentially pose risk to the fetus or the pregnancy, but the highest priority is to save the mother. Risk versus benefit regarding both the woman and her fetus complicates the choice of therapeutic interventions.

The dosages should be based on the standards of adult, nonpregnant persons, but the clinician should be aware that physiological changes during pregnancy sometimes alter the distribution and clearance rate of many drugs, especially those cleared by the renal system. If there is a range of dosage, a higher dose may be more beneficial than a lower one. Duration of treatment must also be weighed. The collective experience of opportunistic infections other that PCP during pregnancy is limited.

Other Medical Problems

Many of the problems encountered in HIV-infected women are not currently classified as AIDS-related. They are problems commonly seen in women of low socioeconomic status and in women who are chemically dependent but whose natural history might be altered by HIV infection; they include abnormal Pap smears, syphilis infections, and persistent vaginal candidiasis (Schrager et al. 1989; Chu, Buehler, and Berkelman 1990; Dattel 1990; Minkoff et al. 1990; Mitchell et al. 1992). Treatment currently is consistent with the guidelines for treatment in HIV-negative women, though Pap smears probably should be repeated every six months instead of yearly. There also have been concerns that the recommended treatment for syphilis has not been effective in treating some HIV-infected people (Musher, Hamill, and Baugh 1990). Because of this concern and the epidemic of congenital syphilis in the same population of women at risk for HIV infection, many obstetrical and infectious disease services suggest hospitalizing pregnant HIV-infected women for ten to fourteen days of intravenous penicillin therapy instead of the recommended three-week regimen of 2.4 million units of benzathine penicillin G (bicillin) IM. Because the woman is HIV-infected, issues surrounding her substance abuse may be overlooked. An article by Chu and co-workers on mortality of HIV-infected women of reproductive age found that conditions related to substance abuse accounted for the second largest number of deaths—26.5 percent—after AIDS-related conditions (34.8 percent). Certain pneumonias, septicemia, and other infections not clearly related to AIDS accounted for 31.1 percent of the mortality in women of reproductive age (Chu, Buehler, and Berkelman 1990). It is clear that the majority of HIV-infected women will present for problems that are not AIDS-defining. In a study from Sloane Hospital for Women on the increasing prevalence of pneumonia during pregnancy, the authors found cocaine use in 52 percent of their study population, compared with 10 percent in the general population. Twenty-four percent of the study group was HIV-positive, compared with 2 percent of the general population (Berkowitz and LaSala 1990).

The recent epidemic of syphilis is also related to drug use. A study from Jackson Memorial Hospital in Miami found that mothers of babies born with congenital syphilis tended to be African-American (67 percent) and substance abusers (71 percent) (Ricci et al. 1989). Researchers from Kings County Hospital in Brooklyn found that if a woman had a urine toxicology positive for cocaine at delivery, she was almost five and one-half times as likely to be HIV-infected and nine and one-half times as likely to have fluorescent treponema antibodies than women whose urine toxicologies were negative (Minkoff et al. 1990).

Many of the women will be on methadone maintenance for their opiate addiction. Pregnancy is known to alter the pharmacokinetics for many drugs in some women, and the same is true for methadone (Pond et al. 1985). The dosage should be adequate to keep the woman free of signs and symptoms of withdrawal. For some women, it may mean an increase in the dosage (Mitchell and Brown 1990). It is important that the fetus not experience withdrawal, which is associated with a high fetal mortality rate.

Pregnancies in chemically dependent women are also associated with high rates of intrauterine growth retardation. Serial ultrasound examinations for growth and other means of antepartum surveillance should be utilized. Protocol 5.3 highlights other issues to consider in the medical management of antepartum care.

Protocol 5.3 Medical Antepartum Care

- In addition to routine prenatal tests, use an antigen (anergy) panel with PPD for tuberculosis (tine test should not be used to screen HIV-infected women).
- Include screening for hepatitis B.
- Include serological test for toxoplasmosis.
- Follow CD4+ count, each trimester at a minimum.
- For CD4+ counts of <200/mm³, follow current NIH and CDC treatment recommendations (antiretroviral and appropriate prophylaxis regimens).
- When CD4+ counts fall between 200/mm³ and 500/mm³, the decision to start medication is left to patient.
- Opportunistic infections should be treated as per standard medical protocols. Undertreatment because of concerns for the fetus may compromise the mother.
- Syphilis may need aggressive therapy.
- Women on methadone may need an increase in dosage.
- Fetal surveillance—ultrasounds, biophysical profiles—optimizes fetal outcome.

Source: Authors.

Intrapartum Period

Numerous seroprevalence studies of newborns have documented that the majority of HIV-infected women delivering at a given institution have not been diagnosed, so the application of routine universal precautions is essential. There are few data concerning the impact of certain obstetrical practices on the transmission of HIV. Minimal use of invasive procedures involving the fetus—like scalp electrodes and scalp sampling—may decrease the risk of transmission (Mendez and Jules 1990). Optimal treatment of the fetus should be the priority, however. Cesarean section has not proved protective to the fetus over normal spontaneous vaginal delivery (Nanda and Minkoff 1989). More important, universal precautions do not require "stirrup delivery." Allowing women to deliver in a more comfortable position, such as in a bed or birthing chair, does not compromise the use of universal precautions for blood and body fluids.

Women who are chemically dependent often have a low threshold for stress and pain. Labor is associated with both. The ideal pain reliever for chemically dependent women in labor is regional anesthesia, which is also not contraindicated for use with HIV-positive women (see protocol 5.4).

Postpartum Period

There are a number of documented cases of HIV transmission through breastfeeding (Lepage et al. 1987; Lifson 1988; Ryder et al. 1991; Newell 1992), but the mecha-

Mitchell, Fennoy, Tucker, Loftman, and Williams

Protocol 5.4 Intrapartum Care

- Continue to monitor the use of Universal Precautions.
- Manage labor to optimize outcomes for both mother and infant.
- Method of delivery presently dictated by obstetrical indications only.
- HIV infection currently not a contraindication to the use of any analgesia or method of anesthesia.

Source: Authors.

nism for transmission is unclear. Although the virus has been isolated from breast milk, many women also have cracks and abrasions on the nipple and surrounding areas. For this reason, breastfeeding is not recommended for HIV-infected women in developed countries. The World Health Organization, however, feels that the morbidity and mortality associated with the use of formula in developing countries outweighs the risk of transmission through breastfeeding.

Prior to the advent of HIV, many advocated breastfeeding for women who had ceased illicit drug use. It promotes mother-child bonding and may promote parenting skills, but for the chemically dependent woman whose HIV serostatus is unknown and who refuses to be tested, breastfeeding should not be encouraged.

It is important that women be provided continual health care that includes treatment of her infection by a knowledgeable primary-care provider. Treatment for drug and alcohol addiction is equally important. Establishing a link to such services prior to delivery facilitates continuity of care.

Initiating discussion of such issues as family planning and safer sexual practices prior to delivery allows the woman (and those she deems important in these decisions) time to consider these issues in the face of HIV infection. Many will have made some decisions, but many will have not. Staff need to be supportive in either instance (see protocol 5.5).

Vertical Transmission

At present it is unclear when the transmission of HIV to the child occurs. The virus has been isolated from the placenta, the amniotic fluid, and the fetal tissue. Infection may occur prenatally, at delivery, or through breastfeeding (Lapointe et al. 1985; Vogt et al. 1986; Mundy et al. 1987; Maury et al. 1989). Additional research is needed to clarify issues of transmission for both pregnancy and breastfeeding.

A critical issue in counseling is the transmission rate and the identification of the fetus who is at the highest risk for infection. The risk in each pregnancy may depend on such factors as how advanced the disease is, the woman's immunological state, or the gestational age of the infant at birth (Goedert et al. 1989; Boue et al.

Protocol 5.5 Postpartum Care

- Current recommendation of the U.S. Public Health Service is that HIV-infected women in developed countries should not breastfeed.
- Continual medical care in an appropriate setting should be ensured.
- Drug and alcohol treatment should be maintained.
- Discussions of family planning issues should be continued.

Source: Authors.

1990; Rubinstein et al. 1990). The rate of transmission, estimated from various studies, ranges widely—from 6.5 percent (Hague, Mok, MacCallum et al. 1991) to 65 percent in earlier studies where women had advanced disease. The U.S. Public Health Service estimates a transmission rate of 25 percent. These odds may be unacceptable to many, but women from cultures where childbearing is highly valued may find a 75 percent chance of having an uninfected child a risk worth taking. This may be the case particularly for drug-using women.

Studies have shown that women with HIV base their reproductive choices on the same criteria used by noninfected women of similar socioeconomic and psychosocial status (Holman et al. 1989; Selwyn et al. 1989b). When providers are able to identify which fetus is infected or will be infected, women can incorporate that knowledge into their decision making. Amniocentesis, cordocentesis, and chorionic villus sampling have all been explored as prenatal HIV diagnostic techniques, but because of the blood-borne nature of the virus they themselves involve risk of transmission.

Pediatric HIV Disease

As reported to CDC through December 1992, 86 percent of children younger than 13 years with AIDS in the United States were infected through vertical transmission (ascribed to a mother with or at risk for HIV). Of these patients, 54 percent were non-Hispanic blacks and 24 percent were Hispanics (CDC 1993). Fifty-seven percent of their mothers were injection-drug users or having sex with an injection-drug user. Many of these drug-using minority families are impoverished, with few resources available to them or to their communities (Mitchell and Heagarty 1991).

Among women who have had problems with substance abuse, histories of sexual abuse and violence are common (Coleman 1987; Amaro, Fried, and Cabal 1990). Clinical depression is frequently seen as well (Weisman et al. 1976; Regan, Ehrlich, and Finnegan 1987). The diagnosis of HIV in a child compounds these problems, as diagnosis of a child almost inevitably means diagnosis of the mother. It is not surprising that family dysfunction is the norm under which providers must labor to provide care to the HIV-infected patient.

Diagnostic Issues

Determining HIV antibody serostatus poses unique problems for the newborn because of the passage of maternal antibodies through the placenta (Arpadi and Caspe 1991). As a consequence, an asymptomatic infant can test positive. The maternal antibodies may take up to fifteen months to clear the serum. Thus, frequent monitoring is necessary for all HIV-positive infants (Mendez 1991): monthly visits through six months of age and visits every two or three months thereafter for the asymptomatic infant. In addition to obtaining a history and performing a physical exam at each visits, providers should administer routine immunizations but substitute inactivated poliovirus vaccine for oral vaccine. Developmental exams should be performed every six months. Monitoring of immunological status should be established by one month of age and every six months thereafter, including repeat HIV serology until results are negative on two consecutive occasions. Children who serorevert—receive two negative antibody tests six months apart—should be retested for HIV annually.

The symptomatic child with HIV antibody will receive all of the above evaluations plus studies to clarify the diagnosis: other HIV tests (p24 antigen, viral culture, or polymerase chain reaction) and studies for opportunistic infections (cytomegalovirus, Epstein-Barr virus, toxoplasmosis, etc.). Serum chemistries and radiologic studies are performed every six to twelve months in symptomatic HIV-infected children or as indicated by the child's clinical condition.

Clinical Issues

Pediatric HIV disease is a complex, multisystem disease increasingly recognized as a chronic disorder (Wiznia and Nicholas 1990). Prognosis has been extremely varied, depending on the age of the child and the manifestations at presentation (Scott and Hutto 1991). For example, 70 percent of patients with pulmonary manifestations of lymphocytic interstitial pneumonitis survive more than sixty months, while only 20 percent of those with Pneumocystis carinii pneumonia survive thirty or more months. As with adults, lymphocyte CD4+ cell numbers have been shown to correlate with likelihood of PCP infection, but at different levels (CDC 1991d). Thus prophylaxis is generally recommended for children younger than one year with CD4+ counts of 1,500 cells/mm^3 or less; for children twelve to twenty-three months old with counts of 750 cells/mm^3 or less; for children two to five years old with counts of 500 cells/mm^3 or less. Beginning at age six children follow adult prophylactic protocol, at levels of 200 cells/mm^3 or below.

One of the manifestations of HIV in children that differs somewhat from those of adults is the high frequency of serious bacterial infections that often precede opportunistic infections (Kline and Sherer 1991; Pelton and Klein 1991). Recent NIH studies have shown a decrease in frequency of infections but no change in mortality among children receiving intravenous gamma globulin therapy each month (Pelton and Klein 1991). Such preventive therapy should be superimposed on the health maintenance schedule outlined above.

Developmental and neurological manifestations of HIV are common in children (Butler, Hittelman, and Hauger 1991). These manifestations include delay or regression in motor skills, progressive bilateral pyramidal tract signs, short-term memory loss and attention deficits, or simply failure to progress because of acquired microcephaly. The spectrum of central nervous system disorders has been classified by Auger et al. (1988) into two groups: one with a fairly delayed presentation of symptoms, suggesting a prolonged incubation period with a median of 6.1 years, and one with a short incubation period and a median of about four months. The manifestations themselves may be either subacute and progressive, plateau, or static in nature (Brouwers, Belma, and Epstein 1991). The management of these children, therefore, becomes more difficult as they fail to develop in an age-appropriate manner.

In addition to the respiratory, immune, and neurological systems, other systems are affected. Cardiomyopathy, gastrointestinal infections, nephropathy, and hematologic abnormalities are some of the effects seen. In fact, the patient usually has a variety of systems involved at once. It is this constellation of abnormalities, with its multiple subspecialty needs, that the family must confront for both the pediatric patient and the mother.

Treatment

Primary therapy for HIV infection centers on medications that interrupt the life cycle of the virus (Pizzo and Wilfert 1991). Because HIV is a multisystem disease involving integration of the viral genome into the host genome of target tissues, these medications must be able to reach all organs and to be safe for prolonged periods and for developing organs if they are to be useful in the pediatric age group.

Research on new therapies is limited by the absence of appropriate clinical and surrogate markers of a drug's effectiveness (Pizzo and Wilfert 1991). This is particularly true for the pediatric age group, in which the norms established in adults must be verified for children. Because clinical manifestations vary, it is not easy to translate a new therapy from adults to children.

These therapies require a high degree of cooperation and compliance with an intense medical regimen. The therapies may have limited applicability in some settings, as the dysfunctional family has difficulty dealing with these demands. In addition, the primary caretaker of the child is frequently infected herself and may be ill or suffering from HIV encephalopathy. Clear understanding and ability to follow through with medical regimens may be limited. Finally, substance-abusing women have been characterized as having multiple problems that require social integration—domestic violence, depression, inadequate housing, limited financial resources and vocational skills. Their ability to cope with the multiple demands of treatment for the infected child as well as for themselves is limited without an integrated approach to care (Mitchell and Heagarty 1991; Tracy and Williams 1991).

Developing such integrated models of care for the woman and family faced with HIV disease is a critical goal for health care systems. It is clear that the numbers of infected women and children will continue to increase until effective ways to change the behaviors that place women at risk are identified. Until an effective vaccine is available, or until societal changes enable women to decrease their risk of infection, systems that provide a range of integrated services to meet the needs of the infected woman and her family must be developed. These should include social services as well as treatments for family disorganization. Healthy families require mental as well as physical health. Reducing the stress associated with seeking medical care will aid in restoring and maintaining the mental health of infected women and that of her family.

6

Neuropsychiatric Aspects of Infection

Kathy M. Sanders

One of the ways women can cope is telling it. Don't hold all
this in. Holding it in is stressful. To alleviate the stress, tell
people. But women—people, period—don't want to tell
because they're worried about how they'll be treated. Lots of
the women I work with are carrying this burden all by
themselves, and no one knows but them. Coming to our
support groups is their only outlet, and they do that because
what's said here stays here. Once you get into a group or
meet someone infected, especially if she's well, you can say,
"I want to do whatever it is she's doin'." Communicate with
each other. Knowledge is power.
—Gwen Green

Kathy M. Sanders

Along with the emotional distress of receiving a diagnosis of HIV infection comes significant neuropsychiatric morbidity. Caregivers who treat women with HIV disease or women who are at high risk for HIV infection need to be educated on the wide range of neurologic and psychiatric complications and prepared to treat and support patients emotionally.

At the time of AIDS diagnosis, 40 percent of patients will have signs of central nervous system (CNS) involvement: primary HIV infection of the brain, spinal cord, or peripheral nerves; opportunistic infections involving the CNS; and primary CNS lymphoma. Psychological complications in the course of diagnosis and treatment of HIV infection show group patterns and individual variation. They include the onset of anxiety and depression and the recurrence of such illness as depression, psychosis, and drug or alcohol abuse. A person with HIV disease is at greater risk of attempting and completing suicide than are uninfected people (Kizer et al. 1988; Marzuk et al. 1988; Rundell et al. 1992). Disruptions in the social support network—loss of jobs, friends, or family—exacerbate a person's difficulties in coping with this devastating illness. Clinical awareness and early intervention are essential to assisting people with HIV disease.

Few published studies have focused on neuropsychiatric implications of HIV in women. But a handful of recent works comparing psychosocial functioning in men and women with HIV disease demonstrate some preliminary gender differences that warrant further investigation (Carey et al. 1991; Quick et al. 1991). Until more research is conducted on women, health care providers must rely on studies of male (primarily homosexual) populations.

Neuropsychiatric Disease Associated with AIDS

AIDS Dementia Complex

Since the beginning of the AIDS epidemic, clinicians have recognized neuropsychiatric impairment associated with HIV disease. As progress was made in serology, virology, and brain imaging, it became clear that a specific dementing illness is associated with HIV. Clinicians and researchers have referred to this primary CNS disorder as AIDS dementia complex (ADC) or HIV encephalopathy (Navia, Jordan, and Price 1986; Navia et al. 1986; Grant et al. 1987; Brew, Sidtis, Rosenblum, and Price 1988; Brew, Sidtis, Petito, and Price 1988; Bridge 1988; Grant et al. 1988; Price et al. 1988; Perry 1990; Tillmann and Wigdahl 1991). It is a syndrome of cognitive, behavioral, and motor symptoms (table 6.1).

Initially these symptoms may be subtle. Cognitive changes include problems with concentration and word finding, memory loss, mental slowing, and mild confusion. Behavioral changes include almost any known psychiatric symptom, giving ADC a reputation as a "great imitator," much like the former reputation of

Table 6.1 Early and Late Manifestations of AIDS Dementia Complex

Early

Cognitive	Behavioral	Motor
Forgetfulness	Anxiety	Imbalance
Memory loss (verbal)	Agitation	Unsteady gait
Impaired concentration	Emotional lability	Motor slowing
Comprehension difficulties	Depressed mood	Tremor
Word-finding problems	Apathy	Clumsiness
Mental slowing	Personality change	Weakness (legs)
Mild confusion	Irritability	Numbness
Thought derailment	Social withdrawal	Speech disturbance (stuttering)
	Mania	Dysgraphia
	Psychosis	Fine-motor incoordination

Late

Cognitive	Behavioral	Motor
Amnesia	Mutism	Myoclonus
Aphasia	Frontal lobe dysfunction	Ataxia
Global cognitive dysfunction	Perseveration	Spasticity
Disorientation	Disinhibition	Dyskinesia
Inattention	Hypersomnolence	Incontinence
Delayed response time	Socially inappropriate behaviors	Seizures
Vacant staring	Severe apathy	

Source: Sanders.

syphilis. Any symptom of personality change (irritability, apathy, social withdrawal), depression, anxiety, mania, psychosis, delusion, or hallucination can be a
manifestation of ADC. Neurologic abnormalities include gait disturbance, weakness, paresthesias, dysarthria (including stuttering), dysphasia, dysgraphia, tremor,
seizure, and impaired coordination. The course and progression are variable and
unpredictable, but by the terminal stages the patient will be demented nearly to a
vegetative state, incapable of performing the basic activities of daily living, inconti-
nent, and mute.

Primary infection of the CNS is a well-established complication of HIV disease
(Navia, Jordan, and Price 1986; Brew, Sidtis, Petito, and Price 1988; Price et al.
1988; American Academy of Neurology AIDS Task Force 1989; Tillmann and
Wigdahl 1991). It appears as an aseptic viral meningitis during the acute infection
stage (see figure 6.1). Later in the course of infection, HIV can be detected in the
CNS (Perry and Marotta 1987; Tillmann and Wigdahl 1991). How HIV actually
infects neural cells is unknown; hypotheses include both direct and indirect routes

Kathy M. Sanders

Figure 6.1 Immune Response and CNS Dysfunction

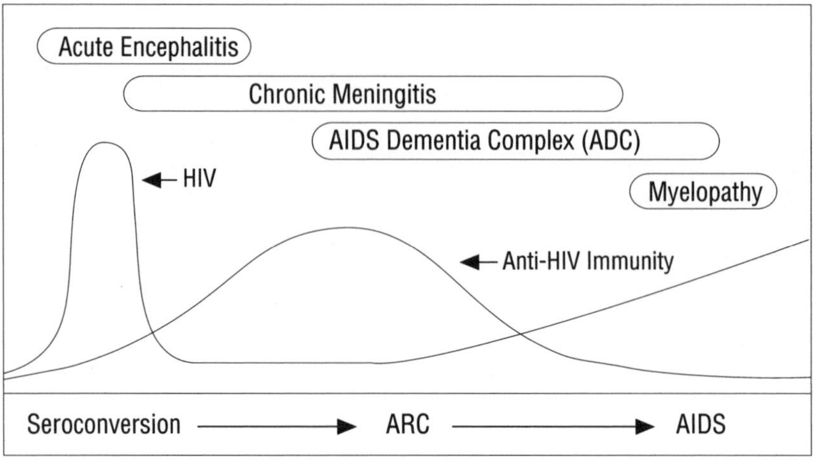

Source: Tillmann and Wigdahl 1991. Copyright W. B. Saunders Publishing Company. Reprinted with permission.

(Brew, Sidtis, Petito, and Price 1988; Price et al. 1988; Tillmann and Wigdahl 1991). HIV may cross the blood-brain barrier directly and interact with specific surface components of glial and neural cells that then allow for entry and infection (Tillmann and Wigdahl 1991). Alternatively or concomitantly, HIV may enter the CNS through HIV-infected monocytes or macrophages at times of blood-brain barrier disruption—the "Trojan horse" theory (Brew, Sidtis, Petito, and Price 1988; Price et al. 1988; Tillman and Wigdahl 1991).

How HIV infection produces neuronal dysfunction and neuronolysis in the CNS is not clear. Mechanisms have been suggested, including the death of neurons or glial cells after direct infection by the virus; the release of neurotoxic substances by infected monocytes and macrophages (cytokines and other viral proteins); the direct neurotoxic action of the HIV envelope glycoprotein, gp120; and autoimmune reactions stimulated by HIV genome incorporation into neural DNA (Perry 1990; Tillmann and Wigdahl 1991).

The neuropathology of ADC at autopsy shows ventricular dilatation and cortical atrophy (Navia et al. 1986). There is white matter pallor with vacuolation. Microscopic examination shows reactive astrocytosis, multinucleated giant cells, perivascular inflammatory infiltrates, and demyelinization. These histopathological changes are most commonly seen in white matter and subcortical gray matter (basal ganglia and thalamus) (Navia et al. 1986; Brew, Sidtis, Petito, and Price 1988; Brew, Sidtis, Rosenblum, and Price 1988; Gray, Gherardi, and Scaravilli 1988; Perry 1990).

The diagnosis of CNS pathology during HIV infection has been aided by high-technology imaging techniques that provide information on structural and functional states of the brain. These techniques are computerized tomography (CT), magnetic resonance (MR), positron emission tomography (PET), and single photon emission computed tomography (SPECT). For patients diagnosed with ADC, CT and MR images show cerebral atrophy and diffuse white matter lesions (Ekholm and Simon 1988; Olsen et al. 1988; Kieburtz et al. 1990; Post, Berger, and Quencer 1991). MR detects more white matter disease than does CT. But not all ADC patients show brain structure abnormalities on CT and MR. When patients are studied with PET and SPECT scans, there is a greater yield of brain metabolism and cerebral blood flow abnormalities that correlate with clinical phenomenology. PET scans measure the glucose utilization or metabolism in different parts of the brain. There may be increased metabolism in subcortical brain tissue, possibly related to inflammation during the acute stage of viral infection (Brunetti et al. 1991; Rottenberg et al. 1987). Later in the course of ADC, decreased areas of metabolism are found in cortical and subcortical areas of the brain (Rottenberg et al. 1987). Cerebral blood flow abnormalities are observed with SPECT (Pohl et al. 1988; Schielke et al. 1990; Brunetti et al. 1991). These cerebral perfusion deficits can be noted without the presence of structural abnormalities on CT or MR and are usually correlated with clinical symptomatology (Pohl et al. 1988; Kuni et al. 1991).

Recognition of new or progressive cognitive, behavioral, and motor dysfunction is imperative in the initial evaluation of HIV infected individuals. Diagnostic tools include neuropsychological testing; brain imaging with MR and SPECT scans; and neurological assessment with lumbar puncture, which involves analysis of the cerebrospinal fluid for presence of HIV or viral products, as well as a search for possible non-HIV causes of the neuropsychiatric syndrome (treponema, opportunistic infections, and lymphoma, for example). HIV involvement in the CNS can precede significant systemic immunosuppression—that is, while CD4+ cell counts are still not below 500 cells/mm^3 (Beckett et al. 1987; Grant et al. 1987; Holtzman, Kaku, and So 1989; McArthur et al. 1989; Marotta and Perry 1989).

AZT, the medication of choice in the treatment of ADC, has been shown to slow the progression of infection and to improve cognitive deficits (Grant et al. 1988; Ostrow, Grant, and Atkinson 1988; Schmitt et al. 1988; Beckett 1990). These clinical improvements are substantiated by the diminution of white matter lesions on MR scans and the normalization of PET and SPECT abnormalities (Brunetti et al. 1988; Grant et al. 1988; Brunetti et al. 1991; Post, Berger, and Quencer 1991). It has also been shown that Dideoxyinosine (ddI) is an effective antiviral agent for HIV infection (Yarchoan et al. 1989; Lambert et al. 1990), though the degree to which CNS benefits accrue has not been documented.

Psychotropic medications can be used for specific psychiatric syndromes in HIV-infected patients (Ayd 1988; Ostrow, Grant, and Atkinson 1988; Fernandez and Levy 1990). Major depressive episodes, which are associated with ADC and HIV disease, can respond to antidepressant medications, as can other organic mood disorders. Such psychostimulants as d-amphetamine and methylphenidate are helpful in treating apathy, cognitive slowing, and depression (Fernandez et al. 1988). Nonpanic anxiety states can be treated with cognitive-behavioral therapy or short half-life benzodiazepines. Brief trials of high-potency neuroleptics in low doses can be useful in treating psychotic symptoms and behavioral dyscontrol (Ostrow, Grant, and Atkinson 1988; Fernandez et al. 1989; Fernandez and Levy 1990; Fernandez, Levy, and Mansell 1990).

Patients with ADC are particularly vulnerable to the extrapyramidal and movement-disorder side effects of neuroleptics. Patients with HIV disease generally are more sensitive to the side effects of psychotropic medications (anticholinergic, alpha receptor blockade). Low starting doses should be increased slowly to the lowest optimally effective dose.

Opportunistic Infections

HIV-related immunosuppression makes the patient vulnerable to a variety of infections. Those that affect the CNS diffusely and may be confused with ADC are cytomegalovirus and herpes simplex virus encephalitis. Metabolic encephalopathies associated with acute systemic illness (such as hypoxia, renal failure, sepsis) and side effects from antimicrobial agents can also mimic or enhance symptoms of ADC.

Opportunistic infections affecting the CNS can also present as focal neurological events, depending on the neuroanatomic location of the lesion. These infections include toxoplasmosis, cryptococcoma, varicella zoster virus encephalitis, tubercular meningitis or tuberculoma, and neurosyphilis. There has been an increasing incidence of primary and secondary syphilis cases in the U.S. population during the past decade (Rolfs and Nakashima 1990). Syphilis infection progresses more rapidly and is more difficult to treat in the immunosuppressed patient with HIV disease (Johns, Tierney, and Felsenstein 1987). HIV-infected patients may go from primary to tertiary syphilis in a matter of weeks or months rather than the usual time frame of years. Evaluation for neurosyphilis must be included in the differential diagnosis for any neuropsychiatric changes in patients with HIV disease.

Personality changes, psychosis, emotional lability, and depression may be the initial symptoms of any of these CNS infections. Neurological and motor changes are common manifestations, with such symptoms as stuttering, paresthesias, tremor, muscle weakness, headache, photophobia, gait disturbance, dysgraphia, and incoordination. Early diagnosis and treatment of the specific opportunistic infection will give the best chance of clinical resolution of the CNS manifestations.

Nonorganic Psychiatric Complications

Psychiatric morbidity of nonorganic origin associated with HIV disease includes grief reactions; adjustment disorders with depressed, anxious, or mixed emotional features; anxiety disorder; major depression; psychosis with delusions of infection; and exacerbation of underlying personality or substance abuse disorders (Fenton 1988; Rubinow et al. 1988; Tross and Hirsch 1988; Tross et al. 1988; Fernandez et al. 1989; Dilley and Forstein 1990; Miller and Riccio 1990).

Three prevalence studies to determine psychiatric disorders in homosexual men (Atkinson et al. 1988), hemophilic men (Dew, Ragni, and Nimorwicz 1990), and women (Brown and Rundel 1990) with HIV disease reflect increased amounts of distress and psychiatric morbidity for all three groups. When noninfected homosexual controls were compared with noninfected heterosexual controls (Atkinson et al. 1988), the prevalence of depression, anxiety disorders, and substance abuse (other than alcohol) was significantly higher in the former group. Because previous psychiatric history is associated with cognitive impairment in HIV-positive patients (Rubinow et al. 1988), this finding increases the clinical concerns in the medical and psychiatric care of patients with HIV disease who have a psychiatric history.

In the male hemophilic cohort studied, the HIV-positive group had higher rates of depression and anxiety even in the absence of personal or familial psychiatric history (Dew, Ragni, and Nimorwicz 1990). The effect of psychosocial factors—educational level, sense of self-mastery, recent losses, and social support of wife, family, and friends—on mental health was explored. Patients with low self-esteem and inadequate social support who had undergone recent losses were more likely than the others to have an increased incidence of psychiatric symptomatology (Dew, Ragni, and Nimorwicz 1990).

In a noncontrolled study, Brown and Rundell (1990) determined the prevalence of psychiatric morbidity among women (N=20) with asymptomatic HIV infection who participated in the U.S. Air Force mandatory screening program. Eighty percent of the women had been infected with HIV by heterosexual sex. Ten women (50 percent) had a Diagnostic and Statistical Manual, Third Edition-Revised (DSM III-R) Axis I psychiatric diagnosis. When minor disorders such as V codes and simple phobias were eliminated, seven women (35 percent of the cohort) had psychiatric diagnoses. The most prominent disorder was hypoactive sexual desire disorder in four (20 percent). Adjustment disorders were diagnosed in three (15 percent) members of the cohort. Organic mental disorder was found in two women (10 percent). Personality disorders (Axis II) were diagnosed in four (20 percent) women. The military cohort consisted of ten African-American and ten Caucasian women who were predominantly middle-class high school graduates with some college who were employed and without histories of injection-drug use (Brown and Rundell, 1990). The women are not representative of the women currently at highest risk for HIV infection in the United States. They may, however, represent an increasingly at-risk population as heterosexual transmission becomes the predominant means of transmission in the United States, as it is in other parts of the world.

In a study of psychiatrically hospitalized AIDS or ARC patients (N=60; 58 males, 2 females), twenty-two were diagnosed with adjustment disorders or major depression, eighteen had dementia, six had schizophrenia, six had brief reactive psychosis, four had bipolar disorder (mania), and four had psychosis related to stimulant use (amphetamine or cocaine) (Baer 1989). Such disorders reflect the variety of serious psychiatric morbidity (other than ADC) that complicates HIV disease.

A study of predominantly heterosexual, Latin, drug-using patients with HIV at Montefiore Medical Center in New York found that the patients did not show significantly higher rates of psychiatric morbidity than non-AIDS patients. They did, however, use psychiatric services at a much higher rate. Females constitute 25 percent of the patient population of the center (O'Dowd and McKegney 1990).

Increased risk for suicide is a commonly accepted clinical concern in work with people with HIV disease (Kizer et al. 1988; Marzuk et al. 1988; Rundell et al. 1992). In a recent study of a military population, Rundell et al. (1992) compared fifteen patients who had attempted suicide with HIV-positive controls who had not attempted suicide. The study found that adjustment disorder, alcohol abuse, personality disorder, history of previous major depression, HIV-related interpersonal or job problems, social isolation, and perceived lack of social support are statistically significant risk factors for a suicide attempt. There was no association with the extent of immunosuppression, abnormal cerebrospinal fluid (CSF) findings, or presence of organic mental disorder.

These findings of dementia, personality disorders, psychosis, mania, and substance abuse among HIV-infected individuals (Baer 1989; Brown and Rundell 1990) underscore the risk factor of mental illness in the spread of HIV infection because of the high-risk behaviors and impaired judgment associated with these diagnoses. Psychiatric comorbidity with HIV disease must be attended to in efforts to contain the spread of HIV and to provide community supports during acute episodes of psychiatric decompensation. Risk for a suicide attempt must be a prominent clinical consideration for HIV-positive individuals, especially those with comorbid psychiatric illness and social isolation. Prevention programs must address the effect of psychiatric impairment on judgment with regard to high-risk behaviors. Comprehensive treatment of mental illness is crucial to containing the spread of HIV.

Gender Differences in Psychiatric Illness

Because a history of psychiatric illness is associated with the development of psychiatric problems during HIV disease, attention to psychiatric comorbidity will remain a prominent feature of the ongoing care of women with the disease. Programs for prevention and treatment of psychiatric comorbidity must be available for individuals at risk, especially for those who perform a complex role in the care and nurturing of others. Psychiatric illness compromises the individual's ability to function in these complex roles, further weakening the social and economic supports needed to cope with HIV disease.

In developing prevention and treatment programs, it must first be acknowledged that the majority of U.S. women with HIV disease are already stressed by limited socioeconomic resources for coping with this disease. An understanding of Latina and African-American women, injection-drug users, limits on access to health care for women of lower socioeconomic status, language barriers, and issues of competency as HIV disease progresses is required in order to serve the needs of American women infected with HIV (Campbell 1990; Minkoff and DeHovitz 1991; Ybarra 1991). In this light it is useful to look at current studies of psychiatric illness in the general American population that do show gender differences in the prevalence of major mental illness. Further epidemiological study of subpopulations with HIV disease will build on this general knowledge in the development of programs to address the mental health needs of HIV-positive women.

During the past decade the National Institute of Mental Health's Epidemiology Catchment Area Program has shown gender differences in prevalence and incidence of psychiatric disorders (Myers et al. 1984; Robins et al. 1984; Regier et al. 1988). The prevalence rates of major unipolar depression, panic, and generalized anxiety disorders are twice as high in women as in men. But antisocial personality disorder and substance abuse disorders are more prevalent in men (Robins et al. 1984). Bipolar disorder shows no sex differences. Schizophrenia afflicts men at a younger age but incidence is not significantly different by sex. Young adults between the ages of twenty-five and forty-four were more likely to have psychiatric diagnoses than adults forty-five or older (Regier et al. 1988).

Prevalence studies of psychiatric disorders in the primary care setting show that almost 30 percent of these patients have depressive and anxiety disorders. A study by Kessler, Cleary, and Burke (1985) showed that 43 percent of women and only 25 percent of men had at least one definable psychiatric disorder. Almost 75 percent of the unmarried (widowed, separated, divorced, or single) individuals were diagnosed with a psychiatric disorder. Recognition of these cases by the primary-care physician was under 10 percent, implying the need for more careful evaluation of mental status in medical outpatient clinics. Barrett et al. (1988) found psychiatric disorders in 26.5 percent of patients in an outpatient internal medicine clinic (10 percent depression, 5.3 percent anxiety, and 11.2 percent ill-defined depressive symptomatology). Women were two to ten times more likely than men to have depression; rates varied with the specific depressive disorder studied. Men, however, were more likely to have generalized anxiety disorder. Unmarried individuals

Kathy M. Sanders

Figure 6.2 Lifetime Prevalence of Comorbid Mental and Addictive Disorders in the United States

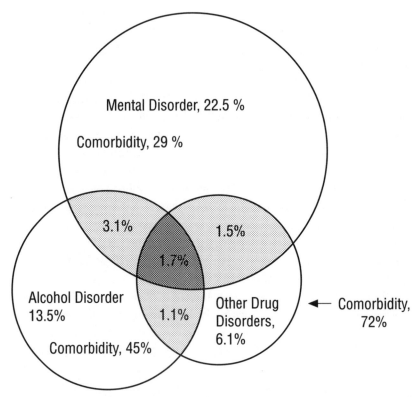

Note: Comorbidity of alcohol disorders with mental disorders is 4.8 percent of the 13.5 percent of people with alcohol disorders. Comorbidity of drug disorders (other than alcohol) with mental disorders is 3.2 percent of 6.1 percent of people with drug disorders.

Source: Regier et al. 1990. Based on Epidemiological Catchment Area data.

were more likely to be depressed, and married individuals were more likely to have anxiety disorder. These findings reflect what is commonly accepted in the literature on depressed patients.

An Epidemiology Catchment Area study found that the median age at onset for anxiety disorders is fifteen; it is twenty-four for major depression; nineteen for drug abuse or dependence; and twenty-one for alcohol abuse or dependence. For the subgroup between 18 and 30 years old who have a diagnosis of major depression or anxiety disorder, the risk of developing drug abuse or dependence doubles (Christie et al. 1988). Looking at comorbidity of mental disorders with alcohol and other drug abuse, Regier et al. (1990) found that 29 percent of those individuals with a mental disorder had a lifetime prevalence of an addictive disorder. Thirty-seven percent of those with an alcohol disorder and 53 percent of those with a drug disorder (other than alcohol) had a comorbid mental disorder (figure 6.2).

Most women with HIV disease (74 percent) are between the ages of twenty and thirty-nine, and 51 percent are injection-drug users (Ellerbrock et al. 1991). Given the increased psychiatric comorbidity for substance abusers, the early onset of psychiatric disorders, and the higher incidence of affective illness in women, recognition and treatment of psychiatric disorders is crucial in the care of women with HIV disease. Important social supports—such as satisfying communication with mate, family, or social networks—are considered to offer significant protection against reactive affective illness (Costello 1982; Miller 1988; Wilhelm and Parker 1989; Genero et al. 1990; Genero et al. in press). Many women at risk for HIV infection in the United States generally have fewer of these support systems (Campbell 1990; Worth 1990; Cohen 1991; Ybarra 1991). The higher rates of isolation experienced by women with HIV (Wofsy 1987) will only increase their expected rates of depressive illness during the course of HIV disease.

Recommendations

The most important first step in the medical and mental care of women with HIV disease is to establish a trusting and warm working relationship so that the challenging and emotionally taxing work of diagnostic evaluation, technological tests, and discussion of treatment can proceed with minimal dropout or noncompliance. It is crucial that the mental status of the HIV-positive woman be monitored attentively for evidence of new symptoms and complaints of memory changes, difficulty in coordinating activities of daily living for herself and her household, and psychiatric distress. When the psychiatric practitioner recognizes clinical changes that may herald an early dementing process, a neuropsychiatric workup is indicated. This evaluation is usually threatening to patients; it requires substantial trust and the ready opportunity to discuss the meaning of a possible diagnosis of ADC.

The Robert B. Andrews Unit—an outpatient clinic specializing in the diagnosis, treatment, and research of neuropsychiatric complications of HIV disease)—at Massachusetts General Hospital recommends the following neuropsychiatric workup for possible ADC or other neuropsychiatric syndromes associated with HIV disease:

1. Evaluation and examination of the patient by a psychiatrist and neurologist.

2. Laboratory data (including EEG, thyroid function tests, serology for syphilis, sedimentation rate, current blood counts including subset analysis

of T-cells, and other tests as warranted) to search for etiologically related hematologic, infectious, or metabolic processes.

3. Lumbar puncture and examination of the cerebrospinal fluid.

4. Neuropsychological testing.

5. Brain imaging with MR and SPECT.

6. Reports, including treatment recommendations, from the psychiatrist to primary care physicians and other medical and mental health care providers.

7. Annual reevaluation, unless more frequent evaluation—as indicated by clinical findings—is recommended.

This comprehensive neuropsychiatric evaluation will aid the HIV-positive woman and her clinician in the diagnosis and treatment of HIV-related disorders. This in turn will allow realistic planning. Early detection and subsequent treatment will delay disease progression, and cognitive deficits will be diminished with the use of AZT. Treatment of depression or paralyzing anxiety will allow practical problem-solving to continue, with the aid of necessary social supports within the system. Socioeconomic issues can be addressed earlier, before the disease prevents the patient's active participation in crucial decisions regarding such subjects as medical benefits, housing, a living will, power of attorney and family needs.

Areas for further research should include longitudinal assessment of the natural history of neuropsychiatric morbidity in a group of HIV-positive women. Special emphasis should be placed on the effect of sex-hormone changes on cognitive functioning through the menstrual cycle, as well as during pregnancy; and on how these hormonal changes may affect the progression of ADC. Other potential areas for research include subset analysis to differentiate among the risk groups for transmission, which would be clinically useful in understanding the needs and problems specific to each woman; evaluation of the impact of enduring substance abuse or recovery from substance abuse on morbidity and on mortality; and implementation of ongoing psychoeducational programs to modify high-risk behaviors. Assessment of premorbid psychiatric status and documentation of personality and coping styles will facilitate the clinical management of life stress, episodes of psychiatric comorbidity, and early detection of cognitive changes associated with primary HIV infection of the CNS or other opportunistic diseases affecting the nervous system. It has also been pointed out (Ickovics and Rodin 1992) that women should be included in psychopharmacological research, including clinical trials of pertinent regimens.

A useful tool for accomplishing these tasks is group therapy based on a supportive and psycho-educational model. This kind of therapy helps establish trusting relationships and reliable participation in studies of neuropsychiatric aspects of HIV disease. Additionally, such counseling serves the social and psychological needs of the women who struggle with the isolation, fear, and emotional distress that accompany their disease.

Women who are still using drugs may require other strategies. Researchers point out that self-help groups of active addicts may be more destructive than helpful, as addicts actually require extensive external ego support from health care and other workers in a highly structured environment (Cancellieri et al. 1988).

Funding for any treatment program must address women's transportation needs, provide day care for children, and establish socioeconomic resources for housing, home heath care, and other medical supports during the progression of HIV disease. Mobilization of community and social supports will be required to supplement the cognitive functioning necessary for maintaining some independence as ADC becomes part of the clinical picture for the woman with HIV disease.

7

Trends in Federally Sponsored Clinical Trials

Joyce A. Korvick

Happily married for only six months, I found myself faced with the horror of being diagnosed HIV-positive. Once I got over the initial shock and developed some sort of acceptance of the news, I found myself in shock again. I could not find any information on women and HIV. I went on a mad search to find out exactly what this diagnosis meant for me. I heard horrible stories through the media that women were dying twice as fast as men with HIV, and that women lived only two to three years after diagnosis. I was thirty-nine years old at the time and definitely not ready to die.

I joined a support group for women with HIV and that was of tremendous help in coping with the mental anguish of my HIV status. But there was a feeling that we (the women in the group) were the few women with HIV and that we were alone, unnoticed, and that there was this fight against HIV for men, but not for women.

We started picking up gay male newspapers to get information and the latest news on HIV. I began to learn the politics, what was new in treatment and the like, but nothing was geared to me, a female. After a couple of months I talked with the group about establishing a newsletter for us, discussing those issues of coping with children and spouses (infected and noninfected), disclosure to family and friends, and, most important, the manifestations of HIV disease in women.

We knew we were having vaginal infections that would not go away, cancer of the cervix, and many other symptoms that were not discussed in gay male literature. We recruited an attorney to write articles on the legal issues for women with HIV—things such as child custody, in the case that we became too ill to care for our children. We recruited a doctor to discuss the manifestations of HIV in women. We needed definitions of pelvic inflammatory disease, dysplasia. We needed to know how it looked and when to expect these problems in relationship to the progression of the disease. We recruited women to write about how they disclosed to their children their HIV status and what types of support our children would need. We gathered nutritionists and holistic practitioners to help us incorporate changes in our diet and to teach us how to blend that into our family meals. All of these were things that were not collected and addressed anywhere for women.

The result was *The Positive Woman,* a newsletter created by, for, and about the woman with HIV disease. In July 1992 we celebrated two years in publication and have grown into a nonprofit organization for women with HIV. We began to connect with women all over the United States, and requests for our publication began to come from faraway places such as England, Germany, France, the Netherlands. We were no longer alone.

Being actively involved in the medical aspects of HIV, along with the politics of the disease, has given us strength

and the recognition we deserved. We were pioneers in every sense of the word. We have begun to come out of our
closets, to dismiss the feeling of shame and embarrass-
ment. We have begun to advocate for ourselves, demanding
that woman-specific research be done and remedies be
found to help us. We are testifying before Congress, the
Centers for Disease Control, and with our state legislative
bodies. We have joined the fight. And with this fight comes
the all-important fight for life. Our message to all women
faced with the challenge of living with HIV is, "Don't quit before the miracle happens."
—Michelle E. Wilson

Clinical trials of HIV therapeutics in the United States are conducted by pharmaceutical companies; federally sponsored multicenter networks; and such nonprofit organizations as the American Foundation for AIDS Research. Most federally sponsored
clinical trials are funded and directed through the National Institutes of Allergy and
Infectious Diseases of the National Institutes of Health (NIAID/NIH). Two multicenter networks—the AIDS Clinical Trial Group (ACTG), initiated in 1986, and the
Terry Beirn Community Programs on Clinical Research on AIDS (CPCRA), established in 1989—are sponsored by the Division of AIDS of NIAID. I focus here on
these two programs, analyzing how they address the research needs of women and
point out future directions.

As of June 1993 the ACTG consisted of thirty-five adult units and twenty-four
pediatric units located primarily in university hospitals. In fiscal year 1992 the units
received $59.8 million; the ACTG network, including the statistical center and its
operations support, had a budget of more than $100 million. There were twenty
protocols (twelve of them for adults) in development, and fifty-two protocols
(thirty-six for adults) open to accrual, or enrollment.

The CPCRA offers community providers and their HIV-infected patients,
especially those underrepresented in HIV-related studies, greater opportunity to
participate in clinical research. The CPCRA has seventeen centers in community
physicians' offices that employ basic data-collection techniques and commonly
available clinical and laboratory methods. As of June 1993 there were five trials in
development and fourteen trials opened to accrual.

The AIDS Clinical Trials Group

As of January 15, 1993, a *cumulative* total of 21,598 patients were enrolled in
ACTG trials, about 14 percent (3,111) of them female and 86 percent male. Of the

Figure 7.1 Percentage of Adult Female Enrollment in ACTG Clinical Trials

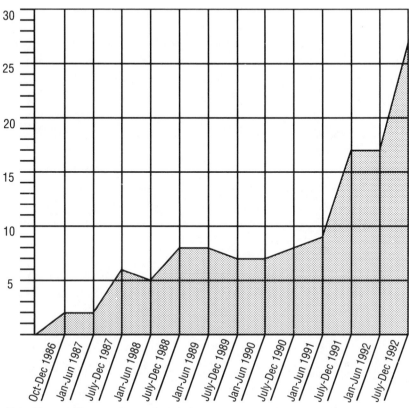

Note: New enrollees per six-month period.
Source: NIAID/NIH June 1992.

total female sample, 1,952 (63 percent) were adult women; 64 (2 percent) were
adolescents; and 1,095 (35 percent) were children. The distribution of pediatric
cases by gender was roughly equal.

The percentage of women enrolled in ACTG trials increased in the past few
years (Cotton, Feinberg, and Finkelstein 1991), especially in summer 1992. As of
August 1992, the last six- to twelve-month accrual of female adult participants was
nearly 20 percent, as shown in figure 7.1 (Spino 1992). A total of 816 women were
newly enrolled in ACTG clinical trials: 26 percent in the perinatal transmission trial
(ACTG 076); 54 percent in a nucleoside combination study (ACTG 175).

Criticisms of the ACTG

Why did the early ACTG studies enroll so few women? Many of the study designs
were rigid and defined very homogeneous groups of patients. Fewer women than

Joyce A. Korvick

men were infected in the early 1980s; in fact, more than half of all AIDS cases in women have been reported since 1989 (Berkelman 1991). Thus, fewer women were likely to fit the stringent entry criteria, which included low CD4+ cell counts or advanced diseases that qualified an AIDS-defining illnesses. Early in the epidemic, clinicians were not as aware that AIDS afflicted women; as a result, many women may have gone undiagnosed entirely. Many women are diagnosed during pregnancy and on that basis have been excluded from trials. Because no national screening for HIV infection exists, it is difficult to predict the actual ratio of infected men to women. But it is fair to say that the number of infected women will continue to grow and that it is incumbent upon those involved in AIDS research to address this group.

The ACTG's efforts to recruit women into clinical trials have been criticized in the past. Enrollment in current studies opened to accrual or in development should reflect the increased participation of women and point to future opportunities for their enrollment. The percentage of women in these trials ranges from 2 percent to 100 percent. One trial, ACTG 175, enrolled 248 (13.9 percent) women in less than six months.

Two large opportunistic-infection trials opened in late 1992: ACTG 196, a study of Mycobacterium avium complex prophylaxis (target enrollment, 1,000); and ACTG 204, a study of cytomegalovirus (CMV) disease prophylaxis (target enrollment, 600). Enrollment criteria for both trials include CD4+ counts of less than 100 cells/mm^3. Because the number of women with AIDS in the United States is increasing, these trials have the potential of enrolling large numbers of women.

Women's Health Activities Within the Federal Agencies

A working group of obstetricians and gynecologists was established by ACTG in March 1990 to discuss issues related to women with AIDS. Members of this group worked with the ACTG Pediatric Committee to develop the first U.S. trial (ACTG 076) for the interruption of perinatal HIV transmission. The study is cosponsored by the National Institute for Child Health and Human Development. During the development of the trial the obstetricians and gynecologists established guidelines for treating HIV-infected pregnant women and conducted a provider survey of women taking zidovudine (Sperling et al. 1992a). Although the major goal of the study was to prevent transmission of HIV to the fetus, the perinatologists addressed the concerns of the women enrolled in the trials and sought to ensure the best standard of care and safety for them as well.

In December 1990 a conference on women and HIV infection was sponsored by the NIH. Participants included health care professionals, women with HIV infection, social workers, government administrators, researchers, and activists. The following April the conference steering committee offered recommendations for research on women with HIV infection to the NIH AIDS Program Advisory

Committee; APAC endorsed the recommendations and urged that they be implemented for future research throughout the public health system (NIAID 1991).

As a result of heightened collaboration within segments of the public health system, the CDC—in collaboration with NIAID and other government agencies—has initiated Women's Interagency Health Study, a large women's AIDS epidemiologic study. By better defining HIV disease in women, information from this study will allow investigators to identify research opportunities that can be applied to therapeutic trials.

In spring 1991 the Women's Health Committee (WHC) of the ACTG was formed to further research of HIV infection in women. This committee has targeted four goals for the ACTG: to help develop and design HIV-associated clinical trials of treatment for pregnant and nonpregnant women; to increase the number of women participating in ACTG clinical trials and to establish uniform criteria that would ensure the inclusion of women; to guarantee that clinical trials evaluate gynecological health and incorporate appropriate gender-specific endpoints; and to participate in the development and design of clinical trials to interrupt maternal-fetal transmission.

The WHC has worked to further refine the research agenda of the ACTG and to address issues related to how AIDS research involving women is conducted. Activities included reviewing all ACTG trials and offering recommendations for future trial design; advising the CDC in its review of the AIDS case-surveillance definition; creating a gynecological assessment form for women in trials; proposing a rationale for the disproportionate enrollment of women in selected trials to study safety, tolerance, and HIV-related diseases; and developing a scientific research agenda for the study of women within the ACTG framework.

The review of current ACTG protocols and procedures by the WHC has highlighted ways to adapt the guidelines to permit and encourage women's participation in clinical trials. For example, women normally have lower hemoglobin levels than men. If the hemoglobin level is set arbitrarily high as an entry criterion, women may not qualify for the study. In addition, doses in many adult trials are not administered according to body weight. This is especially important when the therapeutic range and dose-limiting toxicity are close. A higher dose may actually be more toxic rather than more therapeutic, and a woman (or any individual of small body size) may have to be taken off a study drug prior to obtaining therapeutic benefit. The findings of the WHC will be made available to all investigators in the ACTG.

The WHC has worked with protocol chairs of large studies to justify the disproportionate enrollment of women in selected studies. Although treatment of HIV itself is not likely to be different in women than in men, the associated diseases, toxicities, and safety of the treatment may differ. Review of survival and toxicity differences according to race and gender in two large ACTG studies (ACTG 016 and 019) found no significant differences according to gender, but the small numbers prohibited broad conclusions (Lagakos 1991). Important gender differences may be detected in phase III studies if large enough numbers of women were enrolled.[1]

As one of the ACTG's largest clinical antiretroviral trials (ACTG 175) was being developed, Currier, Spino, and Cotton (1992) reviewed hypothetical power calculations related to sample size and the ability to detect statistically significant differences in toxicity rates. Power calculations for a hypothetical study with a sample size of 2,000 reveal that the ability to detect toxicity differences between men and women (power above 80 percent) varies with the number of women enrolled. For example, with a 10 percent female enrollment one could detect a one-and-a-half-fold increase in toxicities that occurred in 20 percent of the men, whereas with a 20 percent female enrollment one could detect a toxicity that occurred in only 10 percent of the men. That is, the rarer the event in men, the higher enrollment of women that would be needed to discover a one-and-a-half-fold increase in toxicity. The efficacy question was also approached in this model. Enrollment of 10 percent women would allow adequate power to detect a 50 percent increase in disease progression rates; but with a 15 percent female accrual a 33 percent increase might be detectable. On the basis of these arguments, the ACTG Executive Committee recommended "at least" 15 percent accrual of women into ACTG 175.

Retention of women in trials is one of the next big hurdles faced by study teams. The population of women represented today is largely underprivileged, with poor access to health care and few options when it comes to supporting themselves and their children. Nearly 75 percent of all women with AIDS are minority women, and about 50 percent are injection-drug users (CDC 1993). ACTG units are working with community groups to approach this problem in ways that ensure access to trials. Not only must a potential participant be made aware of the existence of a trial for which she may be eligible, but she also must have a way of returning for clinic visits as specified in the protocol. Research regarding motivation and the adherence

[1] Phases of research studies and clinical trials of pharmaceutical studies are defined as follows.

Phase I: Determination of pharmacokinetics (measurements of absorption, half-life, and metabolism of a drug); these studies are often performed on a small number of volunteers. Usually it is the first time the drug is administered to humans.

Phase II: The drug is studied in a target patient population to determine its safety and activity for a specified condition.

Phase III: Large trials involving patients in clinical settings similar to those anticipated for the ultimate use of the study drug. Here the drug is tested against standard therapy (or placebo) to test its efficacy.

Phase IV: Postapproval studies to monitor the safety of the new drug under actual conditions in large numbers of patients.

of women to protocols and medication is important, and coordination with NIMH research in this area is being pursued.

Baseline demographic and gynecological data are being studied in ACTG 175, as are gender-specific toxicities. The gynecologists in the WHC have developed a case report form that targets specific information, including Pap smears, gynecological infections (especially candida vaginitis), and gynecological histories. This form has been piloted in ACTG 175 and will be employed in selected ACTG trials.

Obstetricians in the WHC are working closely with the perinatal group of the Pediatric Committee to develop additional trials for pregnant women. For example, all eligible women from ACTG 076 (a zidovudine trial for prevention of perinatal transmission) were made eligible to enter ACTG 175 after delivery. They have the benefit of continued participation in clinical trials, and ACTG 175 has the benefit of participants who have demonstrated the ability to complete a clinical trial.

Other Research Directions

By the time an agent has been tested in phase I, II, and III clinical trials and has an indication licensed by the Food and Drug Administration (FDA), only limited numbers of women may have received the drug. In addition, studies in pregnant women regarding the safety or dosage of agents are not often undertaken. So the clinician often lacks the important information needed to help a pregnant woman make an informed choice regarding a potential therapeutic agent (Minkoff and Moreno 1990; Wofsy 1991; Sperling et al. 1992b).

The WHC is reviewing ways to increase the participation of women in phase I trials, which study the pharmacokinetic effects of a drug on a small number of volunteers. It has been difficult to reconcile the potential toxicity of a drug that is being taken by a human for the first time with a potential reproductive effect in the individual (see chapter 9). But these studies would add important knowledge of the specific agent concerning size of the individual, pregnancy (the physiology and volume of distribution are strikingly different in pregnant and nonpregnant women), and the influence of such concomitant medications as oral contraceptives. Although these questions are important, necessary studies are rarely performed.

Women-Specific Trials

The first ACTG trial involving the female urogenital system started in late 1992. This is a randomized trial of 5-fluorouracil (5-FU), a topical vaginal maintenance therapy, versus observation after standard therapy for high-grade cervical dysplasia in HIV-infected women (ACTG 200). About 260 women are being studied. Other gynecological conditions under consideration for future clinical trials are vaginal yeast infection, genital ulcer disease, and pelvic inflammatory disease.

Obstacles to performing gynecological trials include a lack of active agents— such as those to counteract human papilloma virus—and a lack of information regarding the epidemiology of certain gynecological diseases in women with HIV. Without this information, a hypothesis cannot be formed. Epidemiologic studies of these conditions that are under way will perhaps provide more data on which to base study designs.

Current Community-Based Research

As of May 14, 1993, CPCRA has enrolled 1,311 women in its research network (19.8 percent of the total). All but two of the trials have enrolled more than 15 percent women. The two that have not involve the testing of antiretrovirals (002, 007). One of the first trials was CPCRA 002: dideoxyinosine versus dideoxy-cytidine in HIV-infected patients who are intolerant of or who have failed zidovudine (ZDV) therapy (10 percent women). Were women underrepresented because they had no access to ZDV? A review of the CPCRA Observational Data Base by Rodriguez and coworkers (1992) did not find gender differences for anti-retroviral drugs at the first six-month followup interview. Were they taking the ZDV long enough to become intolerant or fail? No data were available on duration of prior therapy.

A more striking gender difference is seen in the second trial, CPCRA 007 (nucleoside combination therapy). The study enrolls patients with CD4+ counts below 200 cells/mm^3 or an AIDS diagnosis. Sites began enrolling patients— predominantly males—in late spring 1992. Several sites that traditionally accrue more women are starting enrollment later. The geographic distribution of women by site can influence the ultimate number of women enrolled in a study, even if care was taken to ensure liberal entry criteria.

CPCRA 010 is a randomized, prospective double-blind study comparing flu-conazole with placebo for primary and secondary prophylaxis of mucosal can-didiasis in HIV-infected women. It studies the effect of 200 mg of fluconazole administered weekly on oral, vaginal, and esophageal candidiasis. This protocol has fostered specific gynecological training of clinicians and nurse practitioners within the CPCRA. A baseline Pap smear and gynecological examination are required within sixty days of entry.

The Women, Children, and People of Color Interest Group, along with the Women's Caucus of the CPCRA, is proposing the inclusion of pregnant women in clinical trials of drugs. To date only one treatment trial allows the enrollment of pregnant women (CPCRA 005: INH prophylaxis for anergic HIV-infected people at increased risk for tuberculosis). Again, the issue of therapies during pregnancy is an important one. The ultimate decision rests with the woman, based on the information provided to her by her clinician. Women are permitted to take investigational drugs if the "purpose of the activity is to meet the health needs of the mother and the fetus will be placed at risk only to the minimum extent necessary to meet such needs" (OPRR 1989).

Recommendations for Research

Clinical trials research on women with HIV infection can be divided into several general areas: pregnancy, perinatal issues, and pharmacokinetics; gynecological infections, malignancies, and reproductive health; increased enrollment of women in trials of antiretroviral and opportunistic-infection agents to assess toxicity and activity; Phase I trials for nonpregnant and pregnant women; and motivational and behavioral research.

Scientific interest in research for women with HIV infection will not succeed without financial support, assistance with transportation and child care, and community support for women willing to participate. The informed woman who is willing to come forward may help improve not only her own care but also the care of other women dealing with similar problems. Important findings have led to increased survival for people infected with HIV. As the woman living with HIV disease survives longer, she will need therapies specific to her gender. The challenge to all who endeavor in this field is to ensure her a better quality of life in the years to come.

8

A Community Advocate's View of

Clinical Research

Iris L. Long

My advice to people who work with women: make it
personal. Treat people as if they were your family members,
how you'd like to be treated. At some of these clinics, they
shun you. You go in and they have a mask on, gloves up to
their shoulders, and then they ask you, "How are you doing
today?" I say, "I was doing okay till I came in here."

People have to be more sensitive when they give
women this diagnosis. One young lady I was called in to a
clinic to see was very upset because the doctor just came in
and said, "You're HIV-positive. I'll give you an appointment to
come back in two weeks and we'll get you started on AZT."
Now, he might as well have said, "Can you please get out? I
have more patients to see." So the first thing I did was hug
her, because you want to be held. Places that know they
have a woman coming back who's going to get a positive

> result should arrange ahead of time with a community-
> based HIV group to have a volunteer there, someone who
> can just say, "I know what you're feeling." Don't give medi-
> cines without warning people about side effects and how to
> get through them; don't poke me in the arm with a needle
> and only after I ask explain that it's because my T-cells are
> low. Talk to me first.
> —Gwen Green

A clinical trial may offer a woman new treatment and medical-care options. But a woman who considers participating in an HIV/AIDS clinical trial faces many obstacles—some of them historical and many related to HIV disease.

The shortcomings of clinical research on the effects of drugs on women are not limited to HIV illness. A review of drugs used to treat high blood pressure, for example, shows the extent to which clinical research fails to discover the effects of drugs on women. In 1991 a group of female doctors looked at the data from clinical trials of a common antihypertensive drug and found that major probable side effects of antihypertensive therapies related to fat metabolism and sexual impairment in woman had been inadequately studied (Anastos et al. 1991). In some individuals disturbance of fat metabolism by drugs may be life-threatening. Sexual function disturbance is a quality-of-life issue studied with much concern in men; it is at least equally important to women.

Government-Sponsored Trials: ACTG

The two main categories of drugs used to prevent and treat HIV disease are drugs that fight the virus (anti-HIV or antiretroviral drugs) and drugs that treat HIV-related illness. Two National Institute of Allergy and Infectious Diseases (NIAID) AIDS Clinical Trial Group (ACTG) committees have developed most clinical trials: the Primary Infection (PI) Committee, and the Opportunistic Infection (OI) Committee. The PI Committee develops trials to test such anti-HIV drugs as AZT and ddI, and the OI Committee develops trials to test such drugs as aerosol pentamidine (a prophylaxis for Pneumocystis carinii pneumonia, or PCP) and fluconazole (a treatment for such fungal diseases as cryptococcal meningitis). Almost 90 percent of the patients in ACTG trials have been enrolled for studies of these two treatment categories. About 3,230 people have been enrolled in opportunistic infection trials alone (22 percent of total ACTG enrollment). In January 1993 only 327 (7.65 percent) of the national OI trial enrollees were women (Long 1993).

The definition of *asymptomatic* has evolved with the growing understanding of the disease. In 1986, when the clinical trial program began, asymptomatic simply referred to the absence of symptoms. The results of ACTG 019 indicated that 500 mg per day of AZT can delay the progression of disease during a one-year period from an HIV-positive asymptomatic state to AIDS in some patients. After the Food and Drug Administration extended the labeling of the drug to include all HIV-infected adults with a CD4+ cell count of less than 500, the term was expanded to include people taking AZT and PCP prophylaxis with no symptoms. Now the term may also be applied to people with non-AIDS defining symptoms and to people with positive toxoplasmosis serology. It may also include HIV-seropositive individuals with CD4+ cell counts greater than 1,000 who remain symptom free. Not only is the usefulness of the term *asymptomatic* diminished as its meaning becomes less specific, but the term itself may become a source of confusion.

Some investigators presume that people who are asymptomatic are therefore at an early stage of HIV disease. But a review of the entry criteria for trials admitting asymptomatics shows that some trials admit individuals who are clearly *not* at an early stage.

Classifying patients with marked immune suppression as asymptomatic may well lead researchers to the erroneous assumption that patients termed asymptomatic are at an early stage of HIV illness. Some have suggested that the reason women are mostly in the asymptomatic trials is that they are in an early stage of HIV disease, but available data do not support this conclusion. Ickovicks' 1991 study, for example, showed that 60 percent of the women entering Yale-New Haven Hospital for care had CD4+ cells below 200 at time of entry.

Furthermore, a number of factors significant in the enrollment of women in clinical trials are not always considered. Aside from the fact that females are more likely to be asymptomatic, the large variances in enrollment at ACTG sites and in the quality of linkages to women's pools at certain sites should be considered. Enrollment of women in certain late-phase comparison trials appears to be one of the priorities of the ACTG system. This can be partially explained by the historical exclusion of women of childbearing potential from early-phase trials of medicines, based on the 1977 FDA clinical research guidelines.

In the United States, women's enrollment information as of January 1992 gave this profile of the overall ACTG program enrollment:

• Women have greatest access to anti-HIV trials testing AZT (370 entries) and ddI (177 entries). Trials testing ddC have markedly fewer women (32 entries). In January 1993 there were 1,344 women in trials using AZT, if one includes ACTG 076 and 082 (to interrupt perinatal transmission; Long 1993).

• Women have almost no access to trials testing biological products. Three trials testing, variously, alpha interferon, GM-CSF, and IL-2 have enrolled only two women. By 1993 there were ten (Long 1993).

• A biological product proposed for testing in pregnant women had enrolled eight women. The product, recombinant CD4-IgG, will be tested to determine whether it reduces the incidence of HIV infection among infants with perinatal exposure.

• Women have had access to the following OI trials: PCP prophylaxis (82 enrollees), CMV retinitis (41), PCP treatment (32), serious fungal prophylaxis (19), Mycobacterium avium complex (MAC) (11), cryptococcal meningitis (8), herpes (4), cryptosporidiosis (4), and histoplasmosis (4).

• Women's enrollment is lowest in trials that include only symptomatic patients. For example, only 131 women (5 percent) were in primary infection trials admitting only symptomatic patients as of January 1993.

• Women have low enrollment in anti-HIV trials that are early trials, phase I studies. Women historically have not been recruited into phase I trials.

Opportunistic Infection Trials

People with AIDS die of the disease because of life-threatening opportunistic infections. Many of these deaths could be prevented through the development of the best treatments and preventive therapies. These treatments should be tested to determine their effectiveness in both women and men and across the full spectrum of races and ethnic backgrounds.

While some trials—like those for PCP prophylaxis—come close to enrolling their target numbers of patients, acute OI trials, as a group, enroll only 35 percent of their target numbers. These trials are often conducted at hospitals, where linkages among different departments have not always been developed to help locate patients. Different ways of running these trials must be found. If acute OI trials remain severely underenrolled there is little hope of developing treatments for HIV-related women's illness. Quicker ways of reviewing information from such trials and approving drugs for use by all people with HIV must be developed.

Many priority OI drugs have not yet been tested in women, a situation that many activists find unacceptable. For each of the following drugs, government-sponsored clinical trials have enrolled fewer than fifteen women: ganciclovir, foscarnet and amphotericin B, fluconazole, BW566, pyrimethamine, clindamycin, and itraconazole. One government response to its lack of research on women is that most women with HIV are in the early stage of the disease and have not developed CDC-defined symptomatic disease. In truth, opportunistic infections in women have not been studied systematically. Women have not been sufficiently monitored over the years to determine how their HIV disease differs from that in men.

Primary Infection Trials

Adult PI trials receive the highest priority and the highest number of patients. As of January 1992 the PI group has four trials enrolling asymptomatic patients only; one enrolling asymptomatic ARC patients; and ten enrolling asymptomatic ARC and AIDS patients. PI trials with asymptomatic arms accrued 7,062 participants, including 635 women (9 percent). One trial (ACTG 019) enrolled 3,215 patients, representing more than 47 percent of all women and 42 percent of all men enrolled in PI studies (all data cited are as of January 10, 1992; ACTIS 1992b).

There were twenty-four PI trials for symptomatic participants. By January 10, 1992, these trials had accrued 2,491 patients, including 113 women (4.5 percent). Fifteen were early-phase trials (phases I and I/II) and included females (5.7 percent). Late-phase trials included seventy-eight females (4 percent).

Studies of HIV Transmission to Infants

Two trials—ACTG 082 and 076—study whether AZT can interrupt transmission of HIV to the fetus and, later, to the newborn. They are the only trials restricted to women, yet their primary focus is not on the efficacy of a treatment for women.

ACTG 076, a placebo-controlled trial, had 610 patients, mostly HIV "asymptomatic" pregnant women and their children, by January 8, 1993. The trial had been open for enrollment for more than two years.

Although both trials seek to study AZT's effect on HIV transmission, neither studies the impact of AZT on the general health of the woman. The ethical propriety of both trials may be questioned: the woman is studied primarily as a vehicle for delivering the drug to the child while the 30 percent of infants who would in any event have been HIV seronegative are treated with a toxic drug that could harm them. Pregnant women do not have access to experimental drugs offered in other clinical trials or expanded-access protocols. Furthermore,women who participate in these trials have limited access to other clinical trials.

A pediatric trial scheduled to open in 1993 will test ddI in pregnant women. Also in 1993 the ACTG will test active immunization of HIV-infected pregnant women with recombinant gp120 and gp160 vaccines. The ACTG hopes that the immunization not only will help the mother but will also prevent infection from passing on to the child.

Clinical Trial Enrollment in New York

The ACTG program has sponsored eighty-four AIDS and HIV clinical trials in New York state, where 20.3 percent of all the AIDS cases in the United States had occurred through 1992 (New York State Department of Health 1992; CDC 1993). From information collected through early 1990, New York's AIDS Treatment Registry analyzed the clinical trial system, focusing on the kinds of AIDS trials opened in the state and who entered them (d'Adesky et al. 1990). Women's enrollment in New York trials was low at the time, totaling only 190. By February 1993 the number of women in trials in New York was 594 (Long 1993).

New York state, with 29.8 percent of all female AIDS cases in the United States (New York State Department of Health 1992; CDC 1993), has the greatest number of females in clinical trials—31 percent of the national ACTG female participants as of February 1993 (Long 1993). An increase in women's enrollment was registered in both New York state and New York City. In 1990 women made up 12.2 percent of the 1,553 adult trial enrollees in New York state (Long 1993). In early 1993 women made up 15.8 percent of the 3,763 adult participants in New York state and 16.8 percent in New York City. Despite the improved trial enroll-ments of women in the state, enrollment in ACTG trials throughout the country increased only slightly as of January 17, 1992.

How can tracking such figures help women? First, studies of the trials and fig-ures provided by the ACTG help in the assessment of how well local medical cen-ters within the system are studying HIV disease and its complications in women. A review of trial demographic characteristics also reveals which drugs the system is—and is not—testing in women. Such data stimulate further inquiry about why some drugs are tested in women and about the significance of drug trials for women. This information can help provide regularly updated guidelines on treatment for women.

The ACTG does not provide demographic enrollment information on trials that have opened in an individual state. Demographic information on patient par-ticipation in the Community Programs on Clinical Research on AIDS (CPCRA) in New York state is also not available.

Pharmaceutical Industry-Sponsored Studies

The clinical trial system used by drug companies is almost as extensive as the ACTG trial program. The companies do not readily provide information concerning their trial system, trial enrollment, and drug access programs, however. Demographic information was released by drug companies only once to researchers studying the demographics of AIDS clinical trials participants in New York (see d'Adesky et al. 1990). Women accounted for only 5 percent of the participants in twenty-three industry-sponsored trials conducted in New York state in early 1990.

For example, the Expanded Access Program for a ddI study conducted by Bristol-Myers Squibb could not reveal the gender, race, or ethnicity of its 22,000 participants. In April 1990 a company official gave figures of 7,497 men and 309 women (4 percent), saying that the percentage of women was about the same nationally. No breakdown was given for New York state, where 30 percent of all women with AIDS reside (New York State Department of Health 1992; CDC 1993). Sparse as they are, these figures indicate clear problems of access for women and members of other populations.

Community Programs for Clinical Research on AIDS

AIDS advocates were dissatisfied with the minority representation of adults in AIDS clinical trials, arguing that communities should have input into the choice of drugs tested. In the United States the number of women of color in ACTG clinical trials is in extreme disproportion to the number of people of color with an AIDS diagnosis. Through December 1990, 52 percent of all U.S. women diagnosed with AIDS were black women, but only 23 percent of the female ACTG trials participants were reported to be black (Cotton, Feinberg, and Finkelstein 1991). Tracking gender and race information is difficult for advocates because the government does not regularly provide this information to the public.

Advocates at that time believed that the community should test promising medications that the ACTG would not test and suggested that better representation of minority groups might be achieved by conducting clinical trials in the communities where minorities live. AIDS activists pressured the government to support this approach. In October 1989, NIAID founded twenty-five sites in various communities that were mandated to conduct AIDS clinical trials. They did not test non-AZT drugs, as the advocates wished, but simply extended the ACTG program. In essence, the establishment of CPCRA involved the funding of new sites outside the ACTG program.

The majority of the people participating in CPCRA are enrolled in the observational database (ODB); only about 19 percent are enrolled in the clinical trials. The observational database protocol is a multicenter, prospective, longitudinal study with continuous patient accrual over an indefinite period of time. The trials have mirrored those taking place in the ACTG. They include separate prophylaxis and maintenance trials testing pyrimethamine versus clindamycin as prophylaxis in HIV-infected patients with antibodies to toxoplasmosis (T. gondii); ddI versus ddC in those patients with intolerance to AZT; tuberculosis prophylaxis trial (ACTG 177) in patients with latent TB infection and a positive PPD, a second trial in patients with negative PPDs who might have latent infection, and TB skin testing; combination nucleoside therapy; and fluconazole prophylaxis for vaginal candidiasis.

In the ODB and clinical trials together, female participation accounts for 19.7 percent of the nationwide total. The participation of women in the clinical trials alone (removing the women in the ODB) amounts to 12 percent, but the government usually reports the participation of women in the CPCRA "trials" as 20 percent.

Recommendations from the Activist Community

At a meeting on March 18, 1993, the Food and Drug Administration commissioner, David Kessler, agreed to revoke the 1977 guidelines excluding women of "childbearing potential" from drug trials. Women with HIV may still lack access to experimental and parallel track drugs. The input of women and advocates must be solicited and the following recommendations implemented.

• Drugs under study in clinical trials should be analyzed for their effects on women.

• Women with HIV and their advocates should participate in the design and implementation of the longitudinal study of women with HIV being implemented by the CDC, NIAID, and other agencies (the Women's Interagency Health Study to elaborate the natural history of HIV illness in women).

• Design and implementation of clinical trials of drugs to treat acute opportunistic infections, which have been severely underenrolled for years, must be changed. Problem areas must be identified and solutions implemented. The Women's Health Committee of the ACTG should make this problem a top priority.

• Information on medicines available outside of clinical trials should be analyzed with respect to women.

• A women's network must be developed to publicize treatments—and their side effects and effectiveness—in women.

• The Food and Drug Administration should be encouraged to rapidly implement new policies concerning women with HIV and clinical trials. Women activists should continue to meet with FDA administrators, and the FDA should set up a mechanism for reporting women-specific drug side effects and adverse reactions and interactions.

• Women should develop a coordinated agenda for the ACTG Community Advisory Boards associated with the AIDS Clinical Trial Units (ACTUs) in their areas. There should be networking at the national level to achieve consensus on the best agenda for women in trials. There should be designated women representatives at all ACTUs.

• Local needs should be taken into consideration when an ACTU determines which trials it will conduct. For example, a community with a high level of a certain opportunistic infection should be sited for clinical trials of appropriate drugs. NIAID should be encouraged to release all available information about trial participation of women in each locality.

• Obstetricians and gynecologists, nurse-midwives, and other women's health care providers should be encouraged to take leadership roles along with AIDS activists on issues critical to women with HIV disease (see Denenberg 1991).

• The U.S. government must take responsibility for disseminating information on the special nutritional needs of women with HIV, including requirements for nutritional supplements, vitamins, and minerals.

Implementation of these recommendations will bring closer to fulfillment the right of women to be truly equal partners in research.

9

Ethical Issues

Carol Levine

I wouldn't want to raise kids today. We tell my grandchildren, "You've got to have strong hands and a strong heart," the influences out there are so strong. I do have hope for the future with these kids today, though. They're really handling it pretty well, the ones with any intelligence. But one kid I talked to didn't think he'd get [HIV] because he'd never been in jail. So still, I don't think kids today are getting enough education about this disease. They need to hear

Some of the material in this chapter has appeared elsewhere in different form. The section on reproductive rights is largely drawn from Carol Levine and Nancy Neveloff Dubler, "Uncertain Risks and Bitter Realities: The Reproductive Choices of HIV-Infected Women, *Milbank Quarterly* 68, no. 3 (1990): 321–51. The section on research is an updated version of Carol Levine, "Women and HIV/AIDS Research: The Barriers to Equity," *Evaluation Review* 14, no. 5 (October 1990): 447–63.

about it from people they trust, like rappers, to deal with the issue.

Another kid [who was] using drugs had this "it won't happen to me" attitude. I said it can happen to you—not because you're using drugs but because you're *human,* and this thing is happening to everyone.

—Grace Simons

Using a simple word association test or a sophisticated literature search, what topics link *ethics, women,* and *HIV/AIDS?* Chances are, either method will result in a cluster of issues surrounding HIV counseling and testing, vertical transmission and reproductive rights, and participation in clinical research. The existing literature has focused almost exclusively on ethical choices framed by policy analysts, ethicists, and health care providers *about* HIV-positive women and women at risk of infection, not on ethical dilemmas as the women perceive them. Furthermore, discussions about women and ethics typically view women in isolation from others (except unborn or unconceived fetuses). Because the majority of HIV-positive women in the United States have been poor women of color and either drug users or the sexual partners of drug users, questions of ethics have typically been framed by people of one class about those of another, less powerful class.

Although the discussions are admittedly one-sided, they have not been insensitive to the needs of HIV-positive women, particularly as these women become more outspoken in their own behalf. In this chapter I address current and emerging issues in the realm of ethics and policy, particularly regarding research. I also offer some speculations about women's own perceptions of ethical dilemmas and the social context of decision making.

HIV Counseling and Testing

Discussions about HIV counseling and testing policies for pregnant women and newborns have taken place in the context of a broader debate: Should testing be voluntary with informed consent, mandatory (legally required), or "routine" (usually interpreted to mean that the patient may refuse testing but that the health care provider is not obliged to specifically inform the patient that testing will be done)? With some exceptions—screening of blood donors, military personnel, and immigrants, for example—the debate has been resolved in favor of voluntary testing.

The major organizations and groups that have examined testing policies for pregnant women have concluded that voluntary screening with informed consent is the course most likely to produce the desired effect of education, prevention, and appropriate medical and social service followup. The Institute of Medicine, for example, concluded that "individuals (or their legally recognized representatives) should have the right to consent to or refuse HIV testing (except when such testing is conducted anonymously for epidemiological purposes)." In opposing mandatory newborn or prenatal screening programs, the Institute of Medicine (1991) found "no compelling evidence that women and children should constitute an exception to this principle." Similarly, a working group from Johns Hopkins University and the Kennedy Institute of Ethics rejected mandatory screening and recommended a range of voluntary policies (Faden, Geller, and Powers 1992).

This consensus is eroding, however, because of new evidence about the benefits of early diagnosis and intervention in HIV disease. Although the potential medical benefits apply to adults and children, the most vigorous calls for routine or mandatory screening come from pediatricians, who stress the benefits to newborns. Benefits to mothers are often couched in terms of "referrals to care" or "allowing women to make informed decisions about further pregnancies," which often seems to be shorthand for directive counseling to discourage further pregnancies. HIV-positive pregnant women may be denied the potential benefits of early intervention if their physicians follow Centers for Disease Control and Prevention recommendations that term Pneumocystis carinii pneumonia (PCP) prophylaxis in pregnancy "inadvisable" (CDC 1989; Minkoff and Moreno 1990).

Despite these imbalances, the case for early diagnosis of newborns is strong. All babies carry maternal antibodies for fifteen to eighteen months; about a third are truly infected. With new techniques, seropositive infants as young as three months can be more accurately identified (Quinn et al. 1991). Pneumocystis carinii pneumonia in infants is the most frequent and most lethal manifestation of HIV disease. Prophylaxis in adults can prevent or delay PCP, but there are no studies on prophylaxis with infants. However, the U.S. Public Health Service recommends that prophylaxis be initiated in infants with CD4+ cell counts of less than 1,500 (CDC 1991). In addition, antiretroviral therapy can begin at an early age, and babies can be monitored closely for other infections. These benefits are not a panacea but do have a significant impact on the ethics of the screening calculus.

In the interests of identifying HIV-positive infants and providing them with aggressive early interventions, what are the ethical implications of mandatory or routine screening of pregnant women or newborns? Some proposals for identifying HIV-positive infants have focused on unblinding the anonymous newborn screening programs carried out for epidemiological purposes. Over the past several years the CDC has developed what it calls a family of serosurveys to estimate the prevalence of HIV infection in sentinel areas and groups throughout the country (Pappaioanou et al. 1990). In June 1989 the New York State Department of Health proposed modifying its ongoing blind newborn HIV antibody testing program to permit voluntary notification of mothers whose infants test positive (New York State Department of Health 1989). Under the proposal, new mothers would be given the option of learning their baby's test results. Several objections to the proposal were raised by community-based health care providers and others. One concerned the psychologically traumatic impact on new mothers of learning about their own HIV infection and the possible infection of their babies at a time when they are physically and emotionally vulnerable. Another was the potential for coercion by health care providers who feel that women have an obligation to know their serostatus. A final concern was the lack of health care and support services for women and their children who have been identified as seropositive.

Because of these objections, the Department of Health agreed to postpone implementation of the proposal in favor of a much more aggressive voluntary program, the Obstetrical HIV Counseling/Testing/Care Initiative. This program offers voluntary counseling and testing with counseling at twenty-four sites to women who have given birth without access to prenatal care. Initial results indicate that a growing percentage of these women are being counseled (64.8 percent by 1991), consenting to testing (46.9 percent), and being referred to care (New York State Department of Health, AIDS Institute 1992).

Acceptance of counseling and testing is not universal, however, and pressure to unblind newborn seroprevalence studies persists. Such a policy would compromise the scientific validity of these studies and introduce the possibility of their becoming politicized. Blinded surveys test for HIV in blood samples already collected for other medical purposes; they are devoid of all personal identifiers. This approach to measuring HIV prevalence in selected populations enjoys the broad support of epidemiologists, social scientists, and others in public health, primarily for technical, ethical, and practical reasons. Blinded surveys can generate less biased estimates of HIV prevalence because individuals do not choose whether to participate in serotesting. Because the surveys do not place any participant at risk of identification, issues of privacy and confidentiality are not raised (Bayer, Levine, and Wolf 1986). Consequently, study protocols are exempt from Institutional Review Board review, and individual consent forms and measures to secure the confidentiality of the information obtained are not required. For these reasons, blinded studies are simpler, quicker, and less costly than nonblinded surveys. They have also been remarkably uncontroversial and free of political influence. It is interesting to note that blinded serosurveys have been very controversial in England and the Netherlands, however, where objections were raised regarding the lack of consent (Bayer, Lumey, and Wan 1990).

The use of blinded surveys is compatible with a parallel system of voluntary counseling and testing in settings where individuals likely to be at risk of HIV infection are treated. One of the purposes of blinded serosurveys is precisely to identify where resources and services are needed, including counseling and testing. But, as the Public Health Service itself points out, "the surveillance activity, in the case of an HIV prevalence survey, must not be confused with the public health intervention for which the survey may indicate a need" (Dondero, Pappaioanou, and Curran 1988). Furthermore, guidelines issued by the World Health Organization for unlinked anonymous screening for the public health surveillance of HIV infections state: "Voluntary testing (confidential or anonymous) with counselling should be available wherever possible to populations in which UAS [unlinked anonymous screening] is being carried out, so that those individuals who wish to know their HIV-infection status can do so. This is particularly important if the population is estimated to have a moderate to high prevalence of HIV infection. However, such testing should be offered through a separate system" (Global Programme on AIDS 1989).

Blinded anonymous seroprevalence studies offer the opportunity to sample in an unbiased and nonpoliticized way the level of infection in selected settings, with no risk to participants. The studies cannot also serve the equally important but distinct public health and clinical functions of providing individuals with the opportunity to learn their serostatus so they can be advised about modifying their behavior to prevent transmission and about obtaining medical care for themselves and their children. These activities should continue to operate on parallel but separate tracks.

Reproductive Rights of Women with Inheritable Disorders

In December 1985 the CDC officially recommended that women who are HIV-positive or who have AIDS should "be advised to consider delaying pregnancy until more is known about perinatal transmission of the virus." The materials offered by the departments of health in many states go beyond that advice and recommend unequivocally that HIV-positive women should not become pregnant (Bayer 1991). Nonetheless, many infected women are having babies even when they know they are infected and have been counseled about the risks of perinatal transmission or already have a child with HIV infection or AIDS or have lost a child to AIDS (Selwyn et al. 1989; Williams 1990; Holman et al. 1991). Despite the gravity and consequences of continued perinatal transmission, HIV infection is one of a range of conditions that can be passed from mother to fetus and should not be singled out for moral censure and coercive policies. Other less stigmatized conditions are equally or even more likely to be transmitted, to result in suffering or death for the child, and to be costly to the family and society. Reproductive decisions are crucial to biological and social life, and HIV-positive women must remain free to make choices that are consistent with their cultural, religious, and personal values.

Mothers with HIV have dismal long-term prognoses, and those who have developed AIDS face almost certain death. But many women with chronic diseases—and some who are dying—choose to become pregnant, even at considerable risk to themselves. They are more treasured by their families and admired by society for doing so. In contrast, HIV-positive women are considered irresponsible for having babies who may face early death and whose care may be a burden to society. Surely class and ethnicity play a role in these societal responses and judgments.

Federal and state public health officials who exhort HIV-positive women to forgo pregnancy are responding understandably to what is in their view primarily a problem of disease transmission to newborns. Although there is no cure as yet, and some babies are born dying, for most the affliction resembles a long-term chronic disease like cystic fibrosis rather than a degenerative and fatal illness like Tay-Sachs (see Nolan 1989). Given the current knowledge, there is no way to predict whether an HIV-positive woman will infect her fetus (chances are higher that she will not), no reliable way to determine in utero or at birth whether a baby is infected (unless it is born with symptoms), and no way to foretell the likely course of the disease. This array of uncertainties is weighed very differently by public health officials and physicians and by women at risk.

A child-centered analysis based on only the worst outcomes leads many to conclude that all HIV-infected babies are doomed and therefore should not be born, and that public policies should be developed to prevent or discourage HIV-positive women from giving birth. Mary Steichen Calderone, cofounder of the Sex Information and Education Council of the United States, expressed a typical view in arguing that "innocent" and "grotesque" fetuses born to drug-abusing mothers have a right *not* to be born: "And there is also the fetus infected by an AIDS-carrying mother. Until a cure is found for this wildfire disease, why should the same right not to be born be withheld from this fetus?" (Calderone 1989).

Many HIV-infected babies are no worse off than babies born with other severe and life-threatening birth conditions, yet there are no comparable claims that all such babies should have been aborted. Indeed, as a society we point proudly to expensive and technically elaborate neonatal intensive care units constructed to support the imperiled lives of premature infants, most of them also poor. Adequate prenatal care would have prevented most of these premature births and their attendant disabilities. Moreover, in the extended discussions among ethicists, physicians, and lawyers that followed the Baby Doe and similar cases, a consensus has emerged that babies with serious disabilities should be treated except when they are born dying and when treatment would provide no benefit but would increase pain and suffering. Babies and pregnancy have a special symbolism for many women—a symbolism that may be heightened for women with HIV. Janet Mitchell (1988), chief perinatologist at Harlem Hospital in New York, points out that "Latino and black cultures place great value on a woman's fertility. Having a child elevates the status of the woman in her community." Moreover, she says, "pregnancy may be the only time when drug-using women feel good about themselves. Numerous studies have shown that pregnancy is a strong motive for these women to go 'straight.'"

Carol Levine

For some women who are HIV-positive and can face their own mortality, pregnancy is a better than two-thirds chance to leave someone behind for a mother or husband to care for, a link to immortality that genealogy presents. Ernesto de la Vega (1990) of the Panos Institute comments that "part of [Latinas'] culturally determined mission in life is to assure the life of the male and to provide him with existential continuity—that is, to provide him with a male baby that will inherit and pass on the family name. In addition, because a woman's life is traditionally defined by the presence of her male partner, she may wish to have, in the form of a child, a reminder of him so that she can feel she has a graspable part of him if he should die prematurely of AIDS." One need not accept the concept, prevalent in many minority communities, that there's an active governmental policy of genocide to appreciate the power of the loss of a generation of men through societal neglect and the community's desire to replace them through the birth of a new generation. Another important reason that HIV-positive women may choose to become pregnant or to continue a pregnancy is to replace a child lost through disease, denial of custody, or simply the complexities of life in poverty.

The decision to reproduce or to limit reproduction is a complex one reflecting the personal, cultural, social, economic, and religious values of an individual woman. A society that permits poverty, drugs, and economic dislocation, spends differentially for education of the poor, overlooks truancy and dropping out, and perpetuates neighborhoods with inferior health care and social services is morally responsible, at least on some level, for the consequences of these unleashed societal forces.

Although interference with reproductive choice is a fact of life for most poor women and women of color, these women often experience difficulties in obtaining health care, related to reproductive services or not. Access to health care in the inner city ranges from limited to nonexistent. There are few developed patterns of integrated health care and preventive care use. Prenatal care for drug users is grossly inadequate, and most drug treatment programs do not enroll pregnant women and are not set up to permit a woman with child care responsibilities to comply with the rules (Chavkin 1989). The health care system is complex and entered only in emergency situations or as a last resort.

Sterilization and other attempts to limit reproduction are only one side of the restrictions on reproductive freedom. Abortion rights, given constitutional sanction under *Roe v. Wade* in 1973, have been increasingly threatened. Many women who cannot pay for an abortion themselves cannot obtain one with public funds, either. In 1981 Congress restricted Medicaid payments for abortion to cases in which the woman's life is endangered by her continued pregnancy. Many states have limited further funding at the urging of "right to life" organizations. Five states provide some further services, and only twelve provide for the general funding of poor women's abortions. Because of this, abortion of a possibly HIV-infected child is not an option for poor women in many states. Federal funds were not allowed to be used for abortion or for any counseling or education that mentioned abortion as an alternative (the so-called gag rule).

Women who do decide to terminate a pregnancy are increasingly unable to find services to carry out that plan. Access to abortion is even further limited for HIV-positive women whose serostatus is known or disclosed. A survey conducted by the AIDS division of the New York City Commission on Human Rights found a systematic barrier to abortions for women who reveal that they are HIV-positive. In that study, fourteen of the thirty-three clinics and private doctors called (42 percent) refused to provide services after the caller identified her serostatus. Twelve of the providers indicated that they could not perform the procedure because of inadequate infection control procedures, and not a single provider located in Brooklyn would make an appointment (Franke 1989; see also chapter 10). HIV-positive women— the same class of women who have traditionally been encouraged or coerced to limit reproduction on grounds of benefit to themselves, their families, or society—are now being encouraged to limit reproduction to prevent transmission of disease to their children and costs to society. But at the same time their options for making this choice independently are being restricted. Women placed in this no-win situation, not surprisingly, cannot win.

Women in Drug Trials and Clinical Research

Women—especially those of childbearing age and those who are pregnant—have had least-favored status among groups of potential biomedical research subjects. Regulatory agencies, pharmaceutical companies, and researchers have been wary of involving women in research ever since the thalidomide disaster of the late 1950s and early 1960s, in which a sedative liberally prescribed for pregnant women in Europe and Australia turned out to cause horrific birth defects. (The women whose babies were harmed were not research subjects, however, but ordinary patients.)

Research in general came to be considered a risky venture; vulnerable subjects, including women and their fetuses or potential fetuses, were deemed to need stringent protections. Finally, research questions that pertain specifically to women's health—whether diseases that occur only in women or diseases that occur in both sexes but are mainly studied in men—have had relatively low priority on the research agenda.

But the age of protectionism, the period from the early 1960s to the early 1990s, is giving way to the age of inclusionism. The following are a few indications of the new era:

• In June 1990 the General Accounting Office (GAO) of the U.S. Congress reported that grant applicants and staff members of the National Institutes of Health (NIH) were not complying with the agency's stated policy of "encouraging" the inclusion of women as research subjects. Although NIH disagreed with some of the GAO's conclusions, in September 1990 it established an Office of Research on Women's Health "to strengthen and enhance the efforts of the NIH to improve the prevention, diagnosis, and treatment of illness in women and to enhance research related to diseases and conditions that affect women" (Kirschstein 1991, 291).

The *NIH Guide for Grants and Contracts* has been revised to *require* the inclusion of women. The guide states that:

1. adequate numbers of women *shall* be included in clinical studies proportional to prevalence of the condition under study;

2. *failure* to include an adequate number of women will be considered to affect the investigator's ability to answer the scientific question being posed unless an appropriate justification is provided;

3. any *justification* for not including women in such studies will be evaluated by the peer review group assessing the proposal and . . . factored into the final recommendation;

4. no *application* or proposal for which the justification for exclusion of women is considered inappropriate *will be funded* unless such a justification is compelling (NIH 1990).

• In February 1991 the Congressional Caucus for Women introduced the Women's Health Equity Act of 1991, an omnibus package of twenty-two bills designed to improve women's health in the areas of research, service, and prevention. The caucus also asked the GAO to investigate whether the Food and Drug Administration's practices and policies exclude women from the drug-approval process.

• The Council on Ethical and Judicial Affairs of the American Medical Association (1991) declared that "results of medical testing done solely on men should not be generalized to women without evidence that results can be applied safely and effectively to both sexes. Research on health problems that affect both sexes should include male and female subjects."

Although the signs are clear, the road ahead may not be smooth or the most direct route always apparent. Research involving human subjects is regulated by the Department of Health and Human Services (DHHS) through two parallel (but slightly different) sets of rules. One applies to research conducted by or funded by DHHS itself (45 CFR 46, revised March 8, 1983), the other to drug studies that will result in submissions for marketing approval to the FDA (Federal Register 1981).

The federal regulations require prior ethical review of protocols by institutional review boards, committees created by and responsible to the institutions where research is conducted. The regulations do not exclude women from research, but they emphasize the potential risk to fetuses. Beyond the regulations governing research that employs human subjects, FDA guidelines since 1977 for clinical evaluation of drugs stated that women of childbearing potential should be excluded from large-scale clinical trials until the FDA Animal Reproduction Guidelines have been completed, except in cases of life-threatening illness. In March 1993 the FDA announced that this ban, enacted in 1977 guidelines, would be lifted, but no details were given.

Although concern has escalated about the possibility that birth defects may be caused by drugs taken by pregnant women, there has been little concern that fathers' exposure to chemical agents may also contribute to birth defects. In a book on drug and chemical risks to the fetus and newborn published in 1980 (Soyka and Joffe) the authors reviewed animal and human studies in which only the male partner was exposed to the chemical or drug agent, mostly through occupational exposure. They found reports of "adverse effects on progeny of five species for lead, morphine, thalidomide, caffeine, and ethanol, including decreased litter size, birth weight, survival, and learning ability in a T-maze." In humans, lead, anesthetic gases, cigarettes, and caffeine have been associated with a variety of adverse effects on reproductive outcomes. Although it seems likely that maternal exposure remains a more significant factor, the possibility of male-mediated effects should not be overlooked. Further studies should be done on the male-mediated effects of pharmaceutical drugs and occupational exposure.

In drug trial recruitment, HIV-positive women suffer triple jeopardy. They may be excluded because they are women and either potentially or actually pregnant; because they are members of minority groups and lack access to the health care system in general and to research in particular; and because they are drug users and presumed to be noncompliant subjects. Efforts to include women in HIV/AIDS drug trials may be stymied by several barriers: the protectivist regulatory system; the pharmaceutical industry, which seeks to avoid liability for possible teratogenic effects of experimental compounds; the health care system, which has failed to provide access to primary care for many of the poor, minority women most at risk for HIV infection; and minority communities themselves, which are often suspicious of research that has used (and sometimes abused) their members and failed to provide any compensating benefits.

In redressing the imbalance caused by policies that exclude women it is important to consider that women, particularly those who are or may become pregnant, have moral responsibilities to fetuses they plan to carry to term, as do investigators and those who develop or approve protocols involving women. The ethical obligation not to do harm carries particular force when the potential recipient of the harm is an unconsenting fetus whose future health and welfare may be unalterably affected. Approval of a protocol is not an ethically neutral stance; it is an affirmative statement that the choices to be offered to potential subjects, though perhaps difficult to make, are ethically justifiable. Exposing a fetus to serious risk when there are

Carol Levine

alternative treatments or when the benefits are modest is not, in my view, an ethically justifiable choice.

The potential of harm to a fetus is of course a morally relevant factor to the mother herself. The vast majority of women see their own primary interests as identical to those of their fetuses. Women generally do not lightly undertake any medical intervention that will hurt a fetus; in fact, many women deny themselves optimal medical care to avoid risk. Some, however, may exercise their right to choose medical treatments despite known or unknown risks to the fetus.

The choice of including pregnant women or women of childbearing potential is relatively straightforward at the extremes. Excluding a woman suffering a life-threatening condition from access to a potentially life-saving drug on the grounds of potential harm to an unconceived fetus seems not only unjust but also harsh. If a pregnant woman's life is in danger, her fetus is equally threatened. At the other extreme, exposing women and their actual or potential fetuses to serious harm when there are alternative therapies, or when the potential benefits are only trivial, honors autonomy at the expense of common sense.

Other scenarios, however, are not so straightforward. Thalidomide, the drug that causes devastating birth defects when taken early in pregnancy, is one of the best treatments for a serious complication of Hansen's disease (leprosy) known as erythema nodosom leprosum (ENL). Studies of cancer patients suggest that thalidomide can prevent many of the side effects—including the sometimes fatal graft-host reaction—of radiation therapy given to recipients of bone-marrow transplants (Squires 1989). Thalidomide has been found effective in two AIDS patients as a treatment of severe recurrent aphthous stomatitis (painful, relapsing oral ulcerations), for which conventional treatments had failed. One of the patients was a thirty-seven-year-old woman who had previously been sterilized. The authors state: "To prevent the possibility of teratogenicity, thalidomide should not be used in women of child-bearing age" (Nicolau and West 1990). Thalidomide has also been shown to have anti-HIV activity and will be investigated in clinical trials (see Chemical & Engineering News, July 12, 1993).

Suppose an investigator wants to do further study on this use of thalidomide. The primary benefits would be the acquisition of knowledge, though the subjects might reasonably be expected to benefit. Should pregnant women and women of childbearing capacity be excluded? On the one hand, the potential harm to fetuses is so well known and so severe and permanent that pregnant women in the first trimester and sexually active women who do not use contraception could justifiably be excluded. A woman who has no intention of becoming pregnant at the beginning of a study may fail to appreciate the risks or remember the warnings when her life situation changes. A woman who was enrolled in such a study and became pregnant would be faced with the options of abortion (which she might find morally unacceptable) or of carrying the potentially severely damaged fetus to term. In this view, it would be ethical to include women with childbearing potential in the study only if thalidomide or an experimental drug with known similar teratogenic properties were truly life-saving; if there were no alternatives; and if failure to administer it would result in certain death or irreversible serious physical or mental deterioration of the woman and her fetus.

On the other hand, it can be argued that a nonpregnant woman, a woman who uses contraception successfully, or a woman in the later stages of pregnancy who has suffered oral pain unameliorated by any therapy should be able to choose for herself whether to participate in the study, with full and complete disclosure of all risks and benefits. Fortunately, most protocols do not present such difficult choices. In the vast majority of cases women can be offered the same options as men, with full explanation of the risks and benefits to themselves as well as to their fetuses.

Even if exclusionary barriers related to gender or substance abuse were removed, women would still face problems concerning access to research because of their lack of access to primary health care and their needs for assistance with child care, transportation, and family responsibilities. Recruitment efforts will have to take into account the multiple roles women play as family caregivers and employees (often in marginal jobs with little flexibility). Meeting their own health care needs may not be their highest priority; enrolling in research, an alien concept to many, may seem even less important.

The goal is not to persuade women to become research subjects, either for their own good or for the good of society, but to make more equitable the selection of subjects who will undertake the risks and share in the benefits of research.

Ethical Issues as Women See Them

For many HIV-positive women, survival—their own, their children's, their family's—is the only issue. In this context, debates about testing policies or inclusion in research protocols may seem irrelevant. Yet these women do make ethical decisions in their daily lives, such as whether to disclose their HIV status to a sexual partner, thus being responsible but risking abuse and rejection; and whether to continue a pregnancy knowing there is risk of transmission to their unborn child.

What values come to the fore in these decisions? The evidence so far indicates the primacy of relationships—especially the mother-child relationship—over abstract principles or paternalistic counsel. A baby is a chance to have something concrete to love or to be loved by. It is proof of fertility and the visible sign of having been loved or at least touched by another. One HIV-positive woman at the Women's Center at Montefiore Medical Center in New York poignantly explained why she wanted to have a baby: "Right now, I would have to say it means a lot to me. Because I've had so many disappointing times in my life, so many people have died the past several months that a new baby would be like a new beginning for me, even though it's not myself. . . . Whether I had this man with me or not, I probably would have this baby . . . something I love" (Pivnick et al. 1991).

Women may express opinions that differ from their actions. Women at risk of HIV disease may support mandatory testing policies but be reluctant to be tested themselves (Faden, Geller, and Powers 1992). They may declare that having a baby, knowing one is HIV-positive, is "selfish," yet carry such a pregnancy to term (Williams 1990).

Uncertainty is a central concern for all seriously ill people, and it may be even greater for those with HIV or AIDS because the disease is new and medical knowledge is advancing so rapidly. Because so much attention has been focused on men with the disease, women may be particularly distrustful of medical information and predictions about their own future and that of their children.

A comprehensive approach to the problems inherent in women's lives, with special sensitivity to childbearing and disease prevention, is essential for providing women with a framework in which to make informed ethical choices. Counseling women to refrain from pregnancy without providing alternatives for self-fulfillment or education about sexuality and reproduction may prevent some pregnancies, but it also may drive women away from systems that will be perceived as harsh and condemning.

Meaningful education about sexuality and reproduction should begin in elementary school. In addition to helping to prevent the spread of HIV infection and STDs to women and their children, it may help them avoid sexual abuse as children. Access to medical services should be increased for all poor people so that children develop a rapport with health care professionals and are able to discuss health and reproductive issues. There should be increased access to prenatal care to reduce the number of impaired, non-HIV-infected babies. Pregnant women who choose abortion to prevent the birth of a possibly HIV-infected child should have timely access to services. Improved housing and support services will allow mothers to maintain relationships with their children and reduce separations and loss of custody (Pivnick et al. 1991).

Emphasizing the moral responsibilities of HIV-positive women is the wrong focus with the wrong lens. If fairness and justice are to be of service, the lens must be wide enough to encompass the moral responsibilities of men and society as well.

10

Legal Considerations

Michele A. Zavos

Let me try to tell you how being a mother with this disease
feels. It is an issue I have struggled with over the last three
years. Perhaps the pain involved makes the joy that much
greater. My daughter, seven now, is HIV-negative and in the
clear. She is the center of my life, a wanted child in every
sense of the word. . . . She is completing first grade; we
have both made it through this first year of school. There is
always a nagging thought way down deep: how long will I be
here? Will I be there for her first date, for graduation from
high school, for fourth grade?

    I have been trying to draw up custody papers for my
daughter for quite some time now (her biological father died
of AIDS two years ago). I would not give up custody while I
am well, perhaps not even when I am sick. For now, this is

not an alternative for me. I relate this to you because you
need to know that often the children in our lives are our
survival. I work at staying healthy so that I can raise my
daughter. It is she who keeps me on track, centered in my
will to survive. This is an essential to women, to mothers
living with this disease.

—Anonymous

Women with HIV disease confront many of the same legal issues faced by other
HIV-infected individuals. Men and women both may have problems gaining access
to basic health care, maintaining health insurance, obtaining government benefits,
and receiving treatment and prophylactic care. They also may encounter discrimination in employment, housing, education, and other areas. Moreover, people with
HIV disease, like everyone with a potentially catastrophic illness, need a will,
power of attorney, and health care directives to maintain control over their medical
decisions and other aspects of their lives.

But HIV-positive women also encounter a multitude of legal problems exacerbated or caused by their gender and compounded by their socioeconomic status:
most are poor women of color who become infected through injection-drug use or
heterosexual sex with an injection-drug user. A woman's access to reproductive
services may be hindered by her HIV disease; she may be punished criminally
because of her HIV infection; and, despite the large number of women who have
become infected through drug use, she is not likely to be able to gain access to drug
treatment programs.

In addition, women with HIV are usually mothers and primary family caretakers with special legal needs regarding the care and guardianship of their children.
These women may encounter challenges to their parenting status and require legal
representation to keep their children.

In this chapter I provide an overview of some of the myriad legal issues that
may be raised when women become infected with HIV.

Discrimination

Three statutes give most of the legal protections against discrimination provided by
federal law to individuals with HIV disease, though constitutional claims of discrimination against mandatory HIV testing have also been successful.[1] The Americans with Disabilities Act (ADA) of 1990 (42 U.S.C. Sec. 12101), the Fair Housing

---

[1] A Fourth Amendment challenge to a mandatory testing program, Glover v. Eastern
Nebraska Community Office of Retardation 867 F.2d461 (8th Cir. 1989), cert. denied 58
U.S.L.W. 3287 (Oct. 30, 1989).

Amendments Act of 1988 (FHAA) (codified at 42 U.S.C. of 3601 *et. seq.* as the Fair Housing Act of 1968, as amended), and sections 501, 503, and 504 of the Rehabilitation Act of 1973 (29 U.S.C. Sec. 794) cover all individuals with disabilities, specifically those with HIV and AIDS and those perceived to have HIV or AIDS.

Litigation pursuant to Section 504—which applies to infectious diseases— produced the principle that individuals with HIV and AIDS are protected from discrimination under the general prohibitions against discrimination of "otherwise qualified" persons with disabilities. Individuals with disabilities are defined by the Rehabilitation Act as people having physical or mental impairments that substantially limit one or more major life activities; people with a record of such an impairment; or people regarded as having such an impairment (29 U.S.C. Sec. 706[8][B]). "Otherwise qualified" may mean that an individual with a disability meets essential qualifications for participation in a program or has the ability to participate in a program with or without "reasonable accommodation." "Reasonable accommodation" is a modification of a program that allows an individual with a disability to participate without changing the fundamental nature of the program.

Section 504 applies to entities receiving federal financial assistance and to programs conducted by the federal government. Courts have held that Section 504 prohibits discrimination against people with AIDS and HIV regarding employment (*Chalk v. United States District Court*, 840 F.2d 701 [9th Cir. 1988] and *Shuttleworth v. Broward County*, 639 F. Supp. 654 [S.D. Fla. 1986]), public education (*Martinez v. School Board of Hillsborough County, Florida*, 861 F.2d 1502 [11th Cir. 1988] and *Ray v. School District of DeSoto County*, 666 F. Supp. 1524 [M.D. Fla. 1987]), and access to services, including health-related services (Doe v. Centinela Hospital, 57 U.S.L.W. 2034 [C.D. Cal. June 20, 1988], *Doe v. Howard University*, AIDS Litigation Rptr. 2432, March 24, 1989, and *Rhodes v. Charter Hospital*, AIDS Litigation Rptr. 2393, March 10, 1989; see also *Dallas Gay Alliance v. Dallas County Hospital District*, 719 F. Supp. 1380 [N.D. Texas 1989]).

The Fair Housing Act (42 U.S.C. Secs. 3601 *et seq.*) applies to all public or private residential housing, with certain limited exceptions, and as originally amended, prohibits discrimination on the basis of sex, race, religion, and national origin. The 1988 amendments brought individuals with disabilities and families with children within the purview of the FHA's protections. Individuals with HIV and AIDS are covered under these protections as the 1988 Amendments Act uses Section 504's definition of handicap. This addition may be particularly important to individuals with HIV disease because the Amendments Act extends protections to private residential housing and to the establishment of group homes and hospices. (*See Baxter v. City of Belleville, Illinois*, 720 F. Supp. 720 [S.D. Ill. 1989] and *AFAPS v. Rgs. and Permits Administration*, 740 F. Supp. 95 [D.P.R. 1990], in

Michele A. Zavos

which denials of applications to open AIDS hospices were found to violate the FHA.)

The Americans with Disabilities Act of 1990 also adopts the Section 504 definition of *handicap* and covers those protected by Section 504, as well as those believed to have HIV or AIDS or associated with such individuals. It extends legal protections from discrimination in the private workplace and places of accommodation, public transportation, and the activities of state and local governments. Coverage under the ADA is being phased in over three and a half years, with full coverage due in July 1994. At that time all firms employing more than fifteen employees and engaging in an industry "affecting commerce" will be subject to the employment provisions of the ADA; all businesses that "affect commerce" are subject to the public-accommodations provision of the ADA. The broad public-accommodation section encompasses such organizations as day-care centers, hospitals, schools, libraries, and service establishments.

Discrimination statutes patterned after Section 504 exist in most states, the District of Columbia, and many localities, but the definition of *disability* varies widely. Most of the states have formally or informally determined that discrimination against individuals with HIV and AIDS or those perceived to be HIV-infected is covered by these laws. Moreover such statutes prohibit discrimination in the public and private sectors in most jurisdictions (AIDS Reference Guide 1990, 15). Because of this patchwork of laws, however, there remain significant gaps in coverage.

Government Benefits

Historically, women in particular have been hurt by the narrow AIDS case definition announced by the Centers for Disease Control and Prevention in 1982; the definition was revised in 1987 and again in 1993 (CDC 1982, 1987, 1992). Because such entities as the Social Security Administration had relied in part on the CDC definition to determine Social Security Disability Insurance (SSDI) and Supplemental Security Income (SSI) disability benefits, the 1987 definition essentially prevented many HIV-infected women from obtaining government benefits. It is hoped that the new definition, which includes several diseases many women experience, will expand timely access to these needed entitlements.

SSDI provides benefits to disabled workers (and their dependents) who have paid the necessary amount of Social Security taxes, and SSI provides public assistance for disabled individuals with minimal income and resources. A claimant for either of these disability benefits who has CDC-defined AIDS almost automatically receives such benefits, whereas a claimant with HIV disease that is not full-blown AIDS must provide rigorous proof of disability. Such a process often substantially delays an award of benefits and in many cases may even exclude women with HIV disease from receiving benefits.

The Social Security Administration awards "presumptive disability" benefits to SSI claimants meeting the CDC AIDS case definition, but other claimants with HIV disease must await a final award before receiving benefits. An applicant for SSI may be awarded presumptive disability benefits prior to a complete eligibility investigation on the basis of a physician's diagnosis that matches a disease on a list maintained by the Social Security Administration. Presumptive disability payments are made for six months and are not refundable if eligibility is denied. No infections of the female reproductive tract other than invasive cervical cancer are on the presumptive disability list. Hence, a woman with chronic, intractable vaginal candidiasis or human papilloma virus-related cervical dysplasia—though she may be incapacitated—might not be awarded benefits in a timely manner because her symptoms are not on the list.

Regulatory Changes Affecting Benefit Criteria

The CDC proposed the expanded AIDS definition in late 1991, in large part because of the concerns of AIDS-advocacy group regarding flaws in the national AIDS surveillance case definition. As of January 1, 1993, the AIDS definition includes all adolescents and adults with HIV infection who have laboratory evidence of severe immunosuppression (defined as a CD4+ lymphocyte count of less than 200 cells/mm^3 or a %CD4+ of less than fourteen), regardless of history of other current or previous symptoms. It also adds pulmonary tuberculosis, recurrent pneumonia (within the past twelve months), and invasive cervical cancer to the 1987 list of twenty-three diseases.

Potential problems stemming from the case-definition change extend beyond mere epidemiological concerns. It is possible, for example, that insurance companies will begin using CD4+ T-cell counts (not currently proscribed by HIV antibody testing informed-consent laws) as a proxy for HIV infection. There is concern, too, about the potential privacy consequences of labeling someone with AIDS, as all fifty states require AIDS cases to be reported, though about half already require reporting of HIV infection itself. Finally, there are significant psychological consequences in having to adapt to a diagnosis of AIDS when one is still asymptomatic.

On December 18, 1991, the Social Security Administration (SSA) published proposed rulings that purportedly severed the link between the CDC definition of AIDS and the determination of whether individuals with HIV disease are disabled per se (56 Fed. Reg. No. 243 65702–65716). Although the rulings have not been finalized, they were implemented on an interim basis the same day they were published. The SSA has touted the new regulations as expanding the criteria for disability and as including, for the first time, manifestations of HIV disease in women. Claimants with HIV disease and one of five specific medical conditions[2] or CDC-defined AIDS automatically qualify for presumptive benefits, but individuals claiming disability because of other HIV-related medical conditions must meet two of four "functional capacity" criteria: marked restriction of activities of daily living; marked difficulties in maintaining social functioning; marked difficulties in completing tasks in a timely manner because of deficiencies in concentration or pace; or episodes of decompensation that occur about three times a year, last two or more weeks each, and cause the individual to deteriorate (and may include loss of adaptive functioning).

AIDS activists anticipate that the SSA will issue final regulations in this area by summer 1993. It is hoped that pressure on the SSA and Congress will result in regulations that are more sensitive to the needs of women with HIV. People without primary-care physicians—essentially, the majority of women with HIV disease—will be hard-pressed to prove that they satisfy the functional capacity test. They may therefore continue to be prevented from qualifying for presumptive disability benefits and thereby forced to go through difficult and time-consuming assessments of disability.

A number of other concrete objections were raised to the rulings in hearings conducted by Congress in April 1992. Witnesses testified that any one of the four functional tests would render an individual unable to work. Furthermore, they said, asking individuals to meet two standards for disability (the new SSA standards and the new CDC case definition) is inherently discriminatory, and the stricter level of documentation required does not allow for a presumptive diagnosis. Witnesses also testified that the SSA listing does not include several gynecological impairments, including recurrent herpes, internal organ or body cavity abscesses, chronic genital ulcers, and neurosyphilis. Legal advocates have pointed out that the only HIV-related gynecological conditions in the proposed listing are advanced cervical cancer and recurrent vaginal candidiasis in conjunction with another of the listed conditions *and* a functional impairment. Chronic pelvic inflammatory disease—which the secretary of health recognized as a potentially disabling HIV-related impairment in the introduction to the proposed listing—and other conditions may also have disabling gynecological implications (see MFY Legal Services 1992). Again, the requirement to document HIV-related disability and the stringent functional limitation test will most hurt those with the least access to a primary-care

---

[2] Section 14.08(A)-(L) establishes those medical conditions that will per se qualify an individual with HIV disease who does not have CDC-defined AIDS for a disability determination based upon medical evidence and findings alone. These rules were being revised as this book went to press; for further information the reader is referred to announcements in the *Federal Register*.

physician. The National Association of People with AIDS (1992) has summed up the situation this way:

> As the HIV patient population continues its inexorable shift from privately doctored middle class gay, white males to a poor minority inner-city population (medically served, if at all, by understaffed public clinics, emergency rooms and Medicaid mills), the crushing paperwork burden will collapse of its own weight: doctors and social workers treating the poor simply do not have the time, leisure or resources to prepare customized patient care narratives or assemble the necessary masses of medical records and third party/functional reports. Something must be done now to assist patients, physicians, advocates and [departments of disability services] to meet the towering tidal wave of disability determination paperwork which will shortly drown us all.

The Social Security Administration's former policies have also been challenged in federal court in New York City in *S. P. et al. v. Sullivan* (No. 90 Civ. 6294 [MGC]). Plaintiffs alleged that the secretary of the Department of Health and Human Services arbitrarily and capriciously relied solely on the CDC definition of AIDS to determine disability, thereby abdicating its responsibility to determine whether individuals with HIV disease are disabled. It was further alleged that this reliance bars most women, injection-drug users, and poor people from receiving disability benefits, as these groups were excluded from the surveillance base of the CDC when it created its original AIDS case definition. The plaintiffs sought presumptive disability benefits for claimants who prove they are HIV-infected and unable to work. Plaintiffs also asked that the secretary reevaluate current standards for evaluation of HIV-related disease and instruct claims adjudicators to develop and evaluate such claims rather than dismiss them outright. Such relief would be of specific benefit to women with HIV disease, who often experience disabling medical conditions that are not defined as severe or life-threatening in women who are not infected with HIV. Coupled with HIV infection, however, these conditions often severely limit capacity for work and other major life activities. This recognition on the part of the Social Security Administration would provide substantial numbers of HIV-infected women with SSDI and SSI benefits and access to Medicaid, which is critical for obtaining basic health care. It is unclear what effect the new SSA rulings will have on these plaintiffs' claims.

Legislative Bills Affecting Funding

Three bills have been sent to Congress to address the inequities that prevent HIV-infected women from obtaining the full benefit of federal research on the disease, appropriate prevention and education efforts, and social security benefits.

The Women and AIDS Research Initiative (H.R. Amendments of 1993) would authorize additional federal funds specifically for the National Institutes of Health and the Alcohol, Drug Abuse, and Mental Health Administration to research how HIV is transmitted to women, how HIV disease progresses in women, how HIV-infected women should be treated, and how female-controlled physical and chemical-barrier methods of HIV prevention can be developed. The bill would also expand clinical trials of AIDS treatments to include women and would provide funds for child care and transportation to encourage the participation of low-income women.

Another bill, the Women and HIV Outreach and Prevention Act, authorizes federal funds for HIV prevention and education efforts to health care providers who already serve low-income women. These efforts would be aimed at improving outreach to women and access to woman-focused services.

The Social Security and SSI AIDS Disability Act of 1991 would require the Social Security Administration to change its disability eligibility criteria to include the symptomatology of women and injection-drug users instead of relying exclusively on the CDC definition. Women would no longer be denied presumptive disability benefits because they do not exhibit CDC-defined AIDS symptoms.

Prostitution

Although women have often been viewed as introducing HIV disease into the middle-class heterosexual population, men are in fact much more likely to transmit HIV (CDC 1989). Women in American society are often considered important only in relation to their functions as mothers or wives. On this basis it is not surprising that women with HIV disease may face criminal charges or enhanced criminal penalties based solely on the possibility of transmission of the virus.

A good example of this scenario is in the sex-worker industry. A number of states make prostitution a felony when practiced by someone who is aware of being HIV-infected. Although these statutes apply to both men and women, prosecutions for prostitution occur far more often against women. Under the statutes there is no requirement that transmission of the virus actually occur. For example, in the first test of Section 647.B/647.F of the California Penal Code, which was passed in 1989, Cindy Lee Silva pleaded guilty to felony solicitation and received a one-year county jail sentence—twice the usual maximum sentence under the state's misdemeanor prostitution statute (AIDS Policy and Law 1991). A felony prostitution conviction in California carries a maximum three-year state prison sentence. There was no investigation into whether Silva actually transmitted HIV to anyone.

In *State of Florida v. Sherouse,* 536 So.2d 1194 (App. Ct. Fla. 1989), it was alleged that Elizabeth Kay Sherouse was aware that she was HIV-infected and twice agreed to engage in heterosexual intercourse for pay without informing her prospective clients of her HIV status. She was charged with two counts of attempted manslaughter. The state of Florida vigorously argued that Sherouse's intent to commit the illegal act of prostitution was sufficient to support the attempted manslaughter charge, which requires specific intent to kill. The Florida Court of Appeal upheld the trial court's dismissal of the charges for failure to show intent to kill but pointed out that a charge of attempted second-degree murder might have been proved, as it does not require specific intent.

Similarly, the state's attorney of Illinois charged an allegedly HIV-infected woman for criminal transmission of the virus (under Ill. Rev. Stat. 1989, ch. 38, pars. 111–2, 111–3) based on her alleged agreement to engage in oral sex with an undercover police officer (ACLU 1991). Although the charges were dropped when the woman voluntarily entered medical and counseling treatment, the case is another example of the irrationality of such charges, as there have been no definitive confirmed cases of HIV transmission through fellatio performed by an HIV-infected individual.

In *Brooks v. State of Florida,* 519 So.2d 1156 (App. Ct. Fla. 1988), a trial court departed from Florida's sentencing guidelines to give a lengthier sentence for a grand theft conviction to Julia Brown Brooks, who had AIDS. The trial court reasoned that Brooks' long record of prostitution and related charges provided an appropriate basis for such a departure. The same Florida Court of Appeal that decided *Sherouse* vacated the sentence, holding that Brooks' disease was irrelevant to sentencing for the grand theft conviction.

Twenty-eight states have enacted laws that mandate HIV testing of individuals indicted or convicted of prostitution or sex offenses (AIDS Policy Center 1992). Rarely do these statutes provide for any pre- or post-test counseling or medical care of those tested. And they often provide the basis for further prosecution or enhanced sentencing when a seropositive individual is later arrested for prostitution.

Reproductive Rights

The state statutes described above take the view that women in the AIDS epidemic are vectors of HIV transmission rather than individuals who are experiencing HIV disease. This trend follows the development of "fetal rights" in the courts and legislatures, in which women are often treated as incubators of future human beings rather than as people who should control their own bodies (Gallagher 1987).

This attitude was shockingly displayed in *In re A.C.* Angela Carder, a twenty-seven-year-old suffering from apparently terminal cancer, was forced to undergo a caesarian section at twenty-six weeks over her own objections and those of her husband, family, and physicians (533 A.2d 611 [D.C. Ct. of App., 1987]). (See also *Jefferson v. Griffin Spaulding County Hosp. Auth.,* 247 Ga. 86, 274 S.E.2d 457 [1981]; *Taft v. Taft,* 388 Mass. 331, 446 N.E.2d 395 [1983].) A panel of the Court of

Appeals held that Carder's right against bodily intrusion had to be weighed against the rights of her fetus; it found Carder's right subordinate. In a rehearing *en banc* (granted 539 A.2d 203, D.C. Ct. of App. 1988) the court rejected the panel's balancing analysis, holding that the state's interest must be truly compelling to override a patient's medical decisions (573 A.2d 1235 [D.C. Ct. of App. 1990]).

In a different twist on the same theme, women using drugs during pregnancy have been charged with delivering drugs to minors. On April 18, 1991, a Florida appeals court upheld the conviction of Jennifer Johnson, who was charged with passing cocaine to her newborn baby through the umbilical cord (*State v. Johnson*, 578 50 2d 419 [App. Ct. Fla. 1991]). The Florida Supreme Court, however, reversed Johnson's conviction by a unanimous decision, ruling that the Florida legislature did not intend "to use the world 'delivery' in the context of criminally prosecuting mothers for delivery of a controlled substance to a minor by way of the umbilical cord" (602 50 2d 1288 [S. Ct. Fla. 1992]).

Criminal charges for drug use during pregnancy have been filed against women in New York and California. In the latter case, Pamela Rae Stewart failed to follow her physician's advice to stop using drugs while pregnant. When her baby was born brain damaged and later died, she was charged under an old criminal statute with failing to deliver support to a child (Los Angeles Times 1986). Illegal maternal drug use during pregnancy has been criminalized in at least seven states: Florida, Illinois, Indiana, Minnesota, Nevada, Oklahoma, and Utah (Bader 1990).

Given these trends, it is not unthinkable that HIV-infected mothers who are aware of their serostatus might be prosecuted for bearing children. Such action on the part of government would be only another extension of the punitive approach often taken by the state to control women's behavior. In other cases, women with HIV might be charged under child neglect statutes with transmitting HIV to their children and could face loss of the children as a result. Such prosecutions, like those for drug use during pregnancy, would be focused on poor women and women of color.

In fact, a case similar to such a hypothetical occurred in North Carolina in 1992. There an African-American woman in her early twenties was convicted for "failure to follow public health warnings" to inform her sexual partners of her (alleged) HIV infection and to use a condom during sex. Public health authorities used as evidence against her the fact that she had gotten pregnant. A wealthier woman who was HIV-positive would never have sought governmental assistance and would therefore never have been subjected to prosecution (see Cooper 1992).

Mandatory HIV testing of newborns makes these types of charges more likely. Screening could occur on a uniformly mandatory basis, as is done with select, treatable conditions (such as hypothyroidism), or it may occur when drug use by the mother is suspected. Because the results of antibody tests concerning the actual HIV status of a newborn are inconclusive, child neglect or criminal charges may be brought erroneously.

Many women with HIV have been disenfranchised from the medical care system by their poverty and race. Prenatal care is not always accessible, drug-treatment programs for pregnant women are often nonexistent, and drug-treatment programs for other women are often overcrowded or unavailable. Once a woman with HIV disease becomes pregnant she may be faced with restricted reproductive services because of her HIV disease or coerced into choosing an abortion.

In New York City, where AIDS is the leading killer of black women of reproductive age, the City Commission on Human Rights (1990) found that 42 percent of health care providers surveyed in 1988 refused to make appointments for abortions when potential clients identified themselves as HIV-positive, or else they over-charged for procedures. Most often they stated that their offices were not equipped to provide abortion services to HIV-infected women or that staff members were unfamiliar with uniform infection-control procedures. These spurious rationalizations raise serious concerns that health care providers are not complying with uniform infection-control guidelines. As it is not possible to know the HIV serostatus or other infection status of all patients, these facilities may be endangering both clients and staff members. This survey was repeated in 1990 and 1992. In 1990 sixteen of fifty-one providers (31 percent) either refused an abortion or raised fees when told that the caller was HIV-positive. The New York City Commission on Human Rights issued either a letter or a subpoena to eighteen abortion providers believed to have discriminated on the basis of HIV status. The entire sample was resurveyed in 1992, and this time only two (4 percent) of the abortion providers discriminated; one who had received a subpoena and one new provider. Statistical comparisons indicated that there was a substantial difference in discrimination between 1988 and 1992 and between 1990 and 1992, significantly associated with the intervention (letter/subpoena; p=.0001). The authors of this summary study conclude that HIV-related abortion service discrimination does occur and can be potentially mitigated by active intervention (de Jung, Holman, Carrino, Caplan-Cotenoff, and de Leon 1993).

In *Doe v. Jamaica Hospital* (31248/89, Kings County, New York), in what may be the first case of its kind, an HIV-positive woman challenged a hospital's alleged practice of refusing appropriate prenatal treatment to women with HIV disease and coercing them into abortions. The plaintiff learned that she was HIV-positive only after agreeing to a "voluntary" HIV test at the hospital and had an abortion after being subjected to extreme pressure by hospital staff. Her claims were brought under Section 504, the New York State Human Rights Law, the New York Civil Rights Law, and certain tort principles.

Michele A. Zavos

Personal Legal Planning

Although every woman must consider the possibility that she will not be able to decide about her medical care, take care of her children, or maintain her everyday life if she should become severely ill or injured, these concerns are more immediate and possibly more difficult to confront for women with HIV. For women who are married, husbands usually are authorized by law to take over these decisions. But for lesbians, unmarried women, or women whose husbands are unavailable, it is a challenge to develop legally recognized arrangements that will ensure that their wishes are implemented. Legal documents or court procedures that allow for substituted judgment play a crucial role in helping to see that a woman's wishes will be followed.

Health Care Decisions

Among the most important legal documents for women with HIV is the power of attorney for health care, also known as a health care directive. By executing this document, a woman can delegate a range of health care decisions to a designated person, called an agent. These powers of attorney go into effect if the HIV-infected woman becomes unable to make her own health care decisions because of mental or physical incapacity. The agent is then empowered to make decisions consistent with the infected woman's known wishes.

The powers granted by these documents can encompass decisions concerning life-sustaining treatment, invasive procedures, choice of medical providers, priorities for visitation, and access to medical records. About one-third of the states and the District of Columbia have formally recognized powers of attorney for health care through the specific statutes. In other jurisdictions case law or executive branch opinions have validated this approach (Albert et al. 1991). Even if such documents have not been authorized by law, many health care providers will honor them if they are unambiguous.

A power of attorney may also be used by a woman with HIV disease to delegate control over her financial affairs to her agent if she becomes mentally or physically incapacitated. This control may range from authority to cash checks to the power to transfer real estate. For many women with HIV disease, a financial power of attorney may be an important tool for maintaining access to government benefits.

Living wills allow an individual the right to refuse medical treatment in certain proscribed circumstances, generally when a medical condition is deemed irreversible or terminal. Currently forty-two states and the District of Columbia have living will or "death with dignity" laws (Albert et al. 1991). These statutes usually provide that competent individuals may execute a document that provides for the continuation of care necessary to keep the patient comfortable but allows life-sustaining procedures to be ended when doctors determine the patient to be terminally ill and unable to make such medical decisions. Most states require that two physicians attest in writing that a patient's condition is irreversible or terminal before the living will becomes effective. Individuals who wish to execute a living will must comply with their state law to ensure that the patient's wishes, as expressed in the living will, are honored. In at least twenty-seven of the states and the District of Columbia where living wills are authorized, however, pregnant women are excluded from such protections (Benton 1990; see also Dyke 1990).

Both health care powers of attorney and living wills are particularly important in view of the recent Supreme Court decision in *Cruzan v. Director, Missouri Department of Health*, 1109 S. Ct. 2841 (1990), which held that a competent person has a constitutionally protected liberty interest in refusing unwanted medical treatment but required that her wishes be established by "clear and convincing" evidence. Partly as a result of the national debate spurred by the Cruzan case, regulations were passed in late 1991 mandating that all hospitals receiving federal funds must ask all patients on admission if they have a living will or advanced directives or if they wish information about these documents.

Where a power of attorney and a living will have not been executed or are not recognized and decisions must be made about an HIV-infected woman's medical care or financial affairs, the court will make substituted judgments through conservatorship or guardianship proceedings. The court will appoint the conservator or guardian, who may not reflect the ward's values or agree with her life choices, resulting in unwanted decisions about medical care or finances. (See, e.g., the protracted litigation in *In re Guardianship of Sharon Kowalski*, 478 N.W.2d 790 [Minn. 1991].) These procedures can be avoided only if providers are able to address these issues with HIV-affected women ahead of time.

All of the legal documents and court proceedings discussed above govern a woman's affairs while she is still living. A will determines her affairs after death. Even though most women with HIV disease do not have extensive estates, execution of a will gives them more control over their lives by determining the distribution of their property upon death. In addition, certain provisions in a will may affect guardianship of children. For most women with HIV, execution of the documents discussed here can help them negotiate their way through some of the difficult problems caused by HIV disease. But there are often significant difficulties in getting these documents drafted and signed. First and foremost is access to legal advice. As this is a complex area of the law, it is essential that women with HIV disease consult with someone trained in these issues.

Because of the nature of HIV disease, which can subject an individual to recurring bouts of very serious illness along with with periods of relative health, it is all the more important that these decisions be made. They include considering whether to designate someone to authorize her medical treatment decisions should

Table 10.1 Laws and Documents That May Apply to Women with HIV

	Americans with Disabilities Act	Rehabilitation Act (Sec. 504)	Fair Housing Act	State and Local Discrimination Statutes	SSI	SSDI	Medicaid	AFDC	Healthcare Power of Attorney (Health Care Directive)	Court-Ordered Conservatorships or Adult Guardianships	Living Will	Financial Power of Attorney	Will	Guardianship	Adoption	Foster Care	Court Orders
Discrimination																	
Employment	•	•		•													
Access to health care	•	•		•													
Services (public accommodation)	•	•		•													
Housing	•	•	•	•													
Education	•	•		•													
Insurance	•			•													
Government Benefits																	
Financial aid					•	•		•									
Health care					•	•	•	•									

Personal Legal Planning

- Medical treatment
- Termination of life-sustaining procedures
- Financial affairs
- Property
- Guardianship of children

Care of Children

- Custody
- Support
- Medical treatment

† Upon death

Souce: Author.

Michele A. Zavos

she become unable to do so; to give another person the power to control her financial affairs; to sign a document that would permit the termination of life-sustaining medical treatment; to execute a will so that she can determine the distribution of her property and affect the appointment of a guardian for her children; or to leave all of the above decisions to a court (see table 10.1).

Family Law

The great majority of women with HIV disease are functionally single parents and must provide for their children in some manner regardless of their physical condition. These issues encompass the care and custody of children both while the mother is living and after her death.

Because of the episodic nature of HIV disease, infected women need to be able to designate caretakers for their children without giving up full custody. Most states do not have a simple mechanism for a mother to appoint a temporary guardian for her children. Although informal arrangements can be made during periods of serious illness, such arrangements are highly subject to challenge. A mother may therefore feel it necessary to arrange for a long-term transfer of custody and authority before such actions are truly necessary. Complicating such decisions is the reality that once a child has been placed in foster care or with a permanent guardian through a court appointment, a mother faces difficult and expensive court proceedings to regain custody.

Guardianship

Often parents designate guardians for their children through provisions in their wills. But because most women with HIV disease are poor and without legal counsel they usually do not execute wills. In many situations a woman may nominate a guardian by executing the appropriate guardianship papers. But even if a guardian is nominated the court must make the final appointment decision. A court generally gives the wishes of the nominating person (or testator) great weight, but unless the guardian is appointed prior to the mother's death—something courts are reluctant to do—the mother cannot be certain that her wishes will be implemented. If the father is available, however, he would get custody should he seek it, generally even over the mother's designation of a guardian in a will, absent unusual circumstances.

Practitioners in this area suggest that a new form of guardianship is needed, one that will spring into existence when a mother is unable to care for her children and lapse when she has recovered sufficiently to provide for them (Zarembka and Franke 1991). New York has adopted just such a statute (New York Surrogate Court

Procedure Act Sec. 1726, approved December 12, 1992). Pursuant to this statute, a woman (or any individual) may through a judicial proceeding appoint a "standby guardian" over the person or property of her child by executing a written designation before two witnesses. The guardianship becomes effective upon the written determination of incapacity or debilitation by the mother's physician or upon death. The mother may revoke the appointment by writing to both the court and the standby guardian.

Adoption

More permanent than guardianship is the possibility of adoption of children while their mother is still alive. This is an extremely difficult and emotional decision for a mother because it generally requires her to terminate her rights to the children. Adoption, however, can ensure the mother's control over who has legal responsibility for her children and may therefore give her some comfort about their welfare. When a family member or close friend becomes the adoptive parent, arrangements can be made to continue the mother's relationship with her children, often with no change in their day-to-day lives.

Custody

At times, custody and visitation issues manifest themselves in disputes between an HIV-infected mother and an uninfected father, though the reverse is more likely to occur, as when a gay father has HIV disease. Although a court will employ the "best interests of the child" criterion to make a custody determination, the crucial questions in such disputes center on whether a parent's HIV disease will be transmitted to the children, affect the parent's ability to care for the children, or unduly stigmatize the children. These questions are often raised even though HIV disease is not casually transmitted and should be treated as any other health condition in this context.

Some of the earliest reported cases in this area recognized the fact that HIV is not transmitted by casual contact. *In Jane W. v. John W.*, 137 Misc. 2d 24, 519 N.Y.S. 603 (1987), a trial court allowed a father visitation pendente lite ("during litigation") in spite of his AIDS diagnosis, concluding that AIDS is not casually transmitted. In another case the following year, the maternal grandparents of children in their father's custody petitioned to have him tested for HIV (Doe v. Roe, 139 Misc. 2d 209, 526 N.Y.S.2d 718 [1988]). The court denied the request on the basis that even if the father were HIV-infected he posed no danger to his children.

In *Stewart v. Stewart*, 521 N.E.2d 956 (Ind. 1988), a court of appeals reversed the termination of a noncustodial father's visitation rights because he had AIDS.

Michele A. Zavos

Most recently, in *Steven L. v. Dawn J.*, 148 Misc. 2d 779, 561 N.Y.S.2d 322 (1990), a father petitioned for change of custody on the basis of the mother's HIV-positive status. The court held that the mother's seropositive status did not constitute a "material change in circumstances" warranting a change in custody when the evidence clearly established that she was physically able to care for the child.

Although courts increasingly are rendering decisions in this area that are based on the facts of HIV disease rather than on fears and stigma, there is no guarantee of such an outcome (See, for example, *White v. Brown,* No. DR 92-150.01, Cir. Ct. of Chilton County, Ala., December 7, 1992). Many parents, when faced with the threat of a custody battle that will involve a consideration of their serostatus, may decide that they cannot manage the emotional and financial drain of litigation. These parents may feel forced to capitulate to the demands of the other parent.

Divorce

A woman's HIV status may also be raised in the area of family law through property distribution, alimony proceedings, and fault allegations, though these instances are extremely rare. Most jurisdictions in this country use no-fault grounds as the basis for divorce, but where fault is relevant, a party may raise allegations of adultery and offer the opposing party's positive HIV status in support. HIV status may also be offered as evidence of a party's present and future health to limit or increase alimony based on financial need or to affect property distribution. (See *R.E.G. v. L.M.G.*, 571 N.E.2d 298 [Ct. of App. Ind.], which overturned a decision by a trial court to base its distribution of property on a finding that a husband's homosexual relationships put his wife at risk for AIDS.)

Summary

The legal problems faced by women with AIDS and HIV are universal and unique. They include lack of access to health care, denial of Social Security benefits, lack of education about AIDS and HIV, unwieldy legal mechanisms that are unable to respond to the particular child-care and personal needs of women with HIV, and the continued discrimination and fear engendered by this disease (see table 10.1).

In the short term, women with HIV disease would be helped enormously by passage of the legislation discussed in the previous section that is pending in Congress; revision of the Social Security regulations to include HIV-related illnesses that are particular to women and injection-drug users; enactment of legislation allowing more flexibility for temporary custody and long-term arrangements; repeal of enhanced penalty statutes for crimes committed by women with HIV disease; and availability of attorneys to represent women with HIV disease. To provide truly appropriate care for women with HIV disease and to protect their jobs, families, and futures, the women must be recognized as individuals, not just as mothers, prostitutes, or baby carriers. Legal, political, and policy-setting entities must work with frontline caregivers to ensure that the needs of women with HIV are not overlooked or their rights usurped.

11

Epidemiology and Natural History

Kathryn Anastos and Sten H. Vermund

I know the exact date I was diagnosed as HIV-infected: it was two weeks after Magic [Johnson] made his announcement. I remember watching him and crying for him like he was my brother. My spiritual background is high, so I was watching this and saying, "Lord, what can I do to help these people?"—not knowing it would be me just a few weeks later.

I had applied for life insurance, and that's how I got tested. When my doctor called me with the result, I was devastated. It seemed like I was going to die that night. I called some HIV hot lines, but they didn't really tell me what I needed to hear: that people can live for years before they develop AIDS. No one told me that.

To be honest, I never thought I was at risk. Neither me or my daughter's father were IV-drug users. Whenever I'd

heard about AIDS on TV or whatever, it just went over my
head because I just heard "drugs and homosexuals." No one
ever talks about transmission when you just had one partner.

I really wish they would stress that anyone can get this.
. . . Anybody is at risk who's sexually active. Lots of people
say they don't want to know, but if they're infected, they're
going to find out someday anyway, when it's almost too late.
People need to get the message that they can get
treatment—not a cure, but help to prolong their life.
—Gwen Green

In mid-1981 the first published reports of a newly recognized acquired immune
deficiency syndrome described a disease occurring only in men (CDC 1981; Gottlieb et al. 1981; Masur et al. 1981). In early 1982 women in New York City hospitals
were diagnosed with the same syndrome (Masur et al. 1982), and by 1986 the
officially defined acquired immunodeficiency syndrome was the leading cause of
death for New York City women aged twenty-five to forty-four (New York City
Department of Health 1989). By 1987 mortality statistics revealed that New Jersey
women in the same age group were also more likely to die of AIDS than of any other
cause, and by 1991 AIDS was projected as the fifth most common cause of mortality
for all American women between fifteen and forty-four. And it is now the most
common cause of death for African-American women in the fifteen to forty-four age
group (Chu, Buehler, and Berkelman 1990).

Statistical models suggest that between 90,000 and 125,000 women in the
United States are infected with HIV and that there has been virtually no leveling
of incident AIDS cases in this population, unlike the trends noted among gay
men (Gail, Rosenberg and Goedert 1990; Brookmeyer 1991; Rosenberg et al.
1991).

In sub-Saharan Africa more than half of those with AIDS and HIV infection are
women. Mortality from AIDS in African women may already equal or exceed the
expected number of deaths from all other causes combined (Chin 1990). Thus, HIV
has had a staggering impact on morbidity and mortality in young women in the
United States and worldwide. Nonetheless, large epidemiologic studies of the
natural history of HIV infection in developed countries have included women
primarily in pregnancy-related and perinatal transmission studies (Vermund et al.
1992). Early assumptions that the disease manifests similarly in women and
men may not be correct. In early 1993 there were still no data—published or
unpublished—derived from well-designed prospective cohort studies that compre-
hensively describes the gynecological manifestations and the nongynecological

Kathryn Anastos and Sten H. Vermund

symptoms and complications of HIV infection in women, including the most common opportunistic infections.

In this chapter we review selected features of the epidemiology of HIV infection in women, the increasing impact of heterosexual transmission, and the limited published information describing the clinical course of HIV infection in women. We also suggest an outline for needed research.

Epidemiology

The World Health Organization (WHO) has described broad but distinct epidemiologic patterns of HIV infection and AIDS, which can be distinguished by the predominant mode of HIV transmission and the time period in which HIV spread within a given population (Chin and Mann 1988). The prevalence of HIV infection among women in any population is strongly linked to these patterns of infection. Because transmission patterns can change rapidly, the usefulness of the following classification system may be more limited than when it was originally devised (Mann, Tarantola, and Netter 1992).

In Pattern 1 countries (which include Australia and those in North America and Western Europe) HIV spread extensively in the late 1970s to early 1980s. Men who have sex with men and injection-drug users are the people most commonly infected with HIV in these countries, and the proportion of infected women is smaller—less than 15 percent. Pattern 2 areas include most of sub-Saharan Africa and areas of Asia, the Caribbean, and Latin America. Latin America and much of the Caribbean previously manifested a Pattern 1 epidemic but are now classified as Pattern 1/2 because of rapidly increasing heterosexual transmission (Garris et al. 1992).

In Pattern 2 areas, where the extensive spread of HIV began in the mid to late 1970s, HIV overwhelmingly affects sexually active heterosexuals. Resources for protecting the blood supply are often unavailable in these countries, and the transfusion of infected blood products expands the epidemic. Because more than half of infected individuals are women, perinatal transmission to infants is a major and increasing problem.

General Epidemiology Worldwide

In 1990 the World Health Organization conservatively estimated that more than 3 million women worldwide were infected with HIV, and this estimate rose to 4.5 million infected women by 1992. Higher estimates of the numbers of HIV-infected people—including women—have been made by other AIDS researchers (Mann, Tarantola, and Netter 1992; see table 11.1). Eighty percent of currently infected women (about 4 million) reside in sub-Saharan Africa, the majority of them between fifteen and forty-nine years old. The highest prevalence is often among those

Table 11.1 Estimated Worldwide Prevalence of HIV and AIDS

Figures in thousands	Infected with HIV			AIDS Cases	
	All Adults 1992 (estimated)	Women 1992 (estimated)	All Adults 1995 (projected)	All adults 1992 (estimated)	1995 (projected)
North America	1,167.0	128.5	1,495.0	257.5	534.0
Western Europe	718.0	122.0	1,186.0	99.0	279.5
Australia/Oceania	28.0	3.5	40.0	4.5	11.5
Latin America	995.0	199.0	1,407.0	173.0	417.5
Sub-Saharan Africa	7,803.0	3,901.5	11,449.0	1,367.0	3,277.5
Caribbean	310.0	124.0	474.0	43.0	121.0
Eastern Europe	27.0	2.5	44.0	2.5	9.5
Southeastern Mediterranean	35.0	6.0	59.0	3.5	12.5
Northeast Asia	41.0	7.0	80.0	3.5	14.5
Southeast Asia	675.0	223.0	1,220.0	65.0	240.5
Total	11,799.0	4,717.0	17,454.0	2,018.5	4,918.0

Source: Mann, Tarantola, and Netter 1992.

between thirty and thirty-four, though incidence begins to rise shortly after the age of first coitus. In some Central African cities, more than 30 percent of women between nineteen and thirty-seven and up to 40 percent of women between thirty and thirty-four are HIV-infected (Rwandan HIV Seroprevalence Study Group 1989; Allen et al. 1991). In one study, the prevalence of HIV was more than 20 percent, even among monogamous "low-risk" women, reflecting HIV transmission from a sexual partner who is not monogamous (Allen et al. 1991). Hausermann and Danziger (1991) suggest that women's low social status and their economic dependence on men in virtually all areas of the world have rendered them more vulnerable to HIV infection. (This pattern is discussed in detail in chapter 12.) In these countries, in contrast with Pattern 1 countries, women from higher-income families may have a higher risk of acquiring HIV infection; this is thought to be related to their male partners' financial ability to buy sex from female sex workers. For most women in developing countries, their steady male sexual partner is the most likely source of HIV infection.

There is substantial underrreportage of AIDS from Pattern 2 countries (Mann, Tarantola, and Netter 1992). It has been estimated that through 1988 as few as 10 to 20 percent of all AIDS cases in Africa were reported. In contrast, studies by the U.S. Centers for Disease Control and Prevention have indicated that more than 90 percent of AIDS cases in the United States are reported. Although a cumulative total

Kathryn Anastos and Sten H. Vermund

of 75,100 cases of AIDS in Africa were reported for both men and women through 1990, WHO has estimated that in 1989 alone there were 225,000 *new* cases of AIDS among women. It is projected that 1,367,000 adults in sub-Saharan African will have developed AIDS by 1992—and that in 1992 alone 600,000 women will be diagnosed with AIDS. In the United States the total number of cases since the beginning of the epidemic through 1992, in both women and men, has been about 250,000. The Asian epidemic, which has begun fiercely in Thailand, India, and elsewhere, will prove to be devastating (Chin 1990).

The United States From 1981 through December 1992 a total of 27,485 cases of AIDS in women were reported to the CDC, constituting 11 percent of the cumulative adult and adolescent cases in the United States.[1] Nearly 23 percent of these cases were reported in 1992, the twelfth year of CDC reporting of AIDS statistics. Women represented 12.8 percent of all AIDS cases in adults and adolescents reported in 1991 and 13.5 percent of those reported in 1992, a steadily increasing proportion of the total. Among all cases of AIDS reported for adult and adolescent women from 1981 to 1991, 73.8 percent were among African-American and Hispanic women; the large majority were reported from urban areas of the northeastern United States and Puerto Rico, where there is more injection-drug use (Menendez et al. 1990; CDC 1993). Thus, in the United States, the major burden of the HIV epidemic is located where drug use is most prevalent. As outlined in chapter 13 these areas tend to be inner-city communities of color that already struggle with poverty, all forms of substance abuse, and poor access to both preventive and therapeutic health care services (Coates et al. 1990).

Thus the annual number of AIDS diagnoses continues to increase faster in U.S. women than in men. In addition, the proportion of women in each risk-exposure category is changing. The percentage acquiring HIV through their own injection-drug use has been declining somewhat over the past decade: in 1986, 52 percent of women with AIDS had a personal IDU history in contrast with 45 percent in 1992 (Guinan and Hardy 1987; CDC 1993). There has been a dramatic increase in cases attributed to heterosexual transmission in women—from 21 percent of all reported adult female cases from 1981 through 1986 to 40 percent of reported cases from October 1991 to September 1992.

Heterosexual Transmission in Pattern 1 Areas Although heterosexual transmission has been the predominant mode of HIV infection in Pattern 2 countries since the beginning of the epidemic, the "reality of heterosexual transmission of HIV in the

---

[1] The total includes adolescents but excludes 1,992 girls who were twelve or younger at time of diagnosis.

Table 11.2 Factors Associated with Heterosexual Transmission of HIV

	Male-to-Female	Female-to-Male
Non-use of condoms	Yes	Yes
Anal intercourse	Yes	No
Sex during menses	Possible	Yes
Number of sexual contacts	Yes	Yes
Advanced disease state (as measured by CD4$^+$, p24, antigen, or AIDS diagnosis)	Yes	Yes
Genital sores, infections, or inflammations	Yes	Yes
Use of IUD	Possible	Unknown
Use of oral contraceptives*	Possible	Unknown
AZT use leading to decreased risk	Probable	Probable

*Whether oral contraceptives inhibit or increase the likelihood of transmission is controversial.

Souce: Adapted from Padian 1991.

United States has been accepted slowly" (Allen and Setwell 1991). Common misconceptions about heterosexual transmission of HIV persist among medical professionals, as well as the lay public. For example, many women and men mistakenly believe that heterosexual transmission occurs almost exclusively from anal intercourse and that it is nearly impossible for a woman to infect a man (see table 11.2).

A number of studies indicated that male-to-female heterosexual transmission of HIV may be substantially more likely than female-to-male transmission, particularly in Pattern 1 countries. Padian and co-workers (1991) estimated a nineteenfold excess risk for male-to-female sexual transmission among HIV-discordant monogamous couples. Other studies suggest threefold to fivefold excess risk (Chiodo et al. 1990; De Vincenzi et al. 1990; Nicolosi et al. 1990; Rehmet et al. 1990). But studies done in STD clinics in New York City did not demonstrate significant differences in the risk of heterosexual transmission between women and men in a setting where trading sex for crack and high rates of STDs, including genital ulcer disease (GUD), were common among both women and men (Chaisson et al. 1991; Stoneburner, Chaisson and Weisfuse 1990). The authors suggest that other potential contributing factors need to be examined, including type and duration of sexual contact, number of partners, HIV status of partners, history of syphilis, and substance abuse. The studies of New York City STD clinics suggest that in some industrialized countries female-to-male heterosexual spread might be facilitated by STDs, mimicking the situation found in many developing countries. One study from Africa (Hayes and Schultz 1992) suggests that the presence of genital ulcers markedly enhances female-

Kathryn Anastos and Sten H. Vermund

to-male transmission (making the chances 100 to 2,000 times greater) but has a smaller effect on male-to-female transmission (twenty to fifty times greater).

There are multiple factors that may contribute to more efficient male-to-female HIV transmission. The concentration of HIV is substantially higher in semen than in vaginal secretions, and there is some evidence that antiviral therapy for the index case (that is, infected partner) may reduce heterosexual transmission (Anderson et al. 1992; Massimo et al. 1992). The vagina's reproductive design ensures retention of a reservoir of semen after unprotected intercourse, prolonging the time of exposure to potentially infectious material. Further, the vaginal wall is more friable and permeable than the penis; a mucous membrane is thought to allow greater viral penetration than does skin. The anatomy of the female genital tract also allows infected material to pass through the cervix to the endometrium, which may also present less of a barrier to HIV transmission. Some authorities have also speculated that vaginal intercourse is more traumatic to the vagina than to the penis; mucosal tears may occur, allowing viral transmission.

Female circumcision may well increase HIV risk in the parts of Africa where it is practiced. The most invasive procedure is the infundibulectomy, a removal of the clitoris, labia minora, and labia majora in a nonmedical, nonsterile major surgical procedure. Without her external anatomy the circumcised woman may bleed easily, experience coital trauma, and practice inadvertent or intentional anal intercourse if the vaginal introitus is sewn too tightly or too loosely (Dirie and Lindmark 1992). There do not appear to be any data on HIV risk in circumcised women.

Female-to-female sexual contact may be less likely to spread HIV than male-to-male, male-to-female, or female-to-male contact. Few lesbians have been reported with AIDS who did not also have such risk factors as injection-drug use or high-risk sexual contacts. So few studies have specifically addressed this population, however, that risk among lesbians, particularly among couples, should be studied.

Many other factors that are not specifically gender-related may affect the efficiency of HIV transmission (Vermund et al. 1991a). These include the presence of sexually transmitted diseases, especially ulcerative processes (Stamm, Handsfield and Rompalo 1988; Rodriguez et al. 1992); the number of sexual encounters with an infected partner (Padian et al. 1990); anal-receptive intercourse (European Study Group 1989; Voeller 1991; Lazzarin et al. 1991; Rosenblum et al. 1992); the clinical status of the infected partner (Goedert et al. 1987; Holmberg et al. 1989); and eroded cervix, that is, cervical ectopy (Moss 1991). Ectopy is more common in adolescents (Simonsen et al. 1988) and, possibly, in women who take oral contraceptives (Padian et al. 1990), and it may expose the friable cervical columnar epithelium to semen, thus conferring more HIV infection risk than exposure of HIV to more hardy squamous cervical epithelium.

Sexual customs worldwide generally result in men having significantly more sexual partners than women do. This factor, combined with more efficient male-to-female transmission, has a significant effect on the evolution of the heterosexual HIV epidemic. The result has been declining male-to-female ratios over time in industrialized countries and 1:1 sex ratios in many developing countries, particularly in Africa and Asia. In Uganda, for example, serosurveys of HIV infection from 1987 to 1989 demonstrated female-to-male ratios of 1.42, 1.31, and 1.56 (Berkely et al. 1990). AIDS diagnoses during the same time period—representing infections that occurred several years before—were about equal in women and men (52 percent in women and 48 percent in men) (Berkely, Okware, and Naamara 1989).

In Pattern 1 countries AIDS cases attributed to heterosexual transmission have consistently occurred more frequently in women than in men, presumably because there are many more infected men than women, thus increasing the likelihood that a heterosexual woman will be exposed to HIV by a male partner. But it is likely that the greater efficiency of male-to-female heterosexual transmission also contributes to female risk. The rate of new diagnoses of AIDS in the United States is increasing most rapidly for heterosexual women who are not injection-drug users (Berkelman et al. 1991). In a single year (1990 to 1991), the proportion of AIDS cases in women attributed to heterosexual transmission rose from 31 percent to 37 percent. Thus, for many women in the inner cities and selected rural areas of the United States, the epidemic of heterosexual HIV transmission now resembles in many ways that of a Pattern 2 area (Ellerbrock and Rogers 1990; Ellerbrock et al. 1991).

Although heterosexual transmission of HIV is proportionately less significant in the United States at present (35.8 percent of women and 2.9 percent of men with AIDS cumulatively), on a worldwide scale it is the most common source of HIV exposure for both women and men. Research that can delineate strategies to decrease heterosexual transmission is urgently needed. As observed earlier, antiretroviral therapies reduce semen viral loads and may reduce infectivity as well. Further research must address prevention strategies that can be controlled by women, who are not adequately protected by men's use or nonuse of condoms. These strategies may include female-controlled barrier contraceptives, virucides, microbicides, and, ultimately, vaccines for HIV and STDs (Koff and Hoth 1988; Stein 1990).

Natural History of HIV in Women

To date there is limited information available regarding the natural history of HIV infection in women. Most data describing the disease course in women prior to the use of pharmacologic therapy come from aggregate public health data—information reported to city or state departments of health, the CDC, ministries of health, and WHO. In addition, a few small cohorts of women in individual institutions have been described. Aggregate public health data provide large sample sizes, but their clinical, behavioral, and laboratory data contain biases in reporting and selection and other substantial limitations. Women and men with AIDS may differ in many respects, including socioeconomic status, mode of acquiring HIV, ethnicity, access to and utilization of health care, services received during acute illness, outpatient followup, and responsibility for the care of children and others. Future studies of HIV in women in industrialized countries will, of necessity, study a disease course altered by antiretroviral and prophylactic therapies.

The natural history of HIV in North American men has been studied with notable success in several large cohort studies (Stevens et al. 1986; Kaslow et al. 1987; Winkelstein et al. 1987; Moss et al. 1988; McCusker et al. 1989; Schecter et al. 1989) that continue to investigate the relative frequencies of specific AIDS-defining illnesses, the relationship of surrogate markers to disease progression, the causes of morbidity and mortality, the correlates of long-term survival, and the calculations of patterns of survival. Preliminary information indicates that the disease course may differ in women and men. Women may have different rates of specific opportunistic infections and malignancies, and they have had shorter median survival after a diagnosis of AIDS, especially early in the epidemic, related to later diagnosis, poorer access to health care, or biological cofactors (Rothenberg et al. 1987). In addition, there now exists evidence from small studies that specific gynecological diseases occur more frequently and are more aggressive in HIV-infected women than in uninfected women (Carpenter et al. 1991).

AIDS-Defining Illnesses

Nearly all data sources indicate that Pneumocystis carinii pneumonia (PCP) is the most common AIDS-defining diagnosis for women and men throughout the United States (Ciesielski, Fleming, and Berkelman 1991; Grant et al. 1991; New York City Department of Health 1991; New York State Department of Health 1991; Creagh 1992; Melnick et al. 1992; Szabo et al. 1992; Young et al. 1992; Muñoz et al. 1993). PCP is common in some Pattern 2 areas, such as Latin America, but it is nearly unknown in much of Africa (Lucas 1990; Abouya et al. 1992). Carpenter et al. (1991) and Benson et al. (1992) have described small populations in Rhode Island (forty-four patients) and Chicago (twenty-one patients) in which candida esophagitis was the most common AIDS-defining illness (34 percent and 62 percent, respectively) in women with AIDS seen in a primary-care setting. Similar observations were reported in Rhode Island prior to the widespread use of PCP prophylaxis (Carpenter et al. 1989). Thus prevention of PCP with chemoprophylaxis does not fully explain this distribution of opportunistic infections. No comparison group of men was studied.

Three other studies describe patients cared for in single institutions. Young and coworkers (1992) report that PCP was the most common AIDS-defining illness (48 percent) among 114 women with AIDS in Washington, D.C. Grant et al. (1991) describe AIDS-defining illnesses in 186 women and 512 men diagnosed with AIDS from 1988 through 1991 in the Bronx, New York. The most common AIDS-defining illness in both women and men was PCP (39 percent of women and 34 percent of men). Candida esophagitis occurred in 11 percent of women and 8 percent of men, a difference that was not statistically significant. Excluding Kaposi's sarcoma (which occurs rarely in women), the only significant gender difference found in the Bronx study was severe mucocutaneous herpes simplex disease, which occurred in 2.7 percent of women and 0.4 percent of men. Motyl et al. (1990) report that among 140 febrile patients with AIDS, Mycobacterium avium complex was cultured from the blood of 72 percent of the women and 44 percent of the men, generating the hypothesis that there may be gender differences in susceptibility to that organism.

The CDC has reported (Ciesielski, Fleming, and Berkelman 1991) that among all U.S. cases of AIDS through 1990, the only significant gender differences in AIDS-defining illnesses (excluding Kaposi's sarcoma) were candida esophagitis (occurring 50 percent more frequently in women) and opportunistic herpes virus infections (occurring 32 percent more frequently in women), results similar to those of the clinical study of Grant et al. in the Bronx (1991). Thus, with the exception of the Rhode Island and Chicago series, PCP is overwhelmingly the most common AIDS-defining illness among U.S. women, and it occurs with nearly equal frequency in women and men. Again with the exception of the Rhode Island and Chicago studies (Carpenter et al. 1991; Benson et al 1992), candida esophagitis remains a less common AIDS-defining illness (less than 15 percent of cases), though it may occur with a 30 to 50 percent increased frequency in women. Similarly, there may be a proclivity for women to get Mycobacterium avium complex and opportunistic infections with herpes viruses. Farizo et al. (1992) have documented the tremendous clinical burden of HIV in women even before an AIDS diagnosis is made.

Gender differences of this magnitude, even if they are not the result of bias in data collection, are unlikely to alter clinical practice substantially. Prophylactic regimens to prevent specific opportunistic infections, especially fungal infections (when chemoprophylaxis has been adequately studied and becomes available), will probably need to be offered to all patients without regard to gender. In the absence of definitive guidance from clinical trials, however, a few authors do advocate women-specific fungal prophylaxis with oral ketoconazole or fluconazole therapy for HIV-infected women with CD4+ cell counts of less than 100 cells/mm^3 to prevent esophageal fungal disease (Carpenter et al. 1991). It is likely that prevention of PCP with prophylactic therapy will substantially alter frequencies of opportunistic infections among both women and men and may unmask other clinically significant gender differences in a variety of such infections.

Kathryn Anastos and Sten H. Vermund

Survival with AIDS

"AIDS is a disaster; women die faster" is a slogan popularized by AIDS activists and others campaigning for the allocation of more U.S. federal resources for the study of HIV infection in women. Although there is substantial information suggesting shorter median survival in women, the magnitude of this difference has been decreasing over the course of the epidemic. Several recent studies have found equal survival in women and men. These findings imply that early results suggesting shorter survivals (Rothenberg et al. 1987; Lemp et al. 1990; Moore et al. 1991) were less indicative of a physiologic or biologic gender difference in response to HIV infection than of the disparate socioeconomic and health care access circumstances of early male AIDS cases (predominantly gay and white) compared with female cases (predominantly heterosexuals injecting drugs or sexual partners of drug injectors).

In studies suggesting a shorter median survival among women with AIDS, possible causes include true biologic differences, later diagnoses with consequent suboptimal preventive care, and poor access to care after diagnosis. Later diagnoses may be the result of a health care provider's failure to recognize AIDS in women, a phenomenon noted even in high prevalence areas (Verdegem et al. 1988). Later diagnoses would also occur if HIV-infected women did not seek health care as early as males with HIV. But studies of health care utilization in the ambulatory setting (Mechanic 1976; Gove and Hughes 1979; Cleary, Mechanic and Green 1982), including drug treatment programs (Reed 1987), suggest that women generally seek care earlier and more frequently than do men, though this may not be true for all groups of women. Apparent gender differences in survival may be secondary, then, to recognized or unrecognized sources of detection bias—for example, differences in access to health-care services, socioeconomic-status differences, or delayed recognition and treatment of HIV disease and AIDS-defining illnesses in women.

A major factor confounding the interpretation of gender-specific survival analyses for AIDS is the frequency of Kaposi's sarcoma (KS) as the AIDS-indicator disease, as this has such a marked male predilection. Mucocutaneous KS may occur with much less impairment of immune function than the other AIDS-defining illnesses and has a more indolent course (resulting in longer survival) than other AIDS-defining illnesses. For this reason, most studies that include gender analysis of survival with AIDS now exclude men who acquired the infection by having sex with men or exclude people diagnosed with KS, permitting more suitable biological comparisons of male and female survival data.

Rothenberg and colleagues (1987) compiled one of the first gender comparisons of 5,833 patients with AIDS (5,281 men, 522 women) reported to the New York City Department of Health through 1985; 81 percent of white gay men with KS survived one year, compared with 20 percent of black women injection-drug users with PCP. Median survival for all women was 73 percent that of all men, including those with KS (263 days versus 357 days), but 93 percent that of injection-drug users (263 versus 282 days). Women had a 60 percent higher rate of "zero survival"—that is, subjects who were diagnosed with AIDS at the time of death. These data imply that late diagnosis contributed significantly to a shorter survival in women, particularly in the early 1980s, and that KS is an important feature in differential survival with AIDS.

A similar pattern was documented by Lemp and colleagues (1990) in their description of 4,292 men and 31 women in San Francisco: median survival was 5.9 months in women and 12.5 months in men since AIDS diagnosis. Surprisingly, male injection-drug users had the longest post-AIDS median survival: 15.8 months. In an important followup study, Lemp et al. (1992) extend their survival analyses for 139 female and 7,045 male patients reported with AIDS through May 15, 1991. Men with AIDS lived longer than women with AIDS (14.6 versus 11.1 months). When people receiving antiretroviral treatment were compared, no differences in survival were noted (19.6 months in women and 21.8 months in men). When comparing people not receiving therapy, women's survival after an AIDS diagnosis was far shorter than men's (6.4 versus 14.6 months), probably reflecting both a comparatively later date of AIDS diagnosis and less access to or use of chemotherapy and prophylaxis. The San Francisco Women and AIDS Project found a post-AIDS median survival of 7.4 months in 77 women, excluding transfusion recipients, through May 1990 (Cohen 1990).

Many other sources of public health statistics have demonstrated shorter survival in women with AIDS. The Australian National Health and Medical Research Council (Whyte, Swanson, and Cooper 1989) reported a median survival of 3.8 months among 21 women and 11.4 months among 533 men with AIDS through July 1987. Among 95 women diagnosed with AIDS in Scandinavia through September 1990, median survival was 306 days, significantly less than the median survival of 504 days among men with AIDS (Smith, Hasseltvedt, and Bottinger 1991). The Michigan State Department of Health (Kent 1990) found a median post-AIDS survival of 11.1 months in 195 women and 15.6 months in 1,755 men from cases reported through October 1990. Gender-specific data specifically designed to compare men's and women's survival in Pattern 2 areas are not available, to our knowledge.

Friedland et al. (1991) have reported a well-controlled study of 86 women and 220 men with PCP through 1987 (the pretreatment era) in a single institution in New York City. All patients were of similar socioeconomic status, received care in the same institution, and had PCP as their presenting diagnosis. Women survived an average of 10 months compared to 12 months in men. Paradoxically, male injection-drug users fared better than all other groups, as was noted in the San Francisco study of Lemp et al. (1990). Survival curves did not diverge until four months after initial diagnosis, suggesting that late diagnosis in women does not explain the observed differences in this population.

Thus, through mid-1991, all reports suggest a moderate to marked gender difference in survival with AIDS, with women doing more poorly than men. But in 1991 and 1992 there were several reports suggesting little or no female survival disadvantage. Sherer et al. (1992) found no gender differences in survival among 843 women and 3,359 men enrolled in the Observational Data Base of the Community Programs for Clinical Research on AIDS. Szabo et al. (1992) also found equal survival in 149 HIV-infected women and 111 HIV-infected men in New York City. Review of Medicaid data from New York state (Turner et al. 1991) through 1989 demonstrated a female-to-male risk ratio of 1.1:1 in median survival. Chene et al. (1991) found that male gender conferred a two-and-a-half-fold increased risk of death in 209 patients (49 women, 160 men) with symptomatic HIV disease in Bordeaux, France. The CDC (Horsburgh et al. 1991) also reported that among 819 patients (82 women, 737 men) with HIV in Georgia through 1990, there was equal survival in women and men. Creagh et al. (1992), however, reported shorter survival among African-American women, even when adjusted for CD4+ cell count. In this study, poor survival was strongly associated with not taking antiretroviral therapy even when indicated.

Although information concerning other manifestations of HIV disease progression are rare, two sources of preliminary data suggest that, given near-optimal health care, disease in women does not progress more rapidly than in men; in fact, it may be less fulminant. Carpenter et al. (1991) described the clinical experience with 200 HIV-positive Rhode Island women and found a mean decline of CD4+ cell count of only 50 cells/mm³ per year—less than that reported for men in other studies (Stein et al. 1992). Perhaps this is atypical for women with HIV infection, because all the women were receiving continuous primary medical care with appropriate antiretroviral and PCP prophylactic therapies. The same investigators have reported a small comparative study of 66 HIV-infected women and 57 HIV-infected men in New England suggesting that men were likely to experience a greater decline in CD4+ cell counts (these differences were not statistically significant, however).

Although studies earlier in the HIV epidemic suggested markedly shorter survival in women, the gender gap has apparently narrowed as the epidemic progresses. There is some suggestion that delayed diagnoses contributed to the early findings. More recent information suggests that disease progression, including mortality, is likely to be comparable between men and women of similar social class and risk exposure. Some studies suggest the hypothesis that some women may even fare better in overall survival among HIV-positive people, which must be studied in both a biological and a "health-care accessing" behavioral context. Future studies must accommodate treatment effects in their analyses (Graham et al. 1991, 1992; Moore et al. 1991).

HIV-Related Gynecological Disease

Data concerning the gynecological manifestations of HIV disease are limited. Preliminary information suggests that gynecological infections occur more frequently and are more difficult to treat adequately in HIV-infected women than in uninfected women of similar socioeconomic background. A number of studies have investigated the relationship between HIV disease, human papilloma virus (HPV) infection, and cervical neoplasia.

Cervical Disease Immunosuppression is associated with increased pathological consequences of human papilloma virus (HPV) infection (Halpert et al. 1986; Vermund and Kelley 1990). The cervix is the most common organ to manifest severe HPV-related pathology, though genital warts commonly appear in the vagina, the vulva, or the anus. A dose-response relationship between severity of HPV-induced lesions and increased immunosuppression has been suggested by clinical data (Vermund and Kelley 1990). Exacerbating their risk for further disease progression, immunosuppressed women often respond poorly to conventional treatment for warts (Halpert et al. 1986; Frucher et al. 1992).

Women with HIV infection have been reported to demonstrate a high prevalence of cervical intraepithelial neoplasia (CIN) or squamous intraepithelial lesions (SIL), though only recently have published studies included a comparable uninfected control group (Feingold et al. 1990; Vermund et al. 1990; Laga et al. 1991; Schäfer et al. 1991; Vermund et al. 1991b). These three controlled studies from New York City, Germany, and Zaire clearly document the increased cervical neoplasia risk associated with HIV and HPV coinfection. The Germany and New York studies further suggest the importance of immunosuppression, not merely for HIV, as most relevant for HPV-associated SIL (Schäfer et al. 1991; Vermund et al. 1991). The CDC has recommended cervical screenings of all HIV-infected women at least once a year (CDC 1990). Many clinicians and investigators advocate Pap smears every six months for women with lower CD4+ cell counts, with colposcopy as needed, to ensure that preventable cervical cancer and high-grade precancerous lesions are treated early.

HPV, HIV, and anal dysplasia are associated in studies of homosexual men (Caussy et al. 1990; Palefsky et al. 1990), suggesting a common pathogenic mechanism of HPV-related neoplastic changes in women and men. In women, the magnitude of the association of HIV immunosuppression, HPV, and SIL is dramatic, comparable to the magnitude of the association of smoking and lung cancer in definitive epidemiologic studies. For example, women in the Bronx study with both HIV and HPV infections were about twelve times more likely to have SIL than were women with neither viral infection. Among HIV immunosuppressed people, the association of HPV and SIL is far stronger than among women with better immune

Kathryn Anastos and Sten H. Vermund

Table 11.3 Association of Human Papilloma Virus and Advanced HIV Disease with Cervical Squamous Intraepithelial Lesions

	Symptomatic HIV+		Asymptomatic HIV+		HIV uninfected	
	SIL	No SIL	SIL	No SIL	SIL	No SIL
HPV+	13	11	6	5	3	13
HPV−	0	12	3	22	4	40
	Odds ratio = 29**		Odds ratio = 8.8		Odds ratio = 2.3	

Mantel-Haenszel summary: Odds ratio = 7.0, 95%; Confidence interval = 1.9, 17.0

**Estimated, add 0.5 each cell

Source: Data from study described in Feingold et al. 1990, Vermund et al. 1991b, and Vermund et al. 1990.

capabilities (table 11.3). The mechanism through which immunosuppression may activate and accelerate the pathogenic course of HPV infection is the focus of current investigation.

Alhtough evidence exists for the role of HIV and HPV in cervical SIL, data on cervical cancer per se are limited (Maiman 1991). In developing countries with high baseline rates of cervical cancer, frequency of other causes of immunosuppression and immune activation (malnutrition and coinfections, for example), and prevalence of HIV in women, one might have expected more cervical cancer than has been seen to date. Although women with HIV do not live as long without optimal health care, the incubation period still might be long enough to permit a woman with preexisting cancerous lesions to manifest with cervical cancer. A case-control study of cervical cancer in Africa is needed to investigate whether in fact some cases of cervical cancer are HIV-related but simply have not been reported yet, or whether the cancer now seen in Africa is not HIV-associated. In the United States, controlled studies are needed to supplement worrisome clinical reports from New York City suggesting a growing cervical-cancer problem linked to HIV (Maiman 1991).

There are not currently prospective population-based data to assess the magnitude of risk for progression of SIL. Data are not available yet for judging whether severe or progressive SIL may be comparable, as a prognostic marker, to other opportunistic infections in the AIDS surveillance definition. Further analysis of these issues may be possible now that cervical cancer has been added to the AIDS-defining condition list in the new surveillance-case CDC definition.

HPV may behave like an opportunistic infection predisposing to an opportunistic malignancy. HPV may also behave like an STD by facilitating HIV transmission through disruption of normal mucosal integrity or through altered local immune surveillance. HPV may enhance HIV infection through the equivalent of micro-ulcerations or by creating areas of diminished local immune competence. HPV is so common that even a modest relative risk facilitating HIV entry could result in many infections in the population, making it an important cofactor in transmission. No data are yet available from prospective HIV transmission studies in women to test this hypothesis.

As women live longer in an immunosuppressed state on chemoprophylactic and therapeutic regimens, the association of HIV, HPV, and SIL suggests that cervical disease and HPV infections will become more common among HIV-infected women. With good screening and subsequent care, cervical cancer is a preventable disease, and mortality from cervical cancer should be virtually un-known. Regular Pap smear screening and access to primary care are of the highest priority for HIV-infected women (CDC 1990; Vermund et al. 1991b).

Gynecological Infections Several studies have outlined descriptive data from insti-tutions providing care to HIV-infected women. Even in a population of women receiving gynecological screening (that is, women not symptomatic enough to have sought care), the prevalence of treatable gynecological infections is 50 to 70 percent (Anastos et al. 1992; Clark et al. 1992; Mathur-Wagh et al. 1992). Vaginal can-didiasis, trichomonas, and bacterial vaginosis are the most commonly reported gynecological manifestations.

Vaginal candidiasis is described in case reports as more severe and more frequent in women infected with HIV than in uninfected women. Although the clinical experience of many providers supports this point of view, clinical data comparing rates and severity of vaginal candidiasis in infected and uninfected women are extremely limited. Vaginal candidiasis is a common condition, even in women without immune suppression, and careful study will be required to deter-mine the magnitude and severity of this problem for HIV-infected women. It is accepted that immunosuppression from any cause predisposes to carriage of yeast in the vagina, however. It should also be stressed that refractory vaginal candidiasis, though not life-threatening, is not a trivial condition. Severe itching and excoria-tion, secondary to a condition that may not be easily treated because of underlying immune dysfunction in the host, can be disabling. Extension of candida to the vulvae, crura, and thighs may also occur (see figure 11.1).

In 1987 Rhoads et al. reported that among twenty-nine women with symptoma-tic HIV disease, seven (24 percent) presented with chronic vaginal candidiasis refractory to standard therapeutic regimens. Chronic candidiasis was defined as a history of recurrent episodes of severe vaginal itching associated with a thick curdlike discharge confirmed to be positive for pseudohyphae by potassium hydrox-ide preparation or Gram stain. All patients had required almost constant use of

Kathryn Anastos and Sten H. Vermund

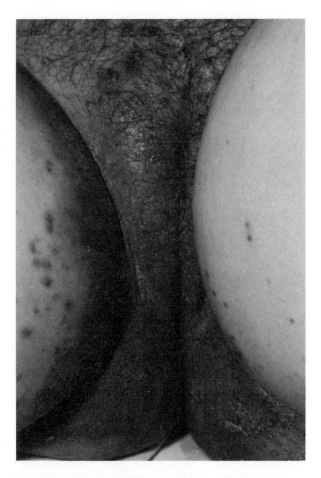

Figure 11.1 Severe genital candidiasis. Patient had vaginal, vulvar, and crural involvement, including centripetal extension to the thighs. Note satellite lesions. Photograph courtesy of Dr. Walter D. Rosenfeld.

intravaginal antifungal agents for at least one year to suppress symptoms. Imam et al. (1990) found that half of sixty-six HIV-infected women in continuing care had noted either new onset or increased frequency of vaginal candidiasis before other signs or symptoms of immune dysfunction were noted. All women with increased frequency of vaginal infection had at least four episodes of vaginal candidiasis per year, and nearly all had noted increased severity and duration of episodes. The mean CD4+ cell count in women with vaginal candidiasis was 506 cells/mm^3, compared with a mean CD4+ cell count of 741 cells/mm^3 among women without vaginal candidiasis. Mayer and coworkers (1991) report that among sixty-six HIV-infected women with a mean CD4+ cell count of 656 cells/mm^3 at diagnosis, 40 percent provided a history of "prior vaginal candidiasis" (not further defined in the abstract). Experience at Bronx Lebanon Hospital has indicated that among 150 HIV-infected women receiving comprehensive screening for gynecological conditions, vaginal candida was diagnosed in 33 women (22 percent) with a median CD4+ cell count of 262, compared with a median CD4+ cell count of 341 in women without vaginal candida infection (Anastos et al. 1992). In our experience, refractory vaginal candidiasis requiring local or systemic suppressive therapy is rare (noted in fewer than 2 percent of patients).

The contribution of HIV-related immunocompromise to the development and severity of vaginal yeast infections remains to be clarified by studies that compare HIV-infected women at various stages of immunosuppression with those who are uninfected. When treated adequately, vaginal candidiasis is a condition of limited clinical consequence, and management strategies for HIV-infected women are already well defined. Short-course therapy should be avoided, and the initial therapeutic approach should be a standard topical antifungal medication with reliance on systemic therapy for treatment failures (Minkoff and DeHovitz 1991).

Clinicians widely feel that pelvic inflammatory disease (PID) is more common and more aggressive in HIV-infected women, though the published data on the condition are limited. Data from San Francisco (Safrin et al. 1990) have demonstrated increasing prevalence of HIV infection among women with PID—from 0 percent in 1985 to 7 percent in 1988, a several-fold higher prevalence than in women having children in the same institution. A study (Hoegsberg et al. 1990) in Brooklyn, New York, demonstrated that women who were HIV-infected and had PID were less likely to have a leukocytosis and more likely to have abscesses requiring surgical intervention. But Malele and coworkers (1991) have reported that among more than 600 female sex workers in Zaire the incidence of PID was low (3 percent per year) and was equal in HIV-positive and HIV-negative women (T. Quinn, personal communication 1992).

As was originally described among men with AIDS, women with HIV infection may develop large nonhealing herpetic ulcers on the genital or sacral area. Women may also have genital ulcers that are not secondary to herpes or other STDs and that may resolve with AZT therapy, implying that HIV itself may be the etiologic agent (Covino and McCormack 1990). In our experience at Bronx Lebanon Hospital in providing care for more than 500 HIV-infected women, more than ten have developed chronic genital ulcers of unclear etiology and with poor response to therapies (Solomon and Denenberg 1992).

Other Gynecological Diseases Clinicians caring for HIV-infected women have begun to suspect that other gynecological disorders may be more prevalent in their patients than in uninfected women. These include other infectious causes of va-

Kathryn Anastos and Sten H. Vermund

ginitis, including trichomonas and bacterial vaginosis; secondary amenorrhea; infertility; and menorrhagia (Bray et al. 1991; Smith et al. 1991; Warne et al. 1991). Many of these conditions, especially amenorrhea and infertility, are known to occur more frequently in women who are injection-drug users and who have had other STDs. Therefore, studies to determine the contribution of HIV infection to the prevalence and severity of these conditions must control for confounding independent associations, including drug use and social conditions. To our knowledge, no such studies have been done to date, though this remains an area of high future research priority.

Research and the Natural History of HIV in Women

In the second decade of the AIDS epidemic we are just beginning to define the appropriate questions to direct research efforts concerning the natural history of HIV infection in women. Protestations that in developed countries there were inadequate numbers of women to study are not tenable. Early case reports of HIV-infected women abounded but were limited in scope (that is, were not organized into a research cohort or network). Through studies of pregnant women and female sex workers, women were studied in their capacities as vectors of infection to their offspring and to their male sexual partners. These research efforts are not ones that resolve critically important issues focused on HIV-positive women themselves. Women-specific manifestations of HIV infection were not studied until the mid-1980s. A recent analysis of the medical literature (Charney and Morgan 1992) indicated that in nineteen articles concerning HIV-infected patients published in 1990, 4,964 men and only 423 women were included; analysis of results by gender was too often omitted.

Specific areas that must be addressed in research efforts include issues relevant for HIV prevention, natural history, and specific gynecological infections (table 11.4).

The methodological problems of conducting necessary natural history research in women are not insignificant but neither are they insurmountable. Because a comparison group of HIV-negative women must be similar in most other ways to HIV-infected women for a sound study, about half of these women will likely be current or former injection-drug users, and a significant proportion will have a history of crack cocaine use. This represents a patient population that has traditionally been very hard to access—both for primary care medical services and for inclusion in research studies. Although one might define part of a comparison group as women receiving care in drug treatment programs, the comparison group for women who became infected through heterosexual contact is more difficult to define. Women seeking medical care in a clinic setting may be systematically

Table 11.4 Areas for Research in Women and HIV Disease

Primary Prevention

- Heterosexual transmission
- Injection-drug use
- Innovative control technologies (virucides, microbicides, HIV vaccines)
- Negotiating safer sex with men

Natural History (nongynecological)

- AIDS-defining illness
- Disease progression by clinical and surrogate markers
- Survival
- Other opportunistic infections and malignancies

Gynecological Manifestations

- Cervical cancer and dysplasia
- Vaginal candida
- Other gynecological infections (pelvic inflammatory disease, etc.)
- Noninfectious conditions
- Gynecological endocrine dysfunction

Source: Authors.

different from women seen in emergency rooms or substance abuse treatment settings.

Examination of other features of the natural history of HIV infection in women will require studies comparing HIV-infected women and men. Such studies will need extremely large numbers of patients (in the thousands) because of the comparatively low likelihood of many of the clinical outcomes: candida esophagitis and other opportunistic infections; severe cervical disease and opportunistic malignancies; death. Alternatively, cohort recruitment can oversample among sicker subjects to ensure higher clinical endpoint results, though clearly such patients will contribute little to the study of earlier HIV manifestations. Women's cohort studies will also require long-term followup.

How large prospective women's studies need to be and how they can be most rapidly effective in addressing key issues are current dilemmas. It is possible that much of the information to be gained from a large prospective women's study can be obtained sooner through other sources, such as cross-sectional studies. Through 1991 there have been only limited analyses of aggregate public health data concerning opportunistic infections and mortality (see Farizo et al. 1992). States with the

Kathryn Anastos and Sten H. Vermund

highest prevalence of AIDS cases could provide analysis by gender of survival and AIDS-defining illnesses. In addition, with some feedback of public health data (specifically, state hospital discharge, tumor registry, and death statistics) to specific institutions that care for large numbers of HIV-infected patients, institution-specific survival analysis could be accomplished. The use of aggregate public health data will not obviate the need for key clinical and laboratory studies to be mounted with less detection and selection bias, but these studies may be coordinated more efficiently than were the many overlapping natural-history studies of men.

Advocates of research on women and HIV must be vigilant to ensure that the research community undertakes and maintains a commitment to study of HIV among women. Two current initiatives may bear mention. First is a collaboration between the CDC and the National Institute of Allergy and Infectious Diseases (NIAID) of the NIH to study 800 HIV-positive and 400 HIV-negative women in Baltimore, Detroit, New York City, and Rhode Island. This study—the HIV Epidemiologic Research Study (HERS)—will address a number of key questions on clinical outcomes. It is anticipated that additional NIAID-sponsored sites (recruiting 1,700 HIV-positive and 375 HIV-negative women) will be added in 1993. These two studies, collectively known as the Women's Interagency HIV Study (WIHS, pronounced "Wise"), have the following research objectives:

• to determine the spectrum and course of the clinical manifestations of HIV infection in women;

• to establish the pattern and rate of decline of CD4+ cells in women, related to key clinical, virological, and other immunological parameters;

• to investigate biological and sociological factors that influence the rate of disease progression;

• to study the factors influencing survival and the quality of life;

• to describe the rates and predictors of HIV seroconversion in the HIV uninfected women;

• to assess the feasibility of intervention research studies, including women-controlled microbicides/contraceptives and HIV vaccines.

Based on research presented at the Ninth International Conference on AIDS in Berlin in July 1993, it would seem that the justification for a women's cohort study is reinforced by the lack of comprehensive information in the above areas. The challenge will be for investigators, advocates, clinicians, women with HIV, and public officials to ensure that WIHS and other analogous studies are run productively and that their lessons are effectively translated into policy for the public good.

12

The Developing World:

Caring for the Caregivers

Kathryn Carovano and Helen Schietinger

When the virus found me, it found an American, a mother of
two children, an artist, a woman with experience in the
media and the government. It found a person whose
lifesong has been an anthem of activity: I am a doer. I take
refuge in action and cannot abide inactivity. It's a family
tradition; my eighty-four-year-old father, who has pursued
the healing of nations, cannot accept the premise that he
cannot heal his daughter. I've discovered that though the
global family is divided by nation and race, gender and
economy, all the differences are flattened by HIV. We share
residence in a global village; I am one with the child walking
the dusty roads of Nigeria, the grandmother tending her
infected family in Manila, the teenage musician in the Hague,
and every HIV-infected mother who longs to see her child
grow into adulthood. I have sometimes feared rejection

Kathryn Carovano and Helen Schietinger

because I am not gay, because I am not an IV drug user, because I am not poor—or even because I am an American. But I have discovered great security in the unity that binds us.

Some months ago I joined the public call for AIDS awareness. But I've come to believe that awareness without action is worse than no awareness at all. This is the message we must bear: That the world cannot love us and ignore us. We cannot love justice and ignore stigma, love our children and keep our silence. Whatever our role, as parents or educators or policy makers, we must act as eloquently as we speak—else we have no integrity.

I have long believed that life has purpose, and my HIV-positive status has not changed this conviction. In all things, I believe, there is meaning. I'd not have chosen to be HIV-positive, but I believe I was chosen for a reason—and I believe that good can come out of this. But I also need those who would understand my pain and be willing to share it. I need courageous models so I will not be discouraged when calling for change that is slow in coming. I need someone to hold me when I can no longer hold myself, to tell me the fight matters when I have no fight left within me. We all need someone to say they understand, they care, they will not forget.

Because HIV asks only one question of those it attacks: Are you human? And this is the right question: Are you human? People with HIV have not entered some alien state of being. They have not earned cruelty and do not deserve meanness. They are people—ready for support and worthy of compassion. I have learned to say to those in positions of power: Do not pity me, listen to me. I am not a victim, I am a messenger. I am not the history of this disease, I am its future. I demand that the world respond to this epidemic not because I may die of it, but because millions of us are living with it.

To the millions of you who are grieving, who are frightened, who have suffered the ravages of AIDS firsthand: Have courage and you will find comfort. To the millions who

are strong I issue the plea: set aside prejudice and politics to make room for compassion and sound policy.
—Mary D. Fisher, speaking at the Eighth International Conference on AIDS and at the 1992 Republican National Convention

Whatever affects women affects the whole family and affects the nation.
—Theresa Kaijage, WAMATA, Tanzania

Everywhere in the world women are suffering and dying from AIDS and bearing witness to death in their families and communities. Throughout the developing and developed world women's risk of acquiring HIV is increasing. For most women the primary risk of infection comes from their—and their partner's—sex lives. But the women who are at greatest risk are so mostly because they are women: their risk is the product both of biological factors and of the social context in which they live. Throughout the developing world and in underdeveloped parts of the so-called developed world, the context keeps women from implementing behavior change to prevent infection by denying them power in society and in their relationships with men.

Little attention has been given to the impact of gender on the HIV epidemic, though it is clearly one of the factors that delineate the abilities of women—and men—to protect their health and well-being and that of their families and to cope with the growing impact of HIV. Gender is determined by social contexts in which status and power combine with biological differences to shape the experience of women and men and girls and boys, and relations between the sexes. More than any other factor, gender determines women's access to information and resources and thus women's ability to protect themselves from HIV infection.

The impact of HIV on women, their households, and their communities is already severe, and it will be exacerbated by the inequality that characterizes relationships between men and women in most societies. It is time to focus on the limits to women's options and to challenge them in order to develop strategies to help women, their families, and their communities confront the epidemic.

Global Disease Distribution

Conservative estimates are that 11 million to 13 million adults and 1 million children have been infected with HIV as of 1993, a total that is expected to rise to 30 million to 40 million by 2000. All estimates assume that an increasing percentage

Kathryn Carovano and Helen Schietinger

will occur in the developing world. It is predicted that there will be more than 1 million adult AIDS diagnoses and deaths per year by the end of the 1990s. Although patterns of transmission vary from region to region, the "feminization" of the epidemic is occurring across the globe.

The countries of sub-Saharan Africa have been the hardest hit by the epidemic. About 6 million people—one of every forty adult men and women in the region— are infected with HIV. The distribution of cases is far from even, however: most cases occur in clusters of population that are usually urban. African men and women are infected in nearly equal numbers, with heterosexual transmission accounting for nearly all cases. One notable variation is that women are infected younger and die younger than their male counterparts. In Uganda the average age of a woman diagnosed with AIDS is twenty-seven; among men it is thirty-five (Obbo 1991). Women also tend to die alone under a stigma of blame.

In Latin America and the Caribbean, HIV initially was a disease that afflicted men almost exclusively, but the the male-to-female ratio of AIDS cases has dropped dramatically in recent years. In Brazil it shifted from 30:1 in 1985 to an estimated 8:1 in 1990. In Mexico the ratio was 25:1 in 1984 and 4:1 by 1990 (Mann, Tarantola, and Netter 1992). In the Caribbean the overall ratio in 1990 was 2:1 (PAHO/WHO 1991). The disease has broadened from one predominantly transmitted through male-to-male sex and blood to one that reaches other segments of the population. Because of uneasiness concerning risky sexual and drug-using behavior in some areas there is a tendency to focus on the more "comfortable" arenas of generalized exhortation regarding heterosexual and perinatal transmission. Heterosexual trans- mission may account for a growing number of HIV infections, but all means of transmission are part of a pattern that remains unique to the region. Trying to normalize the epidemic will cost many lives.

HIV entered South and Southeast Asia through the international drug and commercial sex trades. Though the virus was documented in only a few countries in Asia during the late 1980s, it has spread rapidly in both rural and urban commu- nities. WHO currently estimates that more than 1 million adults may be infected, primarily in Thailand and India. The annual incidence is expected to rise until after the year 2000; as a result, the annual number of HIV infections in Asia is likely to *exceed* the annual number in Africa in the mid to late 1990s (Chin 1991).

All data collected so far point to increasing rates of HIV infection in most developing countries. During the next several decades—if not longer—HIV will be the leading cause of death among young and middle-aged adults and one of the leading causes of infant and child mortality in many developing countries (Chin 1991). The numbers present only one dimension of the impact of HIV on the developing world; we must look much deeper to confront the reality.

Women's Contributions and Community Integrity

In addition to the intrinsic value of their own lives, women's contributions are vital to the health and welfare of their families and communities. As AIDS threatens women it will inevitably threaten the health and stability of those around them. Throughout the developing world gender defines much of the division of labor; as a result, women perform nearly all primary roles in food production and preparation, child care, energy production and use, household management, education, health care, and community organizing. "Women not only prepare and distribute food within the family, but in many countries are themselves substantial food and cash-crop producers. Women are involved in child rearing practices such as breast-feeding, weaning, and immunization, and decision making about family health matters. They often provide home-based care for the disabled, convalescent and chronically sick, contributing essential elements such as affection and compassion" (Panos Institute 1990, 59).

In recognition of these facts the body of knowledge about women in development has gained increasing acceptance since the mid-1980s, particularly in the area of public health.[1] It has been widely recognized that women are key protectors of health and that improving the status of women is a precondition in many societies for improving family health, especially for children. Despite this awareness, the consideration of gender-based benefits and constraints is still frequently excluded from the design and implementation of development programs. AIDS prevention and care programs have proved to be no exception.

The illness or death of any economically active adult results in a decrease in family income. But illness within the family pulls women out of other productive activities, shifting their attention toward caregiving. When a woman becomes ill other family members, probably female, must fill in for her, forfeiting whatever nonessential activities (like school) in which they may have been engaged. For women-headed households (which account for one-quarter to one-third of the world's households), the illness or death of a woman can result in the destitution of the family's dependents. As HIV disease is chronic and disabling, affecting particularly younger women, the impact is considerable. AIDS affects women and men in their most productive years and thus has serious consequences for family income, health, and stability.

[1] In 1973 the Percy Amendment to the Foreign Assistance Act mandated that U.S. foreign assistance integrate women into all development projects. In October 1982 the U.S. Agency for International Development (USAID) issued a policy paper on Women in Development that requires the incorporation of gender in all USAID project and program documents.

Kathryn Carovano and Helen Schietinger

Transmitting HIV to Children

Women's capacity to bear children is perhaps at the root of all gender-defined differences. Because women can transmit HIV to their offspring perinatally, prevention of HIV in women is important for the protection of unborn children. As more women become HIV-infected, the potential impact of HIV on the health of children threatens to reverse child survival gains that have taken years to achieve, particularly in communities with high seroprevalence rates.

In ten Central and East African countries, UNICEF projects that there will be between 250,000 and 500,000 additional deaths of children under five each year because of HIV/AIDS. Those deaths will amount to 1.4 million to 2.7 million additional deaths during the 1990s, increasing the under-five mortality rate to 189 to 259 deaths per 1,000 live births—up dramatically from the UNICEF estimate of 132 and target of 78 under-five deaths per 1,000 (Preble 1990).

The potential inability of a woman to bear healthy children as a result of HIV infection can be a cause of abandonment even prior to the onset of AIDS-related symptoms. Motherhood brings status, security, and validation to many women. There is no social place in many cultures for women who are unable or choose not to have children. Those who are unable to do so may be left by a man who desires a woman who can (Bassett and Mhloyi 1991). M. is a 37-year-old woman living in rural Rwanda who suffers from wasting and fatigue caused by HIV. She was infected with HIV by her husband, her only sexual partner for more than twenty years. Fifteen years earlier she had become infertile and, because she could not bear him any more children, her husband took another wife. It appears that his second wife was HIV-infected and infected him; he in turn infected M. (Schietinger 1992a).

To prevent abandonment, many women with HIV may choose to bear children. A survey of fifty-eight women with HIV infection in Kinshasa, Zaire, reveals that 71 percent of the women interviewed wanted more children within the next two years, and 5 percent were already pregnant (Hassig 1989). Some women who have already lost a child to HIV may choose to bear more children, despite the risk of pregnancy-related complications and the toll that pregnancy can take on their already weakened immune systems.

Women who seek to terminate their pregnancies rather than risk transmitting the virus to their unborn children may also jeopardize their own health status. Accurate data on abortion are extremely limited—especially where the practice is illegal—but it is known that abortions conducted under unsanitary conditions by practitioners with limited training carry significant health risks for women. Each year 200,000 to 500,000 maternal deaths are believed to occur as the result of abortion complications in the developing world (International Center for Research on Women 1989).

The Risk for Women

Women are biologically and socially vulnerable to HIV in ways that are distinct from men. Together these gender-based vulnerabilities present the how and why of women's risk. To understand the potential impact of AIDS on women we examine some of the causes of their susceptibility.

Biological Susceptibility to HIV

For simple biological reasons, women face greater risks of acquiring sexually transmitted diseases (STDs) than men. Not only is a woman more likely to acquire an STD from a male than a male is to acquire an STD from a woman, but she also is likely to suffer more serious long-term consequences of an STD, especially one that is not treated. Overall prevalence rates of STDs in developing countries are thought to be similar for men and women, but STDs are less easily recognized by or diagnosed in women. Because many symptoms are considered normal by uninformed women, treatment is not sought. Finally, because of the heavy stigma attached to STDs and the simple lack of access to diagnosis and treatment, many women suffer from untreated reproductive tract infections—more of which are asymptomatic in women than men. Some STDs and vaginal infections could facilitate HIV transmission. A study conducted among married women attending a family planning clinic in Rio de Janeiro revealed that more than 30 percent had chlamydia during the past year (BEMFAM and AIDSCOM 1992), an affliction that potentially increases women's risk of acquiring HIV infection (Dixon-Mueller and Wasserheit 1991).

Some studies in the United States have suggested that HIV, like other STDs, is more easily transmitted from men to women than vice versa, even without the presence of concurrent infections (Padian et al. 1991). It is unclear, however, whether this applies to men and women in developing countries. There may also be unexpected behavioral implications to this theory: men may feel they have little to worry about and see even fewer incentives to modifying their behavior.

Some women also tend to suffer disproportionately from other conditions, possibly increasing their susceptibility to HIV infection or hastening the progression of HIV disease. Malnutrition is one such condition in many developing countries; some women's diets are deficient when compared with men's because women and girls are fed last and receive smaller amounts and poorer quality food. At the same time, excessive biological and physiological demands are made on their bodies through long work hours, childbearing and lactation, and parasitic disease. One-half to one-third of women of reproductive age in developing countries suffer from iron deficiency anemia. Anemic women are at increased risk of experiencing

Kathryn Carovano and Helen Schietinger

severe blood loss during childbirth. This in turn leads to increased risk of acquiring HIV infection from transfusion, which is a risk for most women who undergo cesarean section (which may be undertaken because the woman's stunted growth makes vaginal passage difficult).

Although their suggestions are not conclusive, some experts speculate that pregnancy may have a negative impact on HIV disease progression if the women's disease is relatively advanced (MacDonald, Ginzburg, and Bolan 1991). Even when it is uncomplicated by HIV infection, pregnancy is one of the greatest health risks for women. "At least one-fourth, and in some countries as many as one-half, of all deaths of women of reproductive age result from causes related to pregnancy and childbirth. This translates to almost half a million women a year who die from pregnancy-related causes in the developing world" (International Center for Research on Women 1989, 20).

In many societies women are assisted in birth by other women, often traditional midwives (Staugaart, Anderson, and Staugard 1986). The midwives are mostly female, often illiterate, and have limited information about or access to barrier protection, such as gloves, to prevent infection and contact with potentially HIV-infected blood. Even nurse-midwives in hospital settings in developing countries have inadequate protection against potential exposure to HIV. A nurse-midwife at a health center in Malawi explains that the maternity facility, which delivers about twenty babies monthly, is issued only five pairs of disposable latex gloves each month. The nurses wash and reuse these until they tear, then save the torn ones for when there are no intact gloves left (Schietinger 1992). A similar situation has been observed at one of the primary hospitals in Guatemala City; health providers will often wear three to five pairs of old gloves in the hope that they will create one intact layer of protection. In these contexts, it is obvious that people assisting in childbirth in either formal or traditional health systems encounter increased risks of acquiring HIV through their work.

Because children are often the first in a family to be diagnosed with HIV infection, a woman's HIV status is often exposed prior to her partner's. The partner of an HIV-positive woman may refuse testing and blame the woman for bringing AIDS into the family, though in most cultures men are more likely than women to have multiple sexual partners and to be exposed to HIV (Bassett and Mhloyi 1991). "If one member of a couple—be it in East Africa or the United States—has AIDS, the coping strategies adopted by the partner may include scapegoating, isolation and violence. The differences in power relations between men and women make it more likely that women will suffer in the scapegoating process" (Nabarro and McConnel 1989).

Social and Economic Vulnerability

Although women's physiological susceptibility to HIV infection is significant, the external social constraints that place women at disproportionate risk in relation to most men are of even greater impact. As Ulin has pointed out (1992), the real causes underlying women's risk of HIV infection "are inherent in the social and economic pressures that leave women with fewer options and little influence on decisions that ultimately determine their place in society" (p. 65).

Because HIV is a sexually transmitted disease, the social norms that influence sexual behavior—norms intimately linked to gender—have a major impact on women's risk of acquiring HIV. The vast majority of women with HIV/AIDS in developing countries were infected through sexual intercourse, often with their steady sexual partner or spouse. Sexual double standards require monogamy on the part of women but accept nonmonogamy as the norm for men. The result is that many women are at risk for AIDS because of the sexual behaviors of their partners, something over which they have little or no influence. A representative sample of 1,458 childbearing women aged nineteen to thirty-seven in Kigali, Rwanda, found an overall HIV seroprevalence rate of 32 percent. Most of the infected women stated that they were themselves monogamous—21 percent of these women reported only one lifetime sexual partner (Allen 1991). It is illustrative to note that the first woman in Mexico diagnosed with AIDS was a fifty-two-year-old housewife whose only known risk behavior was having sex with her husband (Lifshiz 1986).

Women not only have little influence over their partners' sexual behavior outside of the relationship, many also lack control over the sexual activity in their own relationships. Societal norms dictating that men be the sexual decision makers signify that even informed women who are motivated to adopt measures to prevent HIV transmission may be unable to make changes. This is not the case for all women, as AIDSCOM discovered through research in Trinidad and Tobago, where many women reported success in negotiating condom use with their partners (Helquist and Middlestadt 1990). There are, however, many women who fear their partner's mistrust, anger, and possibly even abandonment if they were to raise the issue of condom use (Guimaraes et al. 1991).

Negotiation of change in sexual behavior is based on the premise that women know what to do to protect themselves from HIV—a premise that is far from true for many women, if not most, in the developing world. In many countries efforts to inform women have been limited to attempts to reach them through mass media or to interventions that target sex workers. Consequently, many women have received limited information about AIDS prevention, and even those who know the rudiments often have few of the concrete skills needed to reduce their risk of exposure.

The threat of sexual violence is another reality in many women's lives that raises their susceptibility to HIV infection. Data on rape are limited for two principal reasons: first, it is surrounded with stigma and shame, which may discourage many women from reporting it; and, second, many developing countries provide little legal recourse for rape victims. The data that are available reveal that in such countries as Peru, Malaysia, Panama, and Mexico the majority of rape victims knew their assailants. On average, more than 40 percent of victims were younger than fifteen. At a dormitory of a coed boarding school in Kenya, seventy-one teenage girls were raped by their male classmates and nineteen others were killed on July 10, 1991; the incident was referred to in the *Kenyan Times* as a "common occurrence" (Heise 1992).

For many women, sexual relations within and outside of marriage are linked to economic and social survival (Bassett and Mhloyi 1991). The potential cost of pursuing changes in sexual behavior to decrease the risk of acquiring HIV is very real for women who are financially dependent on their male partners. When women are dependent on their sexual partner's income, any action that might jeopardize the relationship must be avoided. Among the women participating in the study in Rwanda, two-thirds had no income of their own and depended entirely on their partners for economic support; only 13 percent of these women had salaried jobs (Allen 1991). As Ankrah has pointed out, rural African women are particularly limited economically by their lack of land ownership rights or adequate access to land or cash (Ankrah 1991).

Limited economic opportunities also increase vulnerability to HIV infection by leading many women into sex work as a means of survival. Faltering economies and widespread unemployment have led many women to sell sexual services, one of the few income-generating options available (Carovano 1991). For many women, sex work is a choice driven by the need to survive (some are sold by their families), even though it exposes them to more STDs, including HIV. Poor sex workers, as poor women, are less able or likely than their richer counterparts to protect themselves with condoms.

The cumulative effect of the factors defining women's social vulnerability is manifested in the power dynamics between men and women in sexual relationships. It is in the context of the relationship that HIV is transmitted and risk reduction must be addressed. The fact that men are in control of most resources and are responsible for most sexual decision making underlies women's vulnerability to HIV. According to health workers in Brazil, many men infected with HIV did not tell their female partners of their status, nor did they change their sexual behavior; infected women tended to do just the opposite. In essence, women's risk of HIV is a function of women's physiology in combination with their social, personal, and economic subordination to men.

Women and Medical Services

Even though women and men are dying of AIDS throughout the developing world, gender-disaggregated data on HIV disease progression or survival rates is scarce. But lessons from other areas of health suggest that women receive inferior medical care, when they receive any at all, aggravating female AIDS-related morbidity and mortality. This is supported by studies in Uganda that reveal that women AIDS patients are much less likely to receive medical care than men, even when their conditions are the same (UNICEF 1990). And there are women with HIV in Brazil who reportedly seek medical care only after the death of their spouse, often when their disease is at an advanced stage.

Women's multiple responsibilities in the home and limited access to money or transportation often limit their opportunities to visit a health clinic. Women in developing countries report low use of health care services because of a lack of time—their twelve- to eighteen-hour workdays are filled with agricultural labor, housework, and child care—and because of the distance to health facilities (Rutabanzibwe-Ngaiza, Heggenbougen, and Walt 1985, 77). Limited visits to health clinics also restrict women's access to health information, STD treatment, and condom supplies. "Many women raised in male-dominated cultures have to struggle against the impulse to sacrifice their health for the health of the whole" (Bateson 1990).

Abandonment

In the case of AIDS-related illness, fear of abandonment is another very real barrier preventing women from acknowledging their illness and seeking outside care. In Kampala, one study of patterns of caregiving in homes found that when a woman falls ill or shows signs of AIDS-related symptoms before her partner does, she is likely to be sent back to her relatives or to be abandoned (Ankrah 1991), as this case study illustrates: "Anna is a 27-year-old woman who lived in Kigali, Rwanda, until four months ago when her husband discovered she had AIDS and abandoned her; she was forced to return home to live with and be cared for by her parents. She has not received medical care since returning home and her parents do not know that she has AIDS. She is emaciated and weak and her mother says that they cannot afford to buy the foods she would like to eat" (Schietinger 1992a).

For women who are financially dependent on their partners, rejection by the partner or the partner's premature death by AIDS carries with it the prospect of poverty and homelessness. Widows often do not retain control of their spouse's property, especially if they are childless (Endeley 1984). According to UNICEF, in ten African countries women and children make up 77 percent of the population; however, women have the legal right to own or inherit property in only 16 percent of

Kathryn Carovano and Helen Schietinger

the households in those countries. When women head households, incidence of malnutrition and infant mortality are higher; a study from rural Zimbabwe found that risks of childhood malnutrition increased sixfold in households supported exclusively by women (Thiesen 1984).

In Africa, women are caring for sick children, sick husbands, and sick relatives, often in the face of their own impending illness. When twenty-four Rwandan families with a chronically ill family member were interviewed, the primary caregiver was identified as a woman by fifteen of them (65 percent) and a man by six of them (25 percent). The gender of one caregiver was not known, and in two of the families there was no caregiver—the sick women cared for themselves (Schietinger 1992b).

Because most women in developing countries are socialized to put the needs of their husband and children before their own, the first areas to suffer are likely those most directly linked to the women's own health and well-being. Outside employment, education, and training are likely to be set aside as demands increase in the home.

The Impact on Households

According to Freedman's work on household response to economic crisis, "it is women, especially mothers, who bear the responsibility of developing and implementing their family's survival strategies, including almost exclusive responsibility for maintaining the family's health. Yet . . . they continue to be denied the resources, the rights and the decision-making power needed to carry out those responsibilities successfully" (1991, 4). The crisis of AIDS requires households to make adjustments under the same constraints, efforts that in many instances will be further circumscribed by women's own ill health.

The decline of a woman's health and productivity is likely to affect a family's diet and nutritional level (UNICEF 1990), ultimately contributing further to lowered productivity and declining quality of life. One case study from rural Rwanda suggests that the AIDS death of a woman would reduce the nuclear family's agricultural labor input by 50 percent (Gillespie 1989).

A woman's ill health and increased demands on her to provide care in the home limits the time she has available for income-generating activities. Because her limited income is often used for clothing, school fees, and other expenses for the children, if a woman's cash income falls, children will be removed from school. According to Barnett's study on the impact of AIDS in the Rakai district of Uganda, "AIDS-affected households had a higher rate of taking children out of school than other households" (Barnett, Blaikie, and Obbo 1990). Because of the higher value placed on male education in many societies, and because gender-defined tasks fall first to female children as their mothers become ill or overwhelmed as caregivers, girls are likely to be the first affected.

Community-Level Impact

Community development reflects change and growth and, it is hoped, an improved quality of life. AIDS is already challenging that hope in many communities in sub-Saharan Africa, where 30 to 40 percent of certain segments of the adult population are already HIV-infected. In particular communities in other countries, like Peru or Indonesia, the threat of AIDS is just as big a problem.

The provision of care for men, women, and children with AIDS is already having a devastating impact on the health care system worldwide. From Brazil to Tanzania a growing percentage of available hospital beds is being occupied by patients with AIDS, limiting the access of others in already overburdened and underfunded facilities. The development of appropriate and sustainable care strategies for women, men, and children is critical for helping individuals and communities to cope with the potentially devastating impact of HIV.

Care Strategies for Women with HIV

The women who become HIV-infected in the developing world are in many ways in a much more difficult situation than their HIV-infected sisters in wealthier nations. They have many fewer resources to cushion the losses of health and strength, income and ability caused by HIV disease. Health deteriorates faster in the absence of adequate medical care and nourishment.

As bleak as the picture may seem, strategies for caring for HIV-infected women and their families do exist in highly affected communities. We focus here on programs developed in Africa, where the majority of HIV-infected women live. Strategies for caring for these women range from providing income-generating activities, direct material support, direct services, emotional support, and assistance in planning for the future care of their children. Research projects also provide some support services to finite groups of women over a limited period of time. These strategies are being implemented in many locations, including hospital-based outpatient clinics, community-based service agencies, women's homes, churches, and informal community sites, including the street.

Projects that help HIV-infected women generate income through cottage industries are beginning to be developed in several African countries. These programs are particularly important to HIV-infected women, many of whom already live on the edge of poverty and must continue to support their families after they have lost a husband or other adult family member. Income-generating projects are not new with

Kathryn Carovano and Helen Schietinger

the advent of the HIV epidemic, but they may assist in HIV prevention by keeping some young women from being forced into prostitution to support their families.

The limitations of projects of this type can be seen in the rural area of Agomaya, Ghana, where the Catholic church has established a food-processing plant operated by a cooperative of nine women workers (Hampton 1991). This plant processes cassava for local farmers, replacing the labor-intensive process of pounding cassava that is traditionally the woman's role, and processes and sells products made from other locally grown crops. The church has built bread ovens that employ ten women a day and supports other projects such as beekeeping, ceramics manufacturing, and fish-smoking. The goal is to provide employment for women so that they do not have to go abroad to work in the sex industry, a factor that has defined the spread of HIV in Ghana. This project can only provide options to a handful of women, however.

An alternative strategy to producing jobs is that of stimulating entrepreneurship by providing low-interest loans to women who wish to start businesses. WAMATA, a community-based AIDS organization in Tanzania, has identified the need for a revolving loan fund to be used by AIDS-affected families to start such businesses as vegetable production, poultry- and cattle-raising, carpentry, and tailoring (Mukoyogo 1991).

Vocational training, a common church or nongovernmental organization (NGO) activity found throughout Africa, represents a longer-term strategy for enabling women to support themselves. Vocational training is now also seen as a critical strategy for orphans whose parents have died of AIDS. Saint Anne's Vocational Institute, established in Ghana in 1963, is a good example of this strategy. The institute teaches cookery, dressmaking, business affairs, and such crafts as batik fabric-printing (Hampton 1991). Outside funding and support from the government have been crucial for the establishment of these projects in Ghana. In Rwanda, the government provides lessons in needlepoint and basketry to teenage girls to provide them with income-producing skills.

Another much-needed income-producing strategy is the development of policies and laws that enable women to continue supporting themselves and their families by granting them the right to own and inherit land. In countries in which women already have this legal right, a corollary strategy would be to provide legal assistance and advocacy for women attempting to defend their rights to land when challenged by the deceased husband's family.

Although income generation is important for women and orphans who are able to work, communities highly affected by HIV must address the economic plight of HIV-infected women who are too weak or ill to work. Programs designed to provide various types of material support to HIV-infected families in need are being implemented by preexisting social service agencies, NGOs, churches, and in newly developed community-based AIDS service organizations throughout Africa and other parts of the developing world. Support may include the provision of funds for children's school fees and uniforms, emergency cash donations for such one-time needs as funerals and transportation back to the village, food donations to families, or hot meals served in a central location.

The AIDS Support Organization in Uganda (TASO), was one of the first community-based organizations developed to help HIV-infected people. Using external funding, it provides all of the services mentioned above, relying on both paid staff and volunteers (Hampton 1991). Many church-funded hospitals also provide such services to people with HIV infection, both through existing social service structures and through special programs developed to assist people with HIV infection. These services are often provided through informal networks with people in the community. Examples can be found at Kitovu Hospital and Ensambya Hospital, Catholic missions in Uganda, and the religious service agencies Caritas and Good News in Rwanda.

The primary disadvantage of programs providing material support is the scope of the problem it is designed to solve: the need is too great and will not be sufficiently addressed by individual donations to needy people within single communities. Each service is a small drop in a widening ocean of need. In addition, this sort of program depends on ongoing outside support.

As more adults become sick and die, communities hard hit by HIV infection begin to feel the impact as families struggle to support the growing number of children and sick adults in their midst. The underlying problem is the capacity to provide food and shelter and care to increasing numbers of dependent people—including children, who require nurturing and socialization. Generally, women who have come to urban areas to work go home to the villages where they grew up when they lose their means of support in the city, and their families of origin take them in. Exceptions arise in large cities among those who have no roots in outlying villages or who cannot return to those villages. Here women and orphans may find themselves with no means of support and no housing. Some housing programs have developed in direct response to the problem, including orphanages that have opened their doors to AIDS orphans. The Sisters of Charity, who provide shelters for the needy in many cities around the world, have opened a shelter for HIV-infected women and their children in Addis Ababa.

Another care strategy is the provision of medical care to women and their children. Hospitals throughout Africa and parts of Latin America and the Caribbean report high percentages of their patients to be HIV-infected. In 1988, for example, the seroprevalence in Chikankata Hospital in Zambia was 28 percent for all patients, and 49 percent for patients with tuberculosis (Campbell 1990). People with HIV-related disease are usually admitted to the general medical wards of hospitals, though there may be a concentration of people with HIV infection in a particular area.

Kathryn Carovano and Helen Schietinger

The most common outpatient site of HIV-specific medical care is the outpatient department of a hospital—either in an HIV/AIDS clinic, or, even more specifically, an HIV/AIDS clinic for pregnant women and women of childbearing age. It is rare for a health center to have either trained staff or medicines to care for people with AIDS; usually suspected cases are referred to the next level of care for HIV testing and treatment. Some hospitals, however, have extended services directly into the community through AIDS home-care programs, which provide medical monitoring and medicines in the patient's home.

HIV-related medical services often function with the same meager supplies as the rest of the health system of the country, which means the monthly supply of crucial drugs (ketoconazole, penicillin, and aspirin, for example) may last only for a portion of the month, after which patients coming to clinic receive no medicine. The only alternative available in some countries is to give patients prescriptions so they may attempt to purchase medicine in private pharmacies. Most medicines considered vital for HIV treatment in the industrialized world (acyclovir and AZT, for example), are unavailable to people with HIV in most developing countries. Furthermore, pharmaceutical company assistance programs designed to supply drugs like AZT to the indigent do not extend their services to patients outside of the United States.

There are two problems with the concept of providing medical care to individuals with HIV in a developing country. One is that people seek to meet their needs in a hierarchical order, and basic survival needs precede medical care. Unless a woman and her family have adequate nutrition, shelter, and basic physical safety— a need that is not met in many poor communities around the world—they will not seek ongoing health care. Also, as has been pointed out, women often place the needs of their husband and children above their own, neglecting their own needs for medical care.

The other critical problem regarding the provision of medical care in developing countries is the allocation of scarce resources. Because of meager national health budgets, people receive minimal medical care. The health care systems lack physical facilities, trained personnel, and the funds for salaries, medicines, and other medical supplies. Many countries have two to three parallel health systems that work together to attempt to meet these needs: a government-sponsored health system, private sector services, and a health system run by NGOs, usually with outside financial support. In some areas, specially funded programs responding to the HIV epidemic provide quality care and drugs to people within a small geographic area but cannot begin to address the needs of the majority of communities being affected by HIV.

Although some women in developing countries have benefited from research clinics that follow cohorts of women prospectively to study the natural history of HIV in women or to study aspects of perinatal and heterosexual HIV transmission, the majority of HIV-infected women continue to have the same inadequate health care that they had prior to becoming HIV-infected.

In addition to Western medicine, people with HIV infection throughout the world use the expertise of traditional practitioners of many forms of healing: herbs, acupuncture, spiritualism. When used to treat symptoms of HIV infection, many of these methods have been considered to be effective by recipients. Use of healers has been encouraged by many Western medical practitioners as providing emotional comfort and possible palliative relief of symptoms. Although there have been traditional healers who have claimed to be able to cure AIDS, none of these has been proved to be effective.

Throughout the developed and developing world people with HIV infection receive care in the home, usually provided by people who are family members by blood or by affection. Most of these caregivers are women who may or may not receive support from individuals or programs outside the home. In recognition of the inability of hospitals to treat the growing numbers of people with HIV-related illness, home-based care programs have sprung up in communities all over the world, including Africa. By 1989 six home-based care programs had been identified in Uganda and Zambia alone (WHO 1991); there are now home-care programs in many African countries, including Tanzania, Zimbabwe, Zambia, Malawi, Ghana, Uganda, Kenya.

Most of these are hospital-based programs that use medical staff members to provide medical and nursing care and counseling through visits to the person's home. They usually use cars or trucks but often must depend on bicycles or mopeds; they also visit people on foot. The Chikankata Hospital is a rural hospital in Zambia that has developed this model using a multidisciplinary team that includes medical officers, nurses, and social workers. The Kitovu Hospital in Uganda adds community-based volunteers to its home-care team and gives the volunteers bicycles so they may visit families long distances away (WHO 1991).

Home-care programs can provide a range of services. Those that function out of health clinics or hospitals provide medical monitoring, medicines, and transportation to or from the hospital. Both health system-based and community-based organizations can provide emotional and spiritual support; teach families about hygiene, home-care skills, and HIV prevention; and demonstrate by their presence that caregivers will not become infected by providing nursing care to someone with HIV. Some projects provide items for families caring for a person with HIV: bleach, rubber gloves. But they may give the impression that it is dangerous to provide care to a person with AIDS without these supplies, and most people do not have access to them.

Ultimately, the most efficacious home-care model may be that which seeks to be self-sustaining. An example of such a model is the home-care program run by Project Info–SIDA in Rwanda (Schietinger 1992b). This program simply trains Red

Cross volunteers to teach basic nursing care skills to families and sends them back into the community to visit families caring for a chronically ill person. The volunteers teach home-care skills, hygiene, and HIV prevention. Through their visits to the home they also provide emotional support and demonstrate that there is no need to be afraid of the HIV-infected individual. The volunteers live in communities that are themselves poor, so it is not usually possible to provide material assistance to families. But the volunteers often generate additional in-kind contributions from the community for household chores such as carrying water, cultivating, and for such services such as carrying a person to the clinic or hospital or taking food to a hospitalized individual. Red Cross volunteers can also stimulate the community collection of clothes, money for transportation, blankets, and other material goods for personal care.

Many people have questioned the viability of depending on volunteers for community-based services in countries where people are on the whole very poor, but AIDS service organizations such as TASO in Uganda, Pela Vidda in Brazil, MHOL in Peru, WAMATA in Tanzania, and Project Info-SIDA in Rwanda have provided ample proof that some people will reach out to help each other even in very meager life circumstances.

Summary

According to Jacobson (1991), "Few nations, rich or poor, have committed themselves to improving health care for women." The AIDS epidemic gives multiple reasons to continue the push for that commitment and to broaden it to its widest definition. Around the world women with AIDS need health care, but a public health strategy is also needed to protect women *from* AIDS and allow them to cope with HIV in their families.

Another author has said, "In order to develop treatment or prevention strategies for a particular population, it is necessary to first learn to see them and then to become sufficiently visionary to imagine that their lives might be different" (Bateson 1990, 65). An effort to see has been attempted; now is the time for vision.

13

Working with Communities of Women at Risk—

A Chronicle

Helen Gasch and Mindy Thompson Fullilove

Being HIV-positive brings another new task with it, and that is learning a new language. We have all had the experience of going to a doctor, having the doctor tell us what is wrong with our bodies, and then not knowing or understanding, when the conversation is over, exactly what the problem is.

When I come to see you I am dependent on you for your creativity in helping me decide what is best for my situation . . . . I can take in only so much information at a time. You may have to explain issues to me several times before I really understand [them]. You may have to interpret—perhaps simplify—your language for me.

I am one of the women you may be working with. We are all individuals, all engaged in the struggle to live. We need your respect, not your pity. We need your professional judgments, not your personal judgments. We need your

Helen Gasch and Mindy Thompson Fullilove

> expertise to help guide us through this maze we must jour-
> ney alone.
>
> —Anonymous

There is a poster that reads, "We all have AIDS."

The bodies of our leaders, friends, and sisters have become home to HIV. Unable to reach into their cells and strip away viral particles, we watch and grieve and daily learn to rejoice in minutes we once took for granted.

We—women of color who have been working for years in the fight against AIDS—have AIDS in our world. Our dreams of escaping AIDS are dreams of reinventing the world without this plague—the tragic epidemic is our reality—that marks the contours of our lives. We must become the triumphant face of the epidemic, that face that has a story and a name and a proud tradition.

Catastrophe and re-creation is the subject of our text, a text that must reach across cultures and through masks, veils, stereotypes. We have chosen to place this text within a diary of our own lives as women affected by this epidemic. It is our hope that, by linking the personal and the academic, we can reach across barriers and convey some of the reality of poor and minority inner-city communities in the United States attempting to respond to AIDS.

On the streets of the inner city it is common for people to ask of strangers, "Who is you?" This interrogation is a request for credentials and allegiances. The residents of the community want to know, "Is you wit me or is you agin me?" (Thompson and Thompson 1976). Sociologists, among others, share a concern that social allegiances shape research. They point out that researchers with commitments (often concealed) to dominant social norms tend to view subordinate people as troubled, defective, or pathological. Adam (1992, 4) notes, "The resulting scientific images come to be used to invalidate the experiences of the oppressed and to legitimate state domination or professional control, ultimately feeding back into ideologies that blame the victim."

We believe, therefore, that it is helpful to tell the reader something about our work and, more important, about our commitments. We are coworkers at the HIV Center for Clinical and Behavioral Studies, a research group based at the Columbia-Presbyterian Medical Center in New York City. With grant support from the National Institute of Mental Health and the National Institute of Drug Abuse, the center conducts studies of HIV disease, disseminates information on HIV/AIDS, and builds links between the community and the university. It is this last task that is our focus through our work with the Community/Substance Abuse Core. The Core maintains a resource room for the community, offers educational activities, provides technical advice to community agencies, and conducts research, primarily on the relationship between drug abuse and HIV/AIDS. As black women working to understand and prevent the spread of AIDS in communities of color, we see our mission as twofold: first, to provide information to the community about the AIDS epidemic, and second, to ask questions that will deepen our understanding of the epidemic. In each of these roles, we are advocates for people with AIDS. Furthermore, we are advocates for community survival.

March 1986

After a tense week of work, Mindy is planning a quiet Saturday. The phone rings at 8 A.M. Sala Udin, a leader in the fight against AIDS in San Francisco, wants to know if Mindy will head the minority component of an AIDS research unit to be formed at the University of California, San Francisco (UCSF). This seems like a preposterous idea, especially on Saturday morning. "Come talk," says Sala, who is a persuasive man. The plan is powerful. Because of the support of the San Francisco Department of Health, the university researchers have actually accepted, at least in principle, the idea that a portion of a major center grant would be under "minority control." It remains to resolve who will be the minorities and how will they exercise control. Mindy, with a modest track record in research, joins the team. The negotiations are delicate. At one point, Sala slams down his briefcase and threatens to leave the table, a moment that seems to arrive freeze-dried from the 1960s, but the act sways the balance in the right direction. Minorities are recognized and accepted, provided wholehearted support.

In fact, the model that is developed will be a unique and powerful one for AIDS research, a model of true collaboration between university-based and community-based researchers studying AIDS. An important battle had been won, one that shifted the fulcrum ever so slightly in the right direction, affording critical leverage to a trusted community-based organization and away from traditional (white) research centers. At least now there is the promise of sensitive, respectful observation and study of community health problems. To be able to provide the leadership, to pose research questions freely, to own the means of producing "knowledge" for and about communities of color— these are the cherished spoils of war on AIDS in urban communities of color. Perhaps it happens because it is time for it to happen.

In *AIDS and Its Metaphors* Susan Sontag (1988) noted that AIDS is a global phenomenon: "Like the effects of industrial pollution and the new system of global financial markets, the AIDS crisis is evidence of a world in which nothing important is regional, local, limited; in which everything that can circulate does, and every problem is, or is destined to become, worldwide. Goods circulate (including images and sounds and documents, which circulate fastest of all, electronically). Garbage circulates: the poisonous industrial waste of St. Etienne, Hanover, Mestre and Bristol are being dumped in the coastal towns of West Africa. People circulate, in greater numbers than ever. And diseases" (p. 92).

Though it is a global phenomenon, AIDS is not randomly distributed. Particularly in the United States, HIV disease is concentrated in "high-risk" communities. These AIDS epicenters share a recent history of social upheaval that radically affected conventions surrounding sexuality and the use of drugs. War, gay liberation, and "urban renewal"—seemingly disparate processes—have as a common outcome vulnerability to HIV infection. Zwi and Cabral (1991, 1527–28) point out the commonalities of these social contexts:

> Many of these situations occur where there is diminished concern about health, increased risk taking, and reduced social concern about casual sexual relationships. In some circumstances, such as refugee populations and street children, those affected may be struggling to feed themselves, and even if they were aware of HIV it would be considered relatively unimportant. A high turnover of sexual partners, often in exchange for money or goods, may be present. The ability to practice safer sex may be impaired by the use of alcohol and other addictive drugs as well as a lack of information, resources, and power. Those aware of the necessity to protect their health, such as commercial sex workers in many parts of the world, may be unable to ensure that their paying (and even less their nonpaying) partners use condoms. All these social contexts will be exacerbated by homelessness, landlessness, unemployment, rapid periurban settlement, migration, population relocation, and poverty, ensuring fertile ground for sexually transmitted diseases and HIV.

We would argue that these conditions are all unstable processes that are change factors, altering central social behaviors and reshaping the cultures in which the behaviors occur.

Various definitions emphasize that culture is an enduring set of concepts governing individual and group behavior. But in communities affected by AIDS, the received culture has been refined by social change and further reshaped by the epidemic itself. For any group, the culture that existed before the epidemic has become the progenitor of the culture that exists now. Sontag (1988) describes the changes in the culture of gay men in this way: "The view that sexually transmitted diseases are not serious reached its apogee in the 1970s, which was also when many male homosexuals reconstituted themselves as something like an ethnic group, one whose distinctive folkloric custom was sexual voracity, and the institutions of urban homosexual life became a sexual delivery system of unprecedented speed, efficiency, and volume. Fear of AIDS enforces a much more moderate exercise of appetite and not just among homosexual men. . . . After two decades of sexual spending, of sexual speculation, of sexual inflation, we are in the early stages of a sexual depression" (p. 76)

It is the process of social change and its impact on culture that is of concern to us in attempting to understand women's lives in communities affected by AIDS. In particular, it is the process of community disintegration that has been most important in placing women at risk for AIDS.

April 1988

Crack. San Francisco is convulsed by the epidemic. The *Chronicle,* San Francisco's major morning paper, reports that the epidemic may bankrupt the city through the costs of arresting, trying, and retaining drug dealers; the costs of foster care for neglected children; the costs of medical care for crack users. The Centers for Disease Control (CDC) notes that crack is connected to a rise in sexually transmitted diseases (STDs) in major cities. Community leaders tell Mindy and her research colleagues that crack—not AIDS—is *the* issue for minority communities in the Bay Area. "We have to study crack," Mindy says. The team is hesitant. "You know, they shoot strangers in those neighborhoods," a member points out. How to do research safely? Bob Full-ilove, Mindy's husband and coworker, meets a community leader who offers to take them. "Just tell me what you need, how many kids you want to talk to, I'll get 'em for you." It is a new world. This drug, this intensely addictive, eu-phorogenic drug, requires a whole new vocabulary: tossin', tweakin', rocks, pipes. The words are important. They are not just new words for familiar things, they are new words for new things, things not seen before. In 1992 the *Village Voice* will say that the crack epidemic was the most significant cultural event of the 1980s. In 1988, we want to know if it will speed the spread of AIDS. The answer, sadly, is yes.

For all of the communities affected by AIDS, the equilibrium between community growth and death is linked to the community's ability to control the spread of HIV. The social response to epidemics requires resources and energy. Where these are available, communities can mount a vigorous and effective campaign in reaction to a threatening epidemic. Where they are absent, the response will be correspondingly diminished.

Communities of color affected by the AIDS epidemic are disintegrating communities that are already suffering economic and social crisis of massive proportions. The response to AIDS has been slow and painful, limited at every turn by the many problems competing for resources. Minority community leaders have struggled to "add AIDS to the list" of problems, which includes drug abuse, homelessness, teen pregnancy, inadequate education, and unemployment (Weinstein 1991).

Helen Gasch and Mindy Thompson Fullilove

Yet all of these problems have a common source: social disintegration of poor communities.

Because social disintegration is the underlying cause of multiple epidemics, we propose that community-building must be the central response. It is not a short-term activity designed to keep us occupied until a medical cure; rather, community-building *is* the cure. We hope to show that the forces driving the AIDS epidemic in this country are the processes of social disintegration in the inner city.

In terms of economic and political developments in the United States, several forces played out over two decades or more have undermined the quality of life in inner-city communities. For example, as the country's economic base (as indicated by the GNP) shifts from an agricultural and industrial economy toward a service economy, individuals lacking higher education and marketable job skills are displaced and marginalized. The recession that followed the Reagan era—an era characterized by extraordinary growth in private wealth and deep cuts to social and health programs for low- to moderate-income citizens—has hit the have-nots the hardest of all. Urban communities have fallen into a marked physical decay brought on by reductions in investment in infrastructure, in preservation of housing, in delivery of social and health services, and in enforcement of public safety and sanitation services.

The South Bronx "burn-out phenomenon" is in various stages of reenactment in minority areas of large cities around the country. The scenario roughly sketched describes the milestones of urban decay, beginning with the physical demise of housing and leading to the forced migration of residents to surrounding areas, homelessness for many, and finally to the splintering of social networks and a clustering of disease prevalence in affected neighborhoods. In addition, underfunding of social programs and community organizations has weakened or eliminated the ability of poor communities to proactively fight the rapid increase in crime, drug use, and the spread of AIDS. The virus that is spreading most rapidly of all in these communities is one of marginality. Efforts to stimulate involvement of ethnic minorities in the political process, economic viability of minority-run establishments, and government resources directed to preserving social structures can mitigate against the destructive force of the current epidemic.

The real control for the spread of HIV lies in rebuilding damaged communities so that they can function in a health-promoting manner. Without such broad-based, programmatic interventions, the continued deterioration of the inner-city will promote the spread of AIDS and other diseases, like tuberculosis, drug addiction, and violence.

As with drug addiction, which knows no socioeconomic bounds, this spread of disease is not likely to be confined to the inner city alone. As Wallace and colleagues (1992, 1) have argued, HIV infection, "like any other contagious phenomenon, will inevitably diffuse both spatially and socially from present urban epicenters into other communities and social strata at a rate dependent on the prevalence of the disease within the epicenters." Thus, attention to the social foundations of health in the inner city—this process of community-building—is a critical step in protecting the health of the nation as a whole.

February 1989

The Center for AIDS Prevention Studies (CAPS), Mindy's research group at UCSF, has established a home at 74 New Montgomery Street. For more than a year the minority scientists of CAPS have been working on the question, "Why is there excess risk for AIDS in the minority community?" It is clear that blacks and Latins are 20 percent of the U.S. population, but they constitute 40 percent of the people with AIDS. Why? Simple answers don't work. Minorities are not more promiscuous. It can't simply be drug use. There are more drugs in minority communities, but even among drug users minorities are more likely to be infected. "We must continue to search," Mindy tells the audience at the open house. Soon, Dooley Worth will send a copy of an obscure article entitled "A Synergism of Plagues" (Wallace 1988). That article will provide insight. But it hasn't come yet.

Community Disintegration

Although the modern process of community disintegration varies slightly from city to city, the abandonment of urban centers has occurred throughout human history. Wallace and Wallace (1990, 259) note:

Significant contributions in archaeology have traced the rise and fall of several large centers of civilization: Mayan cities, Pella in Greece, Tihuanaco in Peru, Chaco in Southwestern United States, and Ain Ghazal in Jordan. These centers featured populations in the tens of thousands to hundreds of thousands and high cultures. . . . These fell when environmental changes overwhelmed or outflanked the technology and imposed new limiting factors on the enlarged population. For Tihuanaco and Chaco, changes in rainfall and water supply disrupted agriculture over the entire hinterland. For Pella, the closing off of the bay sedimentation created a malarial swamp which eroded public health. In Ain Ghazal, the soil became exhausted by too intense agriculture and ceased producing quantities of crops needed to sustain the population.

Concurrent with the processes of depopulation was a devolution of those ancient cultures, characterized by alcohol abuse, routine cheating by merchants, and official corruption. The Wallaces suggest that observations of the destruction of modern cities shed light on the cultural decline of cities in antiquity. Dear, working in Philadelphia in the 1970s, described a process that he called "contagious housing

Helen Gasch and Mindy Thompson Fullilove

abandonment" (1976, 30). In this process, the burning of a single building increased the risk for destruction of adjacent buildings. Through the deterioration of neighboring houses, whole blocks—and eventually whole neighborhoods—could be destroyed.

Wallace (1988, 1990) extended Dear's work to examine the destruction of the South Bronx, a part of New York City almost destroyed by fire between 1970 and 1980. The most vulnerable houses were those in overcrowded neighborhoods. When occupancy was noted to rise above 1.51 persons per room—a level considered "badly overcrowded" by the U.S. Census—the number of fires increased. Vulnerability to fire was also directly tied to fire services. With adequate resources for fire extinguishment, fires could be contained to a single room or single apartment, and the building could be saved. Without that protection, the building as a whole would be threatened, accelerating the process of "contagious housing destruction," which has serious health consequences. People who are burned out of their homes are forced to move to adjacent neighborhoods, disrupting their social ties and networks.

The mechanism by which social support protects individuals from disease and illness has long been debated. But a substantial body of literature provides evidence that social support is consistently associated with preventive health practices and positive health outcomes for a variety of acute and chronic disorders (see, for example, Hamburg 1982; House and Robins et al. 1982; Broadhead and Kaplan et al. 1983; Berkman et al. 1984, 1983, 1979; Seitz and Rosenbaum et al. 1985). The vehicle for acceleration of HIV spread in damaged communities could take a number of forms. One possible means is through individuals' increased risk behavior owing to substance abuse and the absence of the protective influences of family, friends, and concerned others. Intact social networks, including family relationships and membership in a church, peer group, or other social organization, can help assure the well-being of its members by facilitating the sharing of information, advice, moral support, material goods, and favors. In the case of preventing AIDS, network connections can also mitigate the influence of such destructive elements as crime and drug use, as well as pass along information about risk factors and available health services. Families displaced by loss of affordable housing are often bereft of the social insulation that might protect them from high morbidity.

The growth in the number of AIDS cases in these areas is perhaps largely accounted for by migration patterns of drug users and their subsequent risk behaviors. Formerly stable drug-using networks also reestablish themselves in neighboring communities as they are displaced by burnout. Rates of HIV seroprevalence among injection-drug users who had entered drug treatment programs in New York City from 1984 to 1987 averaged 57 percent (DesJarlais 1989). The spread of HIV is facilitated as infected drug users find new needle-sharing partners or engage in unsafe sexual activity with previously uninfected individuals. The increase in heterosexually transmitted cases of AIDS in inner-city areas has been primarily linked to drug use—smokable cocaine (crack), as well as injection drugs.

The spread of HIV disease throughout the Bronx probably was augmented by the destruction of housing in the poorest sections. Curtailment of this spread was made more difficult by the same processes that rent the social fabric of the Bronx. Levels of HIV infection in the Bronx are now among the highest in the nation—a blinded seroprevalence study of U.S. hospitals observed that one in five young men there is infected with HIV. We learn from the story of the South Bronx that not just infectious disease, but homelessness, infant mortality, violence, and substance abuse are unleashed in the wake of urban decay.

The link between fire services and contagious housing destruction is probably Wallace's most important finding, as it allows us to observe the role of the body politic in the maintenance of the integrity of the urban environment. Maintaining populations at relatively high density requires adequate supplies of pure water, removal of waste, and maintenance of housing, among other services. Without these essential services, city residents will suffer from many kinds of discomfort, including rampant spread of such infectious diseases as AIDS. Yet the control of urban service delivery usually lies outside the minority neighborhoods, and often outside the city itself.

For example, New York—like several other major cities—has over the past decade experienced an increased concentration of poverty, particularly among the young, according to new Census Bureau data (Barringer 1992). By 1990 the number of unemployed teenage dropouts, teenage pregnancies, and female-headed single parent families had all increased in states like New York, where economies have shifted from resource-based industries to technology- and service-based ones, thereby eliminating jobs in the unskilled labor market. Census figures also point out the redistribution of poverty among population groups. From 1979 to 1989 the largest proportion of the 4.3 million increase in people living below the poverty line were children. "One in four of new entrants into the ranks of the poor in the 1980s was under 18 years of age; one in twenty-five was 65 or older" (Barringer 1992); an analyst quoted in the article implied that the federally financed safety net is kept intact for politically vocal constituencies, such as the elderly. A hefty portion of the cost of programs and services for the poor has been transferred in the past decade from the federal government to state and local levels of government and to the private sector. Apparently, federal trickle-down economic policies (flawed in conception) have been stymied by recessions, deficits, and other factors. As AIDS becomes more and more a disease borne by environmental and social conditions inherent to poverty, the questions of who shall pay and what shall be paid for become more urgent.

The disenfranchisement of poor communities—their lack of political clout—underlies their vulnerability when decisions are made to cut services to local areas.

Though an isolated, impoverished neighborhood can't pay for all of the costs of sewage, fire extinguishment, police protection, and health care, these services are not out of reach for us as a nation. If cities are to survive, the larger elements of the body politic must be persuaded to commit resources to the task. The development of a larger political agenda that includes the have-nots is a responsibility at both local and national levels.

Coleman A. Young, mayor of Detroit, said that "the only way we can repel those who would repress the Black people, in my opinion, is to consolidate our ranks and reach out to our potential allies" (Thompson and Thompson 1976, iii). Coalition with allies outside of the minority community, he proposed in 1971, was the path to survival in the years to come.

Meanwhile, internal divisions can continue to threaten community integrity. A community mobilization in New Haven, Connecticut, designed to drive prostitutes off the streets made headlines by covering trees and telephone poles with "John of the Week" posters, listing the names of men arrested for soliciting (Associated Press 1992a). That community protest against "outsiders"—described as drug users, prostitutes, pimps, johns—mirrors attempts around the country. Where such protests are successful, the community is able to continue to function; elsewhere, the introduction of drug use and sales into a neighborhood can initiate or accelerate its decline.

The presence of drugs and drug users poses a significant threat to community life, hence the intensity of the efforts to repel them. The repulsion is fueled by the connection between drug use and AIDS. A resident active in the New Haven protests made this connection, saying, "It is a tragedy [to publicize the names of the johns]. It's also tragic for little schoolgirls to have to wait for the school bus next to hookers. It's a tragedy to find used condoms in the sandbox and in the grass where the kids play outside. These are IV-drug users, and the highest risk category for AIDS" (Associated Press 1992a). The association with AIDS appears to underscore the danger these "interlopers" pose to respectable people and their children. On the other hand, it is an example of people pitted against each other: the insiders (mainstream members) attempting to protect their property from dangerous outsiders (subculture members). Such scenarios offer little hope for the solution to urban problems.

Changing Culture in Changing Times

In 1971 Joyce Ladner published *Tomorrow's Tomorrow: The Black Woman,* a book that describes the circumstances governing girls' development to womanhood in an inner-city community. The girls were all poor and from families struggling to survive in spite of their limited opportunities. As described by Ladner, the complex social structure of the family and the community is critical to survival. Families, for the most part, were made up of three generations, and all members of the family, including very young children, contributed to the survival of the family unit. Families also helped each other. Sharing across families occurred within kinship and pseudo-kinship networks. Despite the ever-present stress of poverty and racial oppression, women had hopes that their children would have a better life than they had.

In the culture described by Ladner, girls were socialized in two primary settings: the extended family and the peer group. Because of economic stress on adults in the networks, the peer group often took on more significance than would have been observed in a more middle-class setting. Peers offered comfort, support, advice and companionship. The influence of peers began at a very early age and increased in significance throughout the preadolescent and adolescent years. From these two sources girls were trained in self-sufficiency as well as interdependence, hostility as well as tolerance. In sum, they were prepared to survive in a world that had little concern for their well-being.

These survival skills have been sorely tested in the intervening twenty years. The social connections that Ladner described depended, in large measure, on the physical cohesiveness of the community. In the context of massive physical destruction owing to burn-out of large segments of the housing stock, unenforced public safety measures, and widespread crime and drug use, residents have been forced out or have moved voluntarily. As a result, whole communities have disorganized and dispersed, their members no longer able to interact as they once had.

Two forces in the community Ladner described have emerged with particular salience under these new conditions. First, increasing violence is more and more an important part of women's daily lives. Second, Ladner emphasizes the role and importance of the peer group in the socialization of girls.

In our own research we have observed the impact on women of their involvement in crack cocaine abuse and the violence and trauma that ravage their lives. The chaos and uncertainty created by cyclical experiences with drug use, violence, and disruption of family life are depicted in the story of "Stephanie," a participant in our Women and Crack study. Following is an excerpted narration to illustrate:

> Stephanie's home life was chaotic and abusive, and her adult relationships followed a similar pattern. For example, the father of her fourth child was a man she met through church. As the relationship progressed, he began to beat her:
>
> 'Then he started getting viler and started hitting me and stabbing me, and he broke my ribs with a pipe, and he broke my jaw. . . . He used to drink too. He used to be in a methadone program. And after that . . . my kids [were] taken away, we had a fight, and drugs and all that.'

Helen Gasch and Mindy Thompson Fullilove

During her fifth pregnancy, she learned of the death by overdose of the father of her first two children. Drug dealers took over her apartment and converted it into a "crack spot" (a place where crack is smoked) with strangers coming and going at all hours of the day and night. Her fifth child, now one year old, was exhausted and frightened by this chaotic situation. When Stephanie asked the dealers to leave, they beat her.

'They started hitting me, punching me in my jaw. The other one would slap me. They had turned the light off, and my son was crying . . . After [pause] they kept coming back. . . . He threatened to kill me and my son. So I left.' " (Fullilove 1992, 280)

The emotional scarring is apparent among the women and children caught up in the cycle of urban decay and the deluge of drugs and violence. Ladner reported that "most" of the children she interviewed could relate directly to some form of violence. She was impressed that the children, who were exposed to violence at an early age, had learned some techniques for managing potentially violent situations.

In the 1990s both of these aspects of girls' lives have been reshaped. By most common measures, violence has increased dramatically in the past two decades. Statistics from the Justice Department's National Crime Survey for 1991 reported estimates of 2.6 million completed violent crimes, an increase of 7.9 percent from the level reported in 1990 (Associated Press 1992b). Including attempted violent crimes, the total was 6.4 million for 1991, up 7 percent from 6 million in 1990. Young children are exposed to gunfire at school, in their neighborhoods, and at home. Carol Beck, a high school principal in New York City, reported in 1992 that half of the students in her school had suffered from puncture wounds. Three murders took place in that school during the 1991–92 school year, raising the level of fear and terror to unprecedented heights (testimony at hearings on Violence and Youth, New York State Assembly, January 15, 1992). In the wake of those murders, city and state officials joined forces to declare April 4, 1992, Domestic Disarmament Day.

December 1989

At an HIV Center colloquium, one of the senior researchers—a white man—cautions the group about providing condom education to poor black women who are sexual partners of drug users. "Many of these women have partners who are violent," he says, "and the women may be at risk for violence if they demand that men use condoms. One can only take assertiveness training so far, and then you risk placing these women at real risk of getting beat up." Helen is outraged. "I think you are perpetuating stereotypes in a careless manner," she tells the speaker. It is not true that all black men are violent. But it is true that some are brutal, some are rapists, some are murderers. That they were victimized and now injure others provides no solace to the women injured by them. Like many black women, Helen will continue to ponder the awful tension created by evoking the victimization of black men as a rationale for the victimization of black women. Since the colloquium, Helen has had to rethink her position several times as more and more women encountered in women's shelters and elsewhere in the community have made her realize that the problem of violence against women, though not "owned" by black men, cannot be ignored. Preventing victimization is integral to the strategy for preventing AIDS in women. The struggle against racism ought not be fought at the cost of sexism.

The peer group, which was always an important socializing force, has taken on even greater importance as orphans reappear on the American scene. Parents' deaths from AIDS have contributed to the burgeoning number of orphans, and the crack epidemic has disabled many mothers and fathers so severely that they are unable to provide adequate care for their young. The peer group is no longer simply an adjunct for parents who cannot provide enough support or guidance; it has become the mainstay of social support for children with no parents at all.

Attitudes and beliefs about life are reshaped by these extreme changes. Violence, some forms of which were always tolerated by the community—physical discipline of children, for example—has now become a major force distorting daily life. In 1991 a young man shot another who bumped into him on a subway, signaling that violence had become, at least for some, a solution for every imaginable problem. As violence escalates, its fallout spreads throughout the community. Violence leaves a mark, in the form of mental disorders, physical wounds, bereavement, fear and more violence. The violence affects everyone.

January 1990

Mindy and Bob arrive at the HIV Center, and Mindy continues to study the crack epidemic. But the Columbia University they both knew as doctoral students is not the same. "You can never step into the same river twice." The medical center is drastically different. People get shot in broad daylight in Washington Heights, which some call Cocaine Central. Guards bar every door to the hospital. The armory that once housed track meets now shelters hundreds of homeless men on cold nights. The Audubon Ballroom, formerly the scene of union meetings and salsa dancing, is boarded up. The streets are littered, the buildings have deteriorated. No chance to say goodbye.

Building Community

On behalf of the U.S. Public Health Service Panel on Women, Adolescents and Children with HIV Infection and AIDS, Surgeon General Antonia Novello presented a poster at the Seventh International Conference on AIDS in which she called for the development of "family-centered, community-based, comprehensive care" to meet the needs of children with AIDS and their families. The panel's full report described the developmental, psychosocial, and psychiatric manifestations of HIV infection and AIDS in infants and children, noting that

> many HIV-infected children belong to single-parent families headed by HIV-infected mothers, women who may have limited social support and poor self-esteem, and who may be too ill to care for the child. If no one can assume the parental role, the child may face multiple disruptions in foster homes or institutional settings. Poverty, homelessness, drug abuse, and un-employment often exacerbate the problems associated with caring for seropositive children and their families. Further, the emotional impact of HIV infection and AIDS affects not only the children who are infected with HIV, but also their noninfected siblings. Additional threats to the family structure include multiple deaths, dissolution of the extended family, incar-ceration, additional illness, abandonment, court removal of children from home, and hospitalization of children or their parents. (Novello and Allen 1991, 11)

Such a range of medical and social problems obviously cannot be addressed by isolated or simplistic solutions. Under the surgeon general's leadership, vital policy and funding decisions have been made to support this comprehensive new approach to treatment. What is colloquially referred to as the "Four Cs"—family-centered, community-based, comprehensive care—has been introduced into many programs for people with AIDS and for the prevention of AIDS. These programs are essen-tially community-building interventions. Within the walls of clinics, day-care cen-ters, hospitals, or drug treatment clinics, staff members and clients rebuild the links that allow survival in difficult times and through life-threatening illness. Successful Four Cs projects are now under way in several major cities across the country, including Atlanta, New York, New Orleans, and Seattle. These projects have been federally funded in recent years by the Health Resources and Services Administra-tion (HRSA) through Pediatric AIDS Demonstration Projects.

This model of health care succeeds not just because it integrates multiple services for affected families, but particularly because it builds connections be-tween the disenfranchised and the health care providers. The impersonal clinic system, through which a woman might see a different provider on every visit, is replaced by a "personal physician." The hours of waiting, during which women form transient social connections, are replaced by support groups and classes of all kinds. As one provider observed, "Women may not spend less time getting care, but they get more care for the time they spend" (Dr. C. Healton, personal communica-tion, October 1991). The women's own peer networks offer advice, guidance, and solace.

From these networks emerge natural leaders who have, in many instances, joined clinic staff as peer counselors or outreach workers. Their first-hand experience and their ability to lead strengthen the link between those who want to serve and those who want service. Instead of hostile and alienating encounters with a seemingly uncaring system, women find friends, support, and useful information in these new settings. Although it may seem that this is little more than reinventing the family doctor, successful family-centered, community-based, comprehensive care in fact accomplishes a task at which the health care system has rarely been effective: delivering care across divides of class, race, and culture.

March 1990

 Helen is writing an article, to be published in the *Journal of Negro Education,* on AIDS prevention in the black community. She is writing about years of health education throughout the black and Latin communities of New York City. Yet it is easier to do than to describe. How do you put into words what happens in a group of women—the sudden laughter when you say what everyone is thinking but won't say; the feeling when women share the pain of fighting for relationships that don't seem to work; and all the feelings brought up around condoms. She struggles to describe her belief that these discussions can make women feel strong and can help women do what they have to do to make their relationships safe. But transforming years of experience into a few principles—how is this to be done?

Social and cultural issues must be resolved in delivering the Four Cs. Staff and clients must develop an effective common language, a set of traditions and rituals, a common history, and a shared hope for the future. In fact, within the context of the center, they must develop a common culture. This view of cross-cultural health care may be at odds with the view of some who believe that the care must be offered in the culture of the client. That would require a level of acculturation that is difficult for most people to make. It is improbable that health care professionals would be able to make that level of adaptation. Therefore, the development of a common culture—which is neither that of the clients nor that of the care providers, but something they invent together—is a more efficient solution to the problem of cross-cultural care delivery.

In the development of this common culture, the key actors on the clients' side are women who can verbalize the wants, needs, and desires of the clients to the provider community. On the provider side, the key actors are those who can listen. Through a slow and arduous process these "translators" help all of those who are engaged in the setting to develop the shared culture.

What does this look like? At the Bayview-Hunter's Point Foundation in San Francisco, the acupuncture clinic offered services for people addicted to crack. As the project developed, it included more family members. One young mother was

Helen Gasch and Mindy Thompson Fullilove

eagerly awaiting the birth of her baby. The acupuncture staff worked closely with her to support her efforts to maintain her sobriety. The other clients organized a shower, collecting much-needed baby clothes, diapers, and bottles. After the baby was born—drug-free and healthy—the clinic celebrated with a welcome-home party for the newborn.

April 1991

Helen has hired two community health educators to provide AIDS pre-vention information in Washington Heights, a New York community composed mostly of immigrants from the Dominican Republic. The two educators pre-pare for a presentation in the women's health clinic across the street. One is a Puerto Rican New Yorker who speaks almost no Spanish, and the other is a newly arrived Dominican woman who speaks virtually no English. Helen goes along to observe the presentation. Has she gone too far with this attempt at cultural appropriateness? The presentation is given in "Spanglish" (one has to be of two worlds to fully understand it). The women worked together well, with humor and lots of visuals. The women in the waiting area were indispensable as translators for the others, supplying the elusive phrases that just didn't translate well. Collective education blurs the lines between the educator and the educatee.

In a methadone program in the Bronx, the Four Cs approach means the devel-opment of a Women's Center. One of the activities of the center is a weekly support group. After about a year of meeting, the women in the group began to discuss HIV. One women tentatively revealed that she was HIV-positive, afraid that she would be rejected by the group. Her disclosure emboldened others to reveal their status, and the group members shared grief and hope. Through a video of the group's meetings, the women are able to share their experience with others around the country.

November 1991

Helen is planning an AIDS seminar for women in a New York City prison. "I'm concerned about helping the women who have women lovers to talk in this session," she tells Mindy. "Why not start there? Be aggressive, put it up front." "The women will understand," Mindy says. When Helen checks her plan with the supervisor of the prison, the supervisor agrees. At the session, some of the women are sitting with their lovers. Helen's opening remarks are unex-pected. Most people act "as if" when they come to the prison. By opening the dialogue with remarks that validated love relationships between women and placed these women's concerns about their risk for HIV foremost, Helen is warmly received. Women are eager to talk about sex—sex with men, with women, pleasures, fears, condoms, rubber dams. Whatever—it's important. But Helen violates a prison rule. She attempts to give the women personal "safer sex kits." The women reach for them rapaciously. The guard moves in. "No personal property here," the guard says, and takes them back.

Conclusion

Communities at risk for HIV are those that experienced rapid social change that altered sexual practices or drug use. The social changes parallel cultural changes. In many instances we have witnessed a disintegration of both social and cultural organization. AIDS services cannot solve all of the problems of disintegrating communities. But the services can play a part in rebuilding community through the development of "family-centered, community-based, comprehensive care." Such services help women suffering from HIV disease to connect to each other and to care providers. These connections replace many social connections that are lost or ruptured in the process of community decline.

These links, fostered by the health care system, provide a model for the rebuilding of community that must take place outside of the treatment setting as well. The effective development of such services will depend on the ability of the care providers to welcome and respect the clients who come to their center. Across barriers erected by class, race, and culture, it is difficult to create an atmosphere that conveys a message of acceptance. Yet those centers that succeed are able to offer healing. They become a model for other centers to emulate. We can and must begin to implement the cure—community building—as we deliver care.

14

Caregiving:

A Matriarchal Tradition Continues

B. Joyce Simpson and Ann Williams

My advice to people who take care of women with
HIV: take a little time out to deal with the person, not
just the disease. See what's hurting inside. They say
men are good at holding things in—women are good
at it, I know. Holding that hurt in will kill. Get to that
core, deal with the inner person. If you do that, you'll
deal with the disease. What we need is more personal
medical care, not just medicine.
—Grace Simons

New and improved treatments have changed the natural history of HIV infection and
AIDS from one of episodic, serious illness requiring tertiary care to chronic illness
that frequently can be managed in an outpatient setting. This change has transferred
much of the responsibility for patient care from the hospital to the family. In
populations affected by HIV, home care is provided predominantly by women. And

because AIDS disproportionately affects persons of color, most of these caregivers are minority women.

The caregivers we describe in this chapter are found in families that are affected by HIV infection primarily attributable to injection-drug use and heterosexual transmission. The problems of caregivers are addressed in the context of family constellations, and the caregiving challenges of the HIV-infected mother and the concerns of the kinship caregiver receive special attention. We identify specific issues and offer recommendations.

Slavery, compulsory migration, and educational and income discrimination historically have disrupted families of color. Matriarchal kinship behaviors, however, countered such disruptions by bonding generations of the disenfranchised (Lerner 1972; Stack 1974). In the prosperous years following World War II people of color migrated in large numbers from rural areas of the United States to large urban centers, where abundant job opportunities existed. As in the years following the Civil War, African-American nuclear families became common in American cities.

In the 1990s income disparity between black and white Americans grew as the U.S. economy slipped into recession. Blacks and Hispanics born since the 1950s experienced large-scale unemployment and underemployment as jobs were lost, particularly in the unskilled and urban sectors. Unlike their parents, these young men and women were unable to secure legitimate employment, and, insidiously, patterns of dependency developed. Men stayed with their parents into adulthood. Women with children, meanwhile, were able to secure entitlements—most often Aid for Dependent Children and Medicaid health insurance—that permitted more emancipated lives. Such arrangements, however, were extremely detrimental to the concept of the nuclear family. Implicit in the receipt of public funds is the agreement that the father of the children never reside with the family. Given such policies and the absence of minority men from the urban setting as a result of incarceration or untimely death from drug abuse, violence, or AIDS, the need for matriarchal tradition intensified (Gross 1989; Finnegan 1990). Such a matriarchal system of social organization is reflected in specific AIDS populations (Gross 1989).

At Yale-New Haven Hospital, for example, fewer than 5 percent of the 300 children born to HIV-infected mothers have their biological father in the home. In only one family in the entire cohort is there a single male head-of-household caregiver (Yale-New Haven Hospital 1992). According to a woman whose two grandchildren, nephew, and daughter-in-law died of AIDS and who now cares for her son and grandson, who are living with AIDS: "When you're dealing drugs and have plenty of money, you have lots of friends, but when you're sick and dying from AIDS, all you have is your mother."

The situation is similar in other large East Coast cities, including New York, Newark, and Washington, D.C. The challenge is to effectively promote family integrity and support the caregiving efforts of both HIV-infected mothers and the kinship foster parents who will provide care after the mother dies.

The Infected Mother

Because more than 99 percent of women with AIDS are heterosexual (Chu 1990) and usually of childbearing age, the needs of many HIV-infected women are inextricably linked to motherhood and family responsibilities. Data from the Centers for Disease Control and Prevention suggest that up to 125,000 American women of childbearing age may be HIV-infected (CDC 1991). If each woman gives birth to two children (on average), at least 250,000 dependent children, many of them HIV-infected, will complicate efforts to meet the needs of infected women. Most women with HIV are caregivers first and patients second.

Traditionally, socially disenfranchised minority women and children in the United States have been disproportionately affected by poverty (Simon 1989). Because about three-quarters of HIV-positive women and children are black or Latina, poverty has a significant impact on the well-being of infected families (Ellerbrock et al. 1991). Most HIV-infected mothers are young, poorly educated, and have few job skills. Obtaining access to entitlement programs, health services, housing, food, and transportation frequently is difficult. For many families, physical and emotional comforts are few, and the pain of poverty exacerbates as illness progresses (West 1988).

> I checked out of the hospital as soon as I could, even though they said I could have bled out. They want me to come in for more tests, but what am I supposed to do with the baby? Do they ever let you bring a baby in with you?
> —Female patient, Yale–New Haven Hospital

The burden of caregiving often delays access to care for HIV-infected women. Such mundane problems as the availability and cost of babysitting and transportation frequently prevent women from obtaining the medical and emotional support they need. Women are reluctant to ask for help from family and friends; a common fear expressed is that they will be questioned about where they're going. Although many women have extended family nearby, the fear of disclosure and rejection prevents them from reaching out for support.

Family Support

Families respond to HIV infection in complex ways. Initial responses often change as illness progresses and as the woman and her family struggle, separately or together, to confront it. For most women with AIDS and HIV-infected children, relationships with their family are complicated by a history of illicit drug use.

A common initial family response to the woman with AIDS is anger at the impending loss of their daughter. This may be compounded by anger at her lifestyle; at her friends, whom they may hold responsible for both the drug use and the HIV infection; and at the health care system, particularly the drug treatment system which has failed to save her. Anger is often driven by guilt. Parents may feel that they have contributed to their daughter's high-risk lifestyle, to her drug use or that of her partner. Well-intentioned and appropriate attempts to set boundaries around drug use in the home may have led to periods of estrangement for which the family now feels responsible. This guilt can lead to enabling behavior on the part of the family if the HIV-infected woman continues or resumes her drug use. It becomes increasingly difficult to limit drug use if the user is a family member dying of AIDS.

Impact of Substance Abuse

Illicit drug use is a major influence in the lives of most HIV-infected women in the United States. Cumulatively, half of the women with AIDS reported to the Centers for Disease Control and Prevention have a personal history of injection-drug use (CDC 1993). An additional 21 percent do not have a personal history of drug injection but are the sexual partners of men who do. Thus, the lives of at least 70 percent of women with AIDS in the United States have been touched by drug use.

As is true for male injection-drug users, the risk of HIV infection for women who inject drugs is increased as they frequent shooting galleries, increase the number of injections, and share injection equipment. Cocaine use is associated with increased risk of HIV among women, whether or not the drug is injected. Women who smoke crack cocaine may be at increased risk for HIV infection as a result of such behaviors as exchanging sex for drugs or money with multiple anonymous partners who are themselves at risk for HIV through injection-drug use. Crack is of particular concern because its use is growing rapidly among younger inner-city women.

Women who use drugs often have high levels of anxiety and depression. They may feel that they have little control over their drug use or their lives. Society's attitude toward and perceptions of addicted women are generally negative, and women who use drugs have limited support networks or backing from male partners. They frequently hold traditional beliefs about sex-role behaviors and see themselves as failures in maintaining these standards.

Often estranged from other family members because of disruptive behavior associated with drug use, women with HIV infection find relationships with their children are frequently the most important connections in their lives. They are deeply involved with and concerned about their children; often their children are the only people with whom they spend significant time. Although they may have low self-esteem, they can take pride in being good mothers. A woman who takes good care of her children despite her drug habit is respected in the subculture of drug use. The AIDS epidemic attacks women in this very vulnerable area: overwhelming guilt at having transmitted HIV infection to their children undermines their self-esteem and compromises their ability to seek appropriate health care for themselves.

As discussed in previous chapters, many women with HIV infection present to the health care system when their disease is at an advanced stage. For example, 60 percent of women enrolled in a medical utilization study at Yale–New Haven Hospital had a CD4+ cell count of 200 cells/mm^3 or less on their first visit to an HIV specialist (Ickovics 1991). It seems most likely that the differences that have been observed reflect the impact of social discrimination on the availability of primary health-care services, as well as a delay in seeking care. Women put off initiating evaluation of their own HIV disease to meet the obligations of family caregiving. Initial care and continuing compliance with recommended medical regimens is also influenced by drug dependence and activity. A woman who is injecting cocaine daily is unlikely to make attendance at a clinic her first priority.

Access to care differs for black and white Americans, and the HIV epidemic is growing most rapidly among those populations of childbearing women who have not been served effectively by the health care system. Numerous psychosocial and economic obstacles may prevent women from seeking care. Many poor women with HIV infection encounter health care providers only regarding family planning, childbirth, and pediatric concerns. It is the experience of many clinicians that women will go to great lengths to obtain care for their children but fail to do so for themselves.

Hospitalizations, frequent clinic visits, and complicated medical regimens for both mother and children increase family stress. The situation becomes more diffi-cult because of the mother's physical and, perhaps, mental deterioration. The quality of family life suffers when the caregiving demands result in chronic fatigue. Feelings of hopelessness can progress into severe depression and even inertia as family members become sick and die (Septimus 1989).

The Kinship Caregiver

Although the majority of caregivers are biological parents, others are adoptive or foster parents. A number of foster parents function under the auspices of Children's Social Services while others care for children from their extended family without any special societal support. The kinship foster parent may be a grandparent, aunt, or older sister who will most likely learn of the HIV diagnosis concurrent with the request to become a foster parent. With little time to ponder the situation and the need urgent and grave, "the immediate impulse of many families is to take in the kids, but as difficulties increase over time, the family may need to rethink their decisions" (personal communication to B. Joyce Simpson from Carol Levine of the Orphan Project, New York City, April 1992).

> I'm not telling my mother about the HIV yet. I'm hoping that by the time I need her to take care of us she will love the baby so much that she won't put us out.

Kinship foster parents of children with HIV experience many difficulties. Interventions that have proved successful in kinship situations involving other sick children—children with cancer, for example—consistently fail to meet the needs of the caretakers of children with HIV. The social stigma of the disease, the lack of resources, multiple infections in a single family, old age, fatigue, and feelings of hopelessness contribute to family difficulties. Some extended families may reject outright any responsibility for infected children. And yet a small but remarkable group of kinship foster parents is committed to caring for their children no matter how difficult. This group has special support needs.[1]

Successful kinship foster parents are self-reliant and competent, display innovative coping skills, find meaning in their lives, and often have strong spiritual beliefs. Such attributes are the components of resiliency (Wagnild 1990). These remarkable caregivers are able to withstand the crises ahead—the losses, grief, isolation, poverty, and discrimination.

The sense of irreconcilable loss—not only of the children's parents to drugs or death, but also of the natural evolution of generational relationships that will never be—is difficult for most caregivers. They expected their relationship with the youngsters to be primarily social, occasional, and distanced. For some, the adjustment to full-time responsibility for the children remains unresolved, and mourning continues for the loss of personal hopes, dreams, and autonomy.

Grief is often cumulative and unrelenting, as family and friends successively succumb to AIDS. Once they have experienced the torment of terminal AIDS, caregivers unanimously voice trepidation as they anticipate the deaths of the children. Many use denial to cope with their grief.

Most caregivers function in isolation. Negative experiences following disclosure of HIV infection leads to excessive secretiveness and mistrust of the few community supports available to them. Rejection by lifetime friends is a painful

---

[1] The following discussion is based on a qualitative study undertaken to better understand the issues of foster care and to identify factors that might explain why these parents choose to do what few other extended families are able to do. B. Joyce Simpson interviewed eleven foster parents, eight black and three white; their ages ranged from fifty to seventy-two (Simpson 1991). Contact with study subjects was made through the Pediatric AIDS Clinic at Yale–New Haven Hospital in New Haven, Connecticut—a city where one out of every forty-two women giving birth is HIV-positive (Connecticut DOHS 1991).

reality. Caregivers often live in constant fear of disclosure and loss of the support of close friends or neighbors. There is frequently an internal conflict between the desire for community support and the fear of potential stigmatization. This self-imposed isolation enhances feelings of helplessness, hopelessness, and depression.

> My next door neighbor helps me a lot. She walks Michael to school in the morning and lets me use her washing machine. I know if she ever found out about his AIDS she would be scared stiff. I'd probably lose a good friend.
> —An elderly grandmother

Self-esteem among caregivers is generally high, but most also experience feelings of shame, failure, and guilt when considering the drug abuse or HIV infection within the extended family. States one great-grandmother, "I came to New Haven newly married. We had a good life, bought a house and a boat, and all our children were college-educated. Drugs and AIDS changed everything. Now I have a daughter, a granddaughter, and a great-grandson with AIDS. It is better my husband is dead and cannot see what has happened. I am afraid one day my great-granddaughter will be the sole survivor in this family. It's sad; we came here with such high hopes." One young woman says, "I had a terrible childhood. My mother was big into drugs. I brought myself up, got a college education, but I just couldn't escape. I had to come back to care for my mother when she got AIDS—she was blind and totally demented during the final months. After my mother died, the doctor recommended HIV testing my six-year-old sister, even though she had never been sick. When her test came back positive, I almost went crazy, but I have to persevere. What choice do I have?"

These families are easy targets for discrimination, an injustice that is often tolerated without complaint (Dalton and Burris 1987). Lacking advocates, they accept a level of humiliation and pain inflicted by an ignorant and fearful society that would not be tolerated by a more politically empowered group.

> Even though we had always been honest with the day-care center about her HIV infection, all of a sudden they wanted her out. They went so far as to include her name and HIV status in letters that they sent to several other day-care centers in town "warning" them that we might soon be applying. We consulted a civil liberties lawyer and were determined to fight back until the day-care people threatened to make our child take the stand. We just could not allow that and so we dropped the case.
> —A kinship foster parent

There are significant differences in the income and medical insurance coverage between kinship foster parents who are supported by Children's Social Services and those families assisted by the probate court system. Social Services-assisted foster parents frequently receive a generous monthly payment plus Title 19 medical insurance for the child, even when he or she is adopted. Children adopted through the probate court system, however, become the sole financial responsibility of the new parents.

The social circumstances of most potential kinship foster parents often reflect those of the HIV-exposed children—that is, primarily low-income with few assets or resources. For this group, the problems lie not in the loss of health insurance and assets experienced by upper-class kinship foster parents, but, rather, in their inability to finance the immediate needs of the newly extended family. The extraordinary and cumulative transitional costs may include the expense of relocating to accommodate and support the surviving children; funeral and burial fees for the deceased parent; probate fees to obtain legal guardianship of each child; and delays of two or three months in the transfer of welfare benefits from the deceased mother to the new parent. In fact, many kinship foster parents experience a lengthy financial crisis as a direct consequence of their child-care commitment. It is unknown how many children may have become wards of the state because of such circumstances. The American Academy of Pediatrics (1989) recognizes this problem: "The burden of caring for a sick child should not be compounded by the threat of financial hardship."

It is common for potential kinship foster parents to resist involvement by Children's Social Services, despite the financial benefits of such an alliance. These agencies are perceived as a threat to the caretaker's autonomy. Foster parents resent any government agency judging their suitability to care for their own kin. The home inspection, fingerprinting, physical examination, and questions are intolerable to some, especially during times of bereavement. Older adults with health problems may be concerned that the state will find them ineligible and remove the children from the home. For all these reasons it is not unusual to find informal foster care occurring, with family members receiving no support monies for extended period of time.

Foster parents are frequently physically exhausted from the demands of caring for their young charges. "My daughter, Sandi, is mad at me, and so is the hospital social worker, but I just couldn't bring her home. I already have her kids, and little Robert wears me out. He needs so much care and twelve doses of medicine every day. It all makes me feel so bad. She's down in North Carolina with my mother now, and they'll manage somehow."

Respite

For many caregivers, the availability of periodic or emergency home-based respite assistance reduces anxiety, stress, and fatigue. Under this arrangement, the family identifies a relative, friend, or neighbor who is paid to provide services that give the primary caregiver relief from the relentless demands of home care. Such state agencies as the Department of Human Resources and local community agencies set aside funds each year for such purposes, though these funds are quickly exhausted.

Reimbursed respite services are supervised in many states by the Department of Human Resources or such providers as the Visiting Nurse Agency or hospice programs. The Connecticut Hospice in Branford, for example, is extending its pediatric home care to an inpatient phase that will offer respite along with terminal care.

Respite support frequently allows a child to remain in a home setting, avoiding costly hospitalizations that are socially driven rather than medically necessary; placing children even temporarily in Children's Social Services foster care is costly and disrupts the child's physical and psychosocial well-being. Many caregivers fear that their exhaustion may be construed as lack of commitment, and they may entertain anxiety that, once placed, their children may not be returned. Trusting relationships and financial supports must be in place if the respite needs of caregivers are to be met.

Despite the myriad difficulties they encounter, kinship foster parents have an admirable capacity to persevere. With great courage they protect and care for their children, providing a stable life at home and unconditional love. They deserve respect for being able to do what so few others are able to do: hold together a young family under the most adverse conditions.

Identification of Foster Caretaker Issues and Recommendations

State and federal agencies, the courts, private enterprises, service providers, and volunteer organizations are not adequately addressing the wide range of difficulties met by families with HIV.

• Medical insurance is lacking for HIV-infected children who do not meet the criteria for Medicaid Title 19 coverage *and* have been denied private medical insurance because of their preexisting condition.

• There is a lack of knowledge in the general community regarding the transmission of AIDS that results in overt rejection and ostracism or subtle discrimination. Such problems have been encountered in churches, pediatric offices, day-care programs, schools, and hospitals.

• There is a lack of early interventions by trained professionals (social workers, psychologists) to help families plan for the adjustments that illness and death will bring.

• Social service agencies are sometimes seen as representing institutional care, so there is a lack of agency support for family-centered care.

• There is a lack of free legal aid to assist families in making wills and designating guardianship.

• The lack of housing assistance for kinship caregivers results in inadequate or unsafe housing. Relocation frequently results in isolation from existing sources of support.

• Community AIDS projects fail to provide culturally sensitive support to minority women, children, and their extended families.

• There is a lack of population-specific statistical projections regarding the extent of the AIDS epidemic.

• Knowledge is lacking concerning the number of orphans cared for by social services that might have remained in extended family care.

• The lack of AIDS antidiscrimination laws contributes to feelings of powerlessness and vulnerability.

The systems identified above should be made aware of the difficulties experienced by families affected by HIV infection. Each system must take responsibility for its own response and develop strategies that work well within the existing organizational structure. Rather than develop policy specifically for children with HIV infection, changes should be made based on existing disability laws and statutes. The following recommendations are in direct response to the problems discussed in the previous sections.

• All HIV-infected children should be eligible for Medicaid Title 19 coverage regardless of family income.

• Aid For Dependent Children funds should be supplemented when a child with HIV infection is placed in kinship foster care.

• All HIV-infected children should be considered medically disabled and therefore eligible for Supplemental Security Income.

• The probate court system should be made aware that the adoption of an HIV-infected child may result in the loss of entitlements and medical insurance and should recommend legal guardianship as preferable to adoption.

• Public legal services should assist families in writing wills and designating guardians for their children.

• The Department of Human Resources should fund home health aides and respite care for parents and kinship foster parents.

• AIDS projects should provide culturally sensitive psychological support services for women, children, and extended family members.

• AIDS education efforts should be intensified so that a knowledgeable public will support families with HIV infection.

• The CDC should continue to provide accurate information and specific projections about the course of the epidemic.

• Courses on AIDS should be included in every medical and nursing school curriculum, with a focus on treating the entire family.

• Federal and state service grants for AIDS internships should be made available to physicians, nurse-practitioners, physician's assistants, medical fellows, registered nurses, social workers, and registered dietitians in areas with a high prevalence of AIDS.

• Direct federal and state service grants or supplemental Medicaid reimbursement should be awarded to institutions that treat people with AIDS, especially those institutions that are absorbing large debts by caring for people with inadequate insurance.

• All institutions should develop an AIDS policy before HIV-infected individuals enter their system. Such policy might address infection control, the individual's right to privacy, and job protection.

• Specific AIDS antidiscrimination legislation concerning housing, employment, and health insurance should be adopted in all states.

• Medical care providers who refuse to treat people with AIDS and HIV infection should be censured by their professional associations and licensing boards.

• Social service agencies should begin planning immediately for the large numbers of children who will be orphaned by the epidemic.

• The related issues of homelessness and inadequate housing that are critical for individuals and families with AIDS should be addressed immediately.

• Culturally sensitive risk-reduction education should be targeted to areas of high prevalence to reduce new cases of HIV infection.

Summary

The number of children likely to be orphaned by the AIDS epidemic in the United States alone is estimated to reach as high as 125,000 by the year 2000 (Michaels and Levine 1992). Thousands of HIV-infected (and HIV-negative) children will survive their parents. Should society fail to promote and support family integrity, the burden of caring for the orphans will likely fall squarely to social services. An expanded system of foster homes and residences may be adequate in the short-term, but the reemergence of large-scale orphanages is not unthinkable. Not only would social services be overwhelmed by the placement needs of large numbers of orphans, but the cost to the taxpayer would be tremendous. Such operational and financial concerns, however, fail to take into consideration the emotional impact of separating young survivors from their extended family at a time of bereavement and loss. If society is to avoid the specter of AIDS orphanages and further disruption of children's lives, then potential kinship foster systems must be adequately supported.

The number of extended families choosing to take responsibility for children orphaned by the AIDS epidemic is small at present. But should the recommendations made here be adopted, a far greater proportion of orphans are likely to remain in the care of the extended family. These changes and adjustments are not extreme.

Much progress may occur once systems become aware of the difficulties to which they inadvertently contribute. As awareness of the issues grows, it is expected that a compassionate response that will support parents and promote kinship foster care will be forthcoming, bringing with it a better quality of life for the families and youngest survivors of the AIDS epidemic.

15

Optimizing the Delivery of Health and Social Services:

Case Study of a Model

Ann Sunderland and Susan Holman

I first found out I was positive after I got pregnant. I wasn't sure how people and doctors were going to react, but they don't treat me any differently than before. That was my second big relief. The first was telling my family. I couldn't keep it to myself.

I told my thirteen- to fourteen-year-old cousins because they're trying to sow their wild oats. I think they won't change, though, till they see me sick. The youngest one—nine years old—came to me and said, "Just cause you have [HIV] doesn't mean you'll get AIDS." These younger ones keep surprising me.

Some family members wanted me to get an abortion when they found out. It took a lot in me to sit down and think about it. Am I heartless to bring a child into the world to die? . . . Hopefully, I'll have the strength to deal with it if she does

> get sick. I'm hoping that if I take care of myself it'll be okay
> for my baby. Can't hurt me for hoping.
> —"Cheryl Smith"

When discussing women with HIV, one is all too often talking about a family with this disease, as partners and offspring also may be infected. One cannot simply address the needs of a woman alone but must also address those of her family (biological family and family of choice). Often, members of the extended family, such as an aunt or uncle, are also infected. The family itself can vary from the traditional nuclear unit to more complex families with children from different relationships and many generations to families separated by immigration or incarceration. Each woman's situation and needs are unique and must be addressed as such.

A composite portrait of the family affected by HIV must reflect the influence of poverty, racial or ethnic minority status, and low socioeconomic status stemming from discrimination, drug abuse, and a host of other factors. Added to this already devastating list is the impact of current fiscal difficulties and cuts in often overloaded health care and social service systems. Bear in mind, however, that HIV infection is an equal opportunity disease, afflicting gay women and straight women, women of means, and women of all races.

In the preceding chapters authors have outlined the requirements of women with HIV and how those needs must be met. Most women have multiple needs that require integration of services. In this chapter we describe a model for service delivery that is in place in an urban medical setting. Case management, which is critical to this model, is detailed subsequently.

Case Study of an Interdisciplinary Model

The setting for this model is a health care center composed of a state medical school and hospital (State University of New York Health Science Center) affiliated with a city hospital (Kings County Hospital Center). The facilities are across the street from each other in central Brooklyn, New York. The overall HIV seroprevalence rate of parturient women in Brooklyn is 1.2 percent; the seroprevalence rate among women of childbearing age residing in the SUNY Health Science Center/Kings County Hospital catchment area is greater than 1.6 percent (Novick et al. 1991).

In 1985 a longitudinal National Institutes of Health study of perinatal HIV transmission was begun. The goals of the study were to determine the rate of transmission of HIV from infected women to their offspring, the natural history of the disease in children, and the effects of HIV on pregnancy and of pregnancy on HIV infection. The study enrolled patients until early 1991, and followup continued into 1993. More than 1,500 pregnant women were approached and offered HIV counseling, and more than 1,000 women were tested; 145 infected women, along with their matched seronegative controls, were enrolled in the study.

The SUNY/KCH study involved providing outreach, HIV testing and counseling, and physical assessment, as well as collecting serologic and other clinical specimens. Data were collected periodically from HIV-positive and HIV-negative pregnant women by means of a questionnaire covering demographic, health, drug, reproductive, and partner information. Periodic followup postpartum examinations included brief physical assessment, interval health history, and repeat blood tests as drawn during pregnancy. The study provided full longitudinal followup of all children, including pediatric care and neurodevelopmental assessments from birth through four years of age. Additionally, all children born to HIV-infected mothers were followed through age six.

The service delivery model was developed to meet the goals of the study and to provide access to care needed by the patients. Outreach was conducted in several clinics, including general obstetrical clinics and a special clinic in a drug treatment center, and through referrals from other hospitals and clinics. New patients in the clinics were approached by study staff and offered enrollment in the study. They could decline or accept the study at any time during their prenatal care, and the care they received was not dependent on enrollment in the study. Patients who chose to enroll in the study were guaranteed confidentiality: test results were not recorded in hospital charts and could not be revealed to any provider without the written consent of the patient. Patients were encouraged to inform their health care and drug treatment providers of their HIV status, however, and the consequences were discussed with them. Patients in the study received a transportation stipend at each study visit.

Staffing

At the height of enrollment the study staff consisted of two nurse-practitioners specializing in adult medicine and women's health, one registered nurse, one physician's assistant, two social workers (an MSW and a BSW), and two physicians. Several staff members had public health degrees. Additionally, a pediatrician specializing in infectious diseases provided care for the children in the study, and an obstetrician specializing in maternal-fetal medicine oversaw the obstetrical component of care. The principal investigator on site was an infectious-disease specialist. Three staff members were Haitians who spoke Creole, two were native speakers of Spanish, and three were conversant in Spanish as well. Other team members had varying degrees of familiarity with these languages.

Training and support for the staff members were ongoing. Everyone received training in counseling and testing as it became available and attended workshops and seminars on the medical and psychosocial aspects of HIV. From the study's inception, case conferences were held weekly to address problems with patients, methods for assistance, staff reactions, and other events of the week. After three years staff members began to participate in a support group run by outside facilitators to address issues that accompany working in this field.

Service Model for Testing

Patients received extensive pre-test counseling that included information about HIV infection, testing, implications for pregnancy, modes and prevention of transmission, personal risk, possibility of positive test results, possible psychological impact, and support mechanisms.

Post-test counseling for all patients was done in person. Whenever possible, two staff members were present when counseling women who tested HIV-positive to provide a support person—because a patient often will tune out the bearer of bad news—and to provide support for the staff.

Post-test counseling for positive women began before the actual counseling session with a staff discussion of implications for the particular patient, assessment of which staff member would be the most appropriate informant, and plans to deal with likely reactions. Test results were given in person, and the length of the counseling sessions varied with the patient. All sessions ended with the patient formulating a plan for informing others and accessing support mechanisms. Followup sessions were scheduled, and post-test counseling remained an ongoing matter for most patients. Partners (sexual, drug) were offered testing, as were other children in the family. For more detail on the counseling process and content used at SUNY see Holman et al. (1989).

Study Protocol

Study visits occurred several times during prenatal care, though study staff was present or available during all other regular prenatal visits. Women who chose to terminate a pregnancy were followed in the same manner as postpartum women. Followup care of the women included monitoring of symptoms and immune status and exams required for data collection (including pelvic exams). With the patient's permission, all of the information was transmitted to the primary-care providers; study and clinic staff worked closely together.

Staff members visited the woman and her baby in the hospital soon after the birth and obtained information from labor and delivery personnel, as well as from neonatal records. The study provided comprehensive well-baby care for all children and monitored for signs and symptoms of HIV disease, offering referrals to pediatric HIV clinics when appropriate. Children were enrolled in either the study clinic or the drug treatment pediatric clinic, depending on where they received their

Ann Sunderland and Susan Holman

Figure 15.1 Service System, SUNY Health Science Center

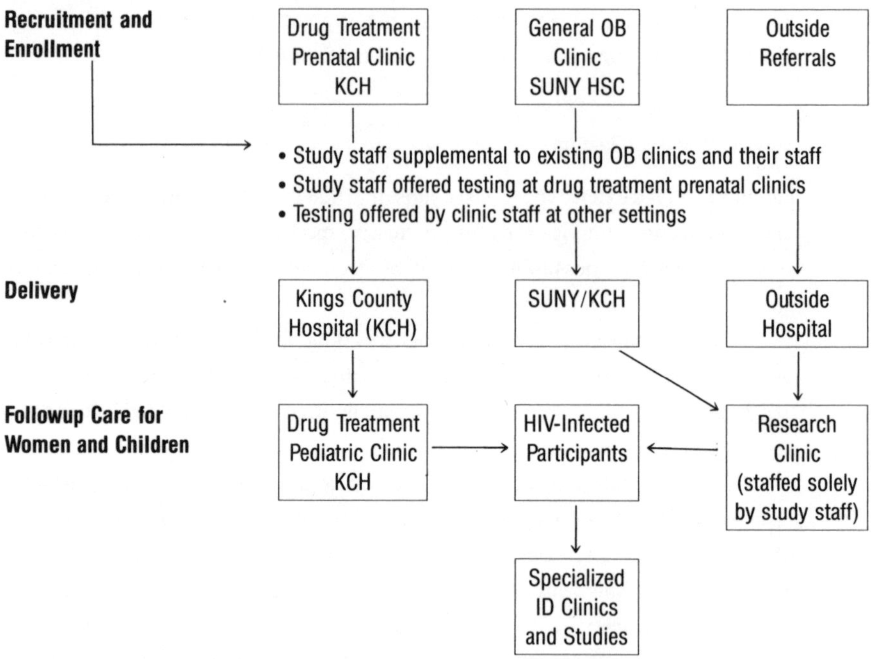

Source: Authors 1992.

prenatal care. Staff members ran the study clinic based in a special research unit and supplemented staff in the drug treatment pediatric clinic (see figure 15.1).

Coordinating Care

Coordination of care for the patient can be divided into three separate yet related groups: clinical care, psychosocial support, and research involvement.

Clinical Care Obstetrical and gynecological care, abortion services, HIV care, treatment for sexually transmitted diseases, and general medical care were all part of clinical care. Because a women entered the study while pregnant, services were initially concentrated on obstetrical and HIV care. We encountered "turf" difficulties with obstetrical services regarding provision of HIV treatment and with infectious-disease services that resisted treatment of pregnant women. Establishing links with both services and designating physicians in each clinic who could consult with the others became important. This became much more of an issue as such treatments as AZT and Pneumocystis carinii pneumonia (PCP) prophylaxis became available to patients with HIV. In our setting, the pregnant woman usually received care from her obstetrician, using the infectious-disease services only for treatment that was unavailable in obstetrics, namely aerosolized pentamidine.

Once the woman delivered she was enrolled in the infectious-disease clinic if she chose. Many asymptomatic women opted to use the monitoring we provided as their primary HIV care and planned to enroll in the HIV clinic only when treatment would be an option. When the study began, there were no treatments available except for opportunistic infections; as options increased, more women chose to enroll in HIV clinics. Women who were already enrolled in an HIV clinic and who became pregnant could, at the discretion of their care provider, continue to receive care in that clinic or have it provided temporarily by the obstetricians.

Related clinical needs also were dealt with, including drug treatment, abortion, tubal ligation, dental, and alternative therapies. Drug treatment services included inpatient detoxification, long-term residential treatment, and a range of outpatient services, including methadone maintenance and drug-free programs. As noted, Kings County Hospital had inpatient drug and alcohol detoxification services, outpatient methadone maintenance, and drug-free programs with a special program focusing on the needs of the pregnant woman. Knowledge of existing programs was essential to link clients with appropriate drug treatment programs. Additional difficulties were encountered in trying to find other programs that accepted pregnant women or women with HIV (see Chavkin 1990). This also was true for locating abortion services.

Because SUNY is a traditional medical center, few alternative or experimental treatments were offered outside of research protocols. (One exception was acupuncture for crack detoxification and other drug treatment.) Many patients were eager to avail themselves of other approaches and appreciated referrals to sites that provided these services. Whenever the patient allowed, study staff were in close contact with the other providers to ensure coordination of care and to avoid duplication of services.

Research Protocols Our involvement was research based, but research was not often the priority of the patient. It was important to be flexible in obtaining data and specimens, particularly with venipuncture. Patients did not want to provide any more blood samples than necessary; to accommodate this we would have the clinic phlebotomists draw extra tubes for us or we would draw the clinically required specimens ourselves, along with the research samples. Thus, close coordination with primary-care providers was necessary. For patients who had complicated care regimens and received services from several clinics, coordination of care often meant accompanying the patient to the various procedures (for example, X-ray and sonography) and indicating to clinic staff what was necessary. Often clinics were unused to seeing pregnant or HIV-infected women, and the intervention by study staff members prevented patients from being re-referred or denied services.

As for many HIV-infected individuals, the only way for our patients to obtain experimental drugs was by entering a research protocol. Most recently, women have been allowed to participate in NIH Clinical Trial 076, which offers AZT late in pregnancy and to the newborn for a specified period to assess safety and transmission interference. Women are also eligible for Women's AIDS Cohort Study (WACS), a newly initiated longitudinal study of the natural history of HIV infection in women funded by the NIH. These studies are available at our site, as is a corollary maternal transmission study, and it is possible that a woman could be enrolled in all four studies. This does not take into account other trials that may be available to the women in the primary HIV clinic or protocols that are offered at different sites. Several women were enrolled in studies conducted at other hospitals and research centers, as were some of the children, including some who went to the NIH for treatment. It was important to be aware of existing protocols and to inform patients of these options, and many did ask for this information.

A major problem of multiple studies is duplication of data, which is further complicated by confidentiality agreements. Multiple release forms were required of patients to allow the transfer of information to the various sites of research and clinical care. We found it critical that staff members be aware of other studies, and study coordinators met with on-site principal investigators weekly throughout the study. Coordination of care became difficult when it was not clear to the patient, or even to the staff, who would be the primary care provider. Moreover, sometimes patients encouraged this duplication of services.

For these women research often provided enhanced services: access to a particular medication, consistency in staffing, more staff available to the patient, stipends toward child care or transportation, and, for some, a sense of making a contribution by helping to further knowledge. Drawbacks to participation included possible public identification of HIV infection and potential stigmatization, the possibility of subtle or overt coercion through offers of monetary compensation or better care, as well as the standard risks of participating in experimental drug protocols. Participation also often necessitated more frequent and longer visits for the patient, which can be especially difficult for working women or women with children at home. Care also became fragmented for women with older children, as those children were not eligible for pediatric care from us and were seen in other clinics. Patients may also suffer when the study ends and they no longer receive the enhanced services that may have been provided to them.

Psychosocial Support A large part of the effort to keep patients in a research protocol involved the provision of psychosocial services. Our team addressed a range of services for patients and their families. This required extensive knowledge of community services and public service systems. The team assessed needs with the patient and provided education regarding HIV and medical issues. Short-term counseling was also provided around a host of issues (relationships, battering, drug use), which often prepared the patient for referral to comprehensive counseling and related services. These issues were addressed on a crisis intervention basis, though our relationship with the patients did allow us to continue to work with them on some of the issues.

Another component of the services we provided was the distribution of material goods. Condoms and spermicides were dispensed to the patients. Items also included standard HIV patient literature, the transportation stipend, lunch, and a copy of a serial videotape of their child from the neurodevelopmental assessments. We also provided diapers and formula in emergencies, and all women received a handmade crib quilt or other gift when their baby was born.

Most referrals were provided for concrete services, such as housing (emergency and permanent), transportation, furniture, telephone service, and food and clothing; government entitlements, such as public assistance, Medicaid, food stamps, heat subsidies, and disability benefits; recreational activities, such as trips and parties; counseling services for individuals, couples, families, and groups; legal services, such as assigning power of attorney, drafting living wills, and planning for guardianship; medical care for family members; and other services, such as job training, respite care, assistance with immigration procedures, home care, child care, schooling, and early intervention programs.

In addition, group counseling was offered on site for HIV-infected adults, including Latinas and Haitians, for children with infected family members, and for caregivers of HIV-infected children. Study staff members were leaders in several such groups and found the service to be especially helpful in bolstering the psychological well-being of the patients. These groups also became a source of concrete help for the patients, who made friends and began to help each other with child care, information sharing, and even housing. Several members became coleaders for other groups begun on site.

It was important to have a good liaison with the foster care system, not only to monitor children who were placed in foster care at birth, but also to assist the biological mother with visitation, and to provide information about her child. Additionally, patients often had other children in foster care and were grateful for help in regaining custody. It occasionally was necessary to notify the authorities of possible abuse and neglect, and it was important to maintain a relationship with the workers about the disposition of the case. Our consent allowed disclosure only in the event that the child would be placed in foster care, and this greatly enhanced our followup and ability to meet research goals.

Our approach to the patient was nonjudgmental, and the only behavior that was unacceptable and resulted in ejection from the study was serious threat of physical harm to the staff members. Only one patient was so discharged. It was important for staff members to remain available to the patient even if the patient was not compliant with the study protocol. Patients often returned to seek staff help with medical or psychosocial problems and then were also willing to resume study compliance.

Psychological issues that were dealt with often stemmed from reactions to learning HIV status; they included guilt, denial, anger, and shame, as well as feelings about death and dying. Many women suffered from low self-esteem. Much of the counseling was focused on empowering the woman by not holding past actions against her and by emphasizing her coping skills and achievements. Family and romantic relationships, as well as general interpersonal skills, were also worked on with many patients.

Our experience, similar to that of other providers (Williams 1990; Anastos and Palleja 1991) showed that many women were best engaged by addressing their concerns about their children. These women grew more able to express their own issues and deal with them. Because of mistrust of the medical setting and the often extreme pressures exerted on the women, it was important for staff members to be able to handle a woman who was acting out or appeared to be out of control and to continue to work with her. It was also important to recognize when a patient's behavior was influenced by drugs or alcohol. On several occasions we found it helpful to have an understanding of psychiatric disorders, and we consulted with psychiatrists when patients exhibited signs of dementia or preexisting psychiatric disorders.

It is critical that the participant in any study-based model of HIV care feel she benefits from participation. For many who are wary of research, the medical profession, or the institution, this benefit can take the form of assistance in some concrete manner, such as help in filling out an application, intervention with a public entitlement problem, or provision of translation. This helps the patients form a stronger relationship with the staff. Many patients lacked the skills to control their lives as much as they wanted to. Thus, much of our supportive counseling was done with the goal of empowering the woman. Support group services were especially helpful with empowerment issues.

Recommendations for Health Care and Social Service Settings

Our model is in many ways particular to our own setting and goals. There are basic elements, however, that pertain to any setting that strives to provide successful delivery of care to women with HIV.

Case Management

We have found the model that best pulls together the elements of care is case management, a well-documented concept that has been "rediscovered" by almost every AIDS policy making body. Definitions vary in degree, but it can be described as a process that attempts to define and meet the biopsychosocial needs of an individual or family and coordinate the delivery of services (Weil 1985). Case management for HIV disease may be oriented to medical care coordination in hospitals (Clark 1988), or it may take place in such community-based settings as Gay Men's Health Crisis in New York, Kupona Network in Chicago, or AIDS Project Los Angeles (see Sonsel 1989). Case management services ideally can take place across agencies so that providers reduce redundancies and gaps in services for people with HIV (Ryndes 1989). The goal of HIV-specific case management has been to provide quality cost-effective services (Beresford 1991) for clients across the entire HIV disease continuum.

No one site can meet all the needs of an individual, so linkage with other service sites is essential. The degree of linkage depends on the patient's needs, the number of services available and the amount of resources allocated to case management. A provider with a caseload of 30 will be able to provide closer management than a provider with a caseload of 300. Case management occurs on a continuum, depending on how acute the clients' needs are. A patient in crisis will be accorded more resources than a patient who is asymptomatic and holding her own.

Accordingly, no one staff person can serve all of a patient's needs. A multidisciplinary approach is necessary and staff members need to be aware of where their own expertise leaves off and when another provider should assist. Flexibility is key, as is the recognition that some skills cross professional borders. Often, a patient will form a stronger bond with a particular staff member who may not have the most appropriate training to deal with the patient's priorities. With proper support for the staff member, this relationship can be very productive and the provider can help the patient become more comfortable with other staff members.

As case management attempts to address the patient's needs, it is important to be clear who defines these needs. Optimally, needs are defined by the patient. This is usually the most effective way to keep the patient in the system, but providers often have their own agendas, of which they need to be cognizant. This is not to say that the provider's agenda is necessarily self-serving or exploitive. For example, a provider may work hard to help a patient deal with a drug addiction problem that the patient chooses to ignore. Providers may differ on what they feel the patient needs. There must be open discussion of agendas and a balance achieved with the patient and among the providers.

Case management requires knowledge of community resources. For HIV infection, this includes a range of biopsychosocial services. In some areas HIV-specific services are readily available, but in other areas existing services—though not geared toward HIV—may be as effective in meeting the patients needs. For instance, many needs—such as home care or drug treatment—are not HIV-specific. With training on how HIV may affect delivery of these services, existing providers can be of great assistance. In New York City, foster care services for children with HIV were initially best handled by an organization designed to meet the needs of these children. Over time, however, more agencies adjusted their delivery of service so they could serve the children as well as the HIV-dedicated program. If providers with expertise in these areas are not available locally or on site, it is imperative to set up links with providers with more experience. In our case, the study obstetrician was available to consult with obstetricians in various prenatal clinics in Brooklyn on HIV management.

In areas where staff members are just beginning to work with HIV disease in women, contacting service providers in high-prevalence areas can help the staffers avoid pitfalls and reinventing the wheel. There are many HIV programs with training components, and most providers are willing to spend some time sharing their experiences with others dealing with the same problems.

Training and Evaluation

Continuous training about the special needs and concerns of patients with HIV is an absolutely essential aspect of service delivery. Provider attitudes about the disease and about people with the disease can range from enlightened to dangerous, and they are greatly affected by overwork and job stress. Organizations that are just beginning to deal with the epidemic have the luxury, if they choose, of planning the style in which they want to approach this illness. This is also the time to plan *proactively* the delivery of care.

It is crucial to have ongoing assessment of how the delivery model is meeting its goals, as no anticipatory training can take the place of serving the population. Mason et al. (1991) illustrate this concept with their account of extensive planning and training around testing contrasted with the reality of the first HIV-positive patient's visit. The Institute of Medicine (1991) recommends that programs be evaluated on process and outcome. The first evaluates whether the program is implemented as planned, whether the infrastructure is in place, and whether services are being delivered as intended. The latter assesses the overall impact of the program, whether goals were met, and what the positive and negative consequences are. Evaluation must be continuous, especially as the knowledge of treatment for HIV and the patient population expands.

Setting and Service Characteristics

The ideal health care setting should be able to provide full medical care for the family at one site. Treatment protocols should be available and medical information freely shared among the patients' providers. One person should be designated the case manager; optimally this would be the person who could provide the closest management. Clinics would take into account child care needs by having staff members (volunteer, perhaps) assist in the waiting room. Clinic times would be sensitive to the needs of women with children in school (they need to pick them up) as well as the needs of working women. One model in the Bronx is experimenting with a family clinic, in which the family stays in an exam room while the providers, adult and pediatric, go from family to family. If clinic appointments cannot be scheduled at the same time or same day, the same place would be helpful. Patients should also be aware of procedures or contact numbers for emergency situations.

There is still controversy about dedicated HIV care units versus mainstreaming of client services. The actual choice of care models is often decided by the available resources but may be influenced by other factors. For example, patients may feel stigmatized by a dedicated unit but can appreciate a staff that has chosen to work there (if that is the case). Close coordination between inpatient and outpatient care settings is essential to maintain followup care. One problem with our model is that as more options became available to women and their families—treatment protocols for women, for children, and specialized clinics—care ironically became more fragmented and complicated for the patient. For this reason efforts to integrate new HIV services into existing services should be undertaken by all involved providers.

Cultural Relevancy

Services provided should consider the special nature of the populations being served, including cultural characteristics, language, and history with the service provider. It was important in our case to be aware of the reputation our institutions had in the neighborhood, and to be able to address this. Having staff members from the community or from the same ethnicity and culture as many of the patients can help provide better insight into concerns and appropriate methods of delivery of services for the patient population. Having staff who can communicate with the patients in their native languages is important; if that is not possible, translation services should be readily available. Staff must make sure that the language used is understandable to the patient and must be familiar with street language and idioms.

The approach to the patient should be client-oriented and nonjudgmental. Patients often are sensitive and defensive about behaviors that are not widely accepted (such as drug use). The patient-provider relationship is greatly enhanced if the patient doesn't feel overtly or covertly attacked. For instance, it was not uncommon for HIV-infected women late in their pregnancies to be asked by hospital staff in a pejorative way why they were having a child (one woman was asked during labor). This is nonproductive and alienating. Training must address awareness of staff members' own feelings around such issues as drug abuse, racial and ethnic differences, sexuality, and lifestyle choices. Patience and perseverance are essential, as many women are preoccupied with the many pressures of day-to-day living and caring for their family, which often take precedence. For these reasons, many HIV-positive women may not be compliant with their own care, as the following description (Instone and Fraser 1991) confirms: "Obtaining health care for the infected child often becomes the primary focus of a woman's available energy. . . . The unpredictable nature of HIV requires that she bring her child to frequent clinic appointments and hospitalizations. At home, she is expected to give her child multiple daily medications. . . . She is told to maintain close telephone contact with her child's HIV health care providers . . . [and] has little opportunity to experience even one day without a reminder of her child's (and her own) infection. Consequently, it is not surprising that many of these mothers have neither the time nor the energy to seek health care for themselves . . . [and that] the health of many women deteriorates while that of the child stabilizes" (p. 108).

These are facts that systems must accommodate. In our study it was not unusual for a woman to drop out of contact only to return up to more than a year later requesting assistance. Often women needed many scheduled appointments before they would show up for HIV care, drug treatment, or HIV counseling because of fears and other demands on them. It was crucial to pick up where the patient was, addressing the gap in followup as matter of factly as possible.

Issues to Consider in Planning

In planning delivery of services, each setting must be aware of access to care issues that affect their goals. Method of payment can become a major issue as insurance may not pay for some treatments and some patients may not be able to pay for their care. It is important to define who is going to be served and be able to provide referrals for those who can not be served. In many instances institutions may have to develop new services before goals can be met. In our case, we were instrumental in developing several services, including group counseling, training for HIV counselors, and recreation events.

In areas of low prevalence, regionalization of HIV services may be necessary. Having centralized services can provide efficiency through economy of scale; it can also alleviate the problem of confidentiality that many women in rural areas and smaller towns face in trying to access care. Drawbacks to regionalization include distance and, often, overburdened services. Linking with existing women's health providers, such as domestic violence and rape units, infant mortality and prenatal care programs, and other area providers may also help maximize resources.

Providers also need to consider whether they should be involved in research, as this can have a strong impact on service delivery. For example, research monies can provide added staff and transportation funds for patients, contribute additional services to existing clinics, or lay the foundation for developing services. Moreover, research funds can sometimes be used to help develop programs that would otherwise be difficult to establish within the existing system of clinical care and administration. Providers also need to look to many sources for funding those services. Of necessity, grants management becomes an important part of delivering HIV-related services.

It may also be necessary to advocate for the patients' needs and to help the patients advocate for themselves. Through our group services, mothers became empowered and formed an advocacy group. This group, ACTUAL (AIDS Children Teaching Us About Love), addresses the needs of children and families. Its members have testified at public hearings and have advocated for themselves at meetings with community service providers, leading to enhancement of services in several cases. Patient input into advocacy is necessary as their needs may not be the same as the needs perceived by the staff. Several members of ACTUAL were participants at a national pediatric AIDS conference at which they learned about treatment protocols available elsewhere. These mothers returned angry that their children were denied services. They helped coordinate a meeting with hospital administrators and physicians to address these needs. As a result, access to different treatment options improved at SUNY and elsewhere because mothers shared information about the referral process to other sites, such as those at NIH.

Outreach to potential patients must also be carefully considered in trying to meet service delivery goals. Much of the effort to reach women has been concentrated in obstetrical and gynecological services because this is where most women interface with the medical setting. But this will not reach women who avoid medical treatment because of payment issues, drug use, immigrant status, or other reasons, and service delivery models need to be organized accordingly. Outreach may have to take place in the community in places ranging from day-care centers to laundromats to street corners. Members from the community that has been targeted can be trained as highly effective outreach workers. Weissman (1991) more thoroughly discusses these issues of outreach and service needs (table 15.1).

Summary

We have described a system for providing research and care to women and children affected by HIV disease. This model may have limited applicability, but it illustrates

Table 15.1 Areas of Consideration in Providing Services for Women with HIV

Access to care	• Method of payment
	• Language
	• Transportation
	• Child-care needs
Case management	• Linkage with broad range of services
	• Multidisciplinary, flexible staffing
Training and evaluation	• Appropriate, ongoing training for staff
	• Continuous assessment of how goals are being met and of unforeseen problems, results, and needs
Cultural relevancy	• Awareness of and sensitivity to concerns of populations to be served
	• Client-oriented approach
Research involvement	• Benefits
	• Disadvantages
Advocacy for clients	• Intra- and inter-agency
Outreach	• Who is to be reached, and by whom
Low-prevalence areas	• Regionalization of services
	• Linkage with existing women's health providers and providers in highprevalence areas to avoid "reinventing the wheel"

Source: Authors

many important concepts for the ongoing care of families with HIV infection. Our focus is on the health care setting, but the broad concepts can be applied to the social service setting as well. Based on this experience, we have outlined several recommendations for case management, training/evaluation, cultural relevancy, service characteristics and other areas.

The literature, while limited, can provide further information about particular types of policies and programs for various populations. Our overall approach in providing services is to consider the special needs of the population, as well as the special demands that HIV infection makes on care delivery. Providers must understand both the strengths and the limitations of their particular service delivery system. They must know how to link patients whose needs are beyond the capabilities of the system to providers who can meet them. Because the knowledge base for care is increasing, with resource availability ever-changing, continuous evaluation and adjustments are essential for successful delivery of services to HIV-positive women and their families.

16

Programs and Policies for Prevention

Krystn Wagner and Judith Cohen

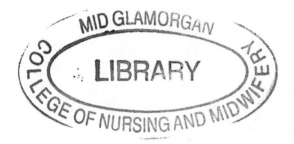

> I have lived with this disease for four years. How long will
> it take for something to really be done? What is it going to
> take? Does it have to come home with your son or your
> daughter to get some attention?
> —Frankie E. Mason

Even under the best of circumstances it will likely be several years before an effective and affordable vaccine or medical cure for HIV disease is widely available. Until then, prevention of HIV transmission is the only available means of limiting the further spread of the pandemic. Programs and policies for the prevention of HIV and AIDS will be needed even after the arrival of an AIDS vaccine, particularly if early vaccines are not completely effective. It is, therefore, essential that sufficient resources and attention be devoted to the development of effective prevention programs and messages at the same time that vaccine and drug development are pursued.

Globally, the vast majority of HIV infections in adults are estimated to have been transmitted through heterosexual intercourse (WHO/GPA 1992; Haseltine 1992). As a result, there is increasing attention worldwide to the prevention of the sexual transmission of HIV and AIDS. The number and proportion of HIV infections and AIDS cases resulting from different modes of transmission varies significantly, however, in different geographic regions and among different populations. This is a fact that must be taken into account when interventions are designed. Women injection-drug users, for example, represent half of all cumulative transmission categories in women in the United States (CDC 1993). Prevention policies and programs must consider such variations when addressing specific communities and individuals at risk.

To date, the focus of HIV and AIDS prevention programs has been on educating and encouraging individuals and communities to change risk behaviors or adopt risk-reduction strategies. Building on experience from the previous decade, it is possible to design and implement effective prevention programs. Successful programs, however, generally require more than communicating basic information about HIV and AIDS. Programs in many areas of the world have succeeded in educating people about HIV and AIDS, including the modes of HIV transmission and the means for prevention. An increase in knowledge alone, however, often does not result in significant changes in risk behaviors (see, for example, Lindan 1991).

The most successful HIV prevention programs and messages address those variables that are most relevant to an individual's willingness and ability to change her or his behaviors, including economic, social, and physical needs, attitudes, beliefs, behaviors, skills, access to information and services, and social norms. A woman who is knowledgeable about HIV and AIDS and condom use is less likely to adopt safer sex behavior if she does not perceive herself to be at risk; cannot afford to purchase condoms; believes condoms imply infidelity or promiscuity; does not know how to use condoms correctly or how to negotiate their use; cannot afford to purchase condoms; or, ultimately, if her sexual partner refuses to use them. These variables can best be identified and understood with the participation of individuals and communities at risk.

Prevention programs and messages need to be developed for specific audiences. Such programs will differ in their emphasis on and treatment of the variables that are relevant to HIV transmission and behavior change: the specific knowledge, attitudes, beliefs, and behaviors of the target group, as well as the social, cultural, and economic context in which these behaviors take place. Thus, one would expect that programs and messages for secondary school students will differ from programs for people attending family planning clinics or programs for injection-drug users. Likewise, prevention programs for gay men in São Paulo or Bombay need to differ, perhaps in significant ways, from programs for gay men in San Francisco or Amsterdam. Programs to reach women have to be as individualized as the communities in which the women live, whether that is an African city or an Iowa farming community.

Finally, it has been observed that community-based or grass-roots organizations have developed many of the most successful prevention programs to date, particularly when the organizations have been involved in both the program's design and implementation. This success is due, in part, to their understanding of and concern for the community, which is reflected in the program messages and services. As a result, community-based interventions are more likely to receive the attention and acceptance of their target audience.

The Need for Prevention Programs for Women

All available epidemiological data indicate that women worldwide are at increasing risk of HIV infection and are in urgent need of programs and policies for HIV and AIDS prevention.

To date, a number of programs worldwide have been developed for commercial sex workers, with the understanding that these women are at high risk of becoming HIV-infected and of subsequently infecting their sexual partners and children. More recently there has been increased attention on targeting prevention programs and messages to men who engage in high-risk behaviors, including clients of prostitutes and injection-drug users. In a recent review of fifteen HIV prevention projects carried out in thirteen countries, the World Health Organization identified specific interventions that have been effective in producing significant changes in people's sexual behavior. Several of these projects, including interventions in Mexico, Tanzania, Thailand, Zaire, and Zimbabwe, target female prostitutes and their male clients (WHO 1992).

Globally, much less emphasis has been placed on developing education and prevention programs for women who are not sex workers. This lack of attention is based on the belief that women in the general population are not the "core transmitters" of HIV infection. Instead, women are infected by male partners who engage in high-risk behaviors: having sex with multiple partners or injecting drugs. It is assumed that if prevention programs successfully change male behavior, then most women will no longer be at significant risk for infection. This focus on changing male risk behaviors is reinforced by the fact that women in the general population are assumed to have little control over the use of the only widely available prevention commodity, the male condom.

Programs that encourage and support men in changing their risk behaviors are essential to HIV and AIDS prevention and to reducing women's risk of infection. Nevertheless, it is important to consider the possible limitations of prevention efforts focusing disproportionately on educating men and changing male behaviors. First, it must be acknowledged that little is known about women's and men's risk behaviors, particularly in the area of human sexuality, as well as women's options for reducing risks. It may be, for example, that more women engage in risk behaviors than is commonly self-reported (Betrand et al. 1989), particularly in cultures where there are social sanctions and penalties (often more draconian for women than for men) concerning such behaviors.

Second, it is important to recognize the tremendous diversity of women worldwide: they are of different ages, marital status, and educational levels, and of different socioeconomic, cultural, and religious backgrounds. These variables are likely to be important determinants or correlates of women's risk behaviors, their perceptions of risk, and their ability to reduce their risk of HIV infection—including determining the use of condoms. Until such factors are better understood, caution should be exercised when prevention programs are developed on the basis of unexamined assumptions or generalizations about women's lives. The heterogeneity of risk must be recognized and incorporated into prevention campaigns. Many middle-class women in India, for example, would not consider themselves sex workers and would be unlikely to perceive as relevant messages aimed at prostitutes. Yet sex for some of these women is not a matter of choice but one of economic survival—and with some of them beginning to discreetly sell sex out of their homes to make ends meet, they are in fact at risk.[1] Thus, although it is important that appropriate messages reach the appropriate audience, it is also important not to enforce stereotyping of risk groups rather than behaviors. Cindy Patton, for example, analyzed WHO documents on HIV prevention that were sent to African countries and found that the dominant ideology of these papers was that HIV transmission is linked to "deviant sexuality." Many women simply will not identify with this framing of risk for their own lives.[2]

Finally, it is important to consider women's possible roles in prevention efforts beyond those of reducing personal risk. The roles of women as mothers and workers, writers and researchers, health care providers and educators, and community members and leaders are generally not discussed in connection with HIV and AIDS prevention. It is important to consider how women in these varied spheres, who are themselves knowledgeable and concerned about HIV and AIDS, may contribute to or lead other education and prevention efforts in the family and community. Thus, prevention policies and programs that focus disproportionately on men may miss an opportunity to educate and mobilize influential and committed women in the fight against HIV/AIDS.

[1] As related by Nalini Singh, participant in a seminar on gender, power, and HIV, at the Eighth International Conference on AIDS, Amsterdam, July 22, 1992.

[2] Cindy Patton, seminar participant, Eighth International Conference on AIDS, Amsterdam, July 22, 1992.

The Need for Gender-Sensitive Interventions

In some cases, the target group for a prevention program is of a single gender; for example, those who attend family planning clinics usually are women. In other cases, the group includes both women and men, as in a class of university students or in an entire community. Whether an intervention is targeted to a group of uniform or mixed gender, it is critical that the plan's policies and programs be gender-sensitive: that is, they must consider those gender-specific variables that are relevant to HIV transmission and those that will enhance or constrain risk-reduction behaviors. Women and men have a number of gender-specific biological and behavioral risk factors for HIV transmission, as well as unique opportunities and constraints for HIV/AIDS prevention. The following are a few examples that illustrate the importance of gender-specific variables in HIV transmission and the need to develop gender-sensitive interventions.

• Women generally do not wear condoms.[3] Strategies that aim to increase the effective use of condoms must address a woman's potential need to negotiate condom use with her partner and the possible difficulties she may encounter, including refusal, rejection, or violence. Messages that simply urge condom use are likely to be seen as inadequate or irrelevant to many women.

• Sexually transmitted diseases (STDs), including chlamydia and gonorrhea, are often asymptomatic or unrecognized in women. While STDs enhance both men's and women's susceptibility to HIV transmission, STDs are more often symptomatic in men, prompting them to seek diagnosis and treatment. Meanwhile, STDs may go undiagnosed and untreated in women, particularly women in resource-poor settings. In addition, STD clinics are unacceptable to women in the general population in many cultures; thus, women often lack access to appropriate diagnosis and treatment services. Gender-sensitive programs should address the unique STD prevention, diagnosis, and treatment needs of women.

• Women in many developing countries have lower literacy levels than men. In such settings, fewer women than men will be reached through written AIDS educational materials. In general, prevention programs for women and men must consider what percentage of each group can be reached through a particular communication channel or access point.

• Women's role in childbearing is closely associated in many cultures with status. Because condoms prevent conception, as well as HIV infection, women of reproductive age may have a distinct set of attitudes and concerns about their use. Women likewise may face difficult pregnancy decisions and consequences regarding perinatal transmission. Therefore, prevention programs need to consider the

---

[3] The availability of the female condom is limited by geography (it's sold mostly in a handful of developed countries) and price (about U.S. $2.50 per condom at time of printing).

particular issues of women with regard to childbearing and perinatal HIV transmission (Carovano 1991).

• Women in many societies have primary responsibility for the health of the family. As a result, women may be uniquely attentive and responsive to health messages, including those concerning HIV and AIDS. Women of reproductive age interact with the health care system through maternal and child health and family planning clinics, potentially important sources of information on HIV and AIDS. In some settings and circumstances, however, women have less access than men to health services and information. Therefore, HIV/AIDS policies and programs should consider women's and men's distinct relationships to the health care system and their respective roles and responsibilities for family health.

These examples illustrate the variety of gender differences significant to HIV transmission and to risk reduction strategies. Effective intervention must take into account the biological, cultural, and socioeconomic factors that put women at risk of HIV infection. The variety and respective weight of these factors may not be known or well understood, however, and research must be undertaken to assess these factors. One example of such an approach can be seen in a Women and AIDS research program undertaken by the International Center for Research on Women. This three-year, U.S. Agency for International Development-funded program supports descriptive and operations research through fifteen projects in developing countries. For example, peer educators will be used among workers in Mauritius, Thailand, Jamaica, and South Africa; traditional sexuality advisers convey information on STDs and AIDS to women in Malawi and Senegal. Ethnographic studies in India, Brazil, New Guinea, and Zimbabwe assess perceptions of gender roles, sexual decision making, partner communication, and other factors. College students in Nigeria, street youth in Brazil, and women attending reproductive health clinics in Guatemala City are targeted in other research interventions (International Center for Research on Women 1992). These and other data-based educational interventions will begin to fill in the sketchy picture of those factors, context, and behaviors that put women at risk around the world.

Other specific intervention strategies for women in the United States are described in the next section. These projects further illustrate the need for gender-sensitive policies and programs, as well as the importance of interventions targeted specifically to women.

Intervention Strategies in the United States

Although prevention and intervention strategies for women are necessarily reflective of their transmission circumstances, these programs need to differ from those for men in two crucial aspects. First, the context of behavior change for women is generally less under their direct control than is the case for men. Second, prevention of HIV transmission for women is concerned with both vertical and horizontal transmission.

Because most HIV transmission to women in the United States occurs through injection-drug use or sexual contact with an infected partner, intervention efforts have primarily been directed at these kinds of transmission. There has been extensive effort to develop mass-media drug prevention messages, but these messages have not been specific to women users, except as bearers of children. Even less information is available to women users who are not currently in treatment.

One exception is the Association for Drug Abuse Prevention and Treatment (ADAPT), a street outreach program that began in 1985 in the Puerto Rican community of Williamsburg in New York City (Serrano 1990). Founded and run by recovering and former injection-drug users, ADAPT carries prevention and support messages to women who use drugs. In addition to education and prevention, ADAPT's facilitators provide sterilization kits and condoms to users and to shooting galleries in the neighborhood. The staff and volunteers are living examples of positive behavior change in urban areas where day-to-day survival is the most pressing issue for women.

Most intervention-oriented treatment programs have been developed from knowledge about men's drug use patterns and needs. Thus, most drug treatment programs are for heroin users; much less is available for polydrug or crack users, who are more likely to be women (NIDA 1992). Similarly, virtually no prevention or treatment programs of the most effective kind, including residential treatment, accept women with children. The relatively few programs that are woman-focused, and the even more scarce ones that serve women without separating them from their families, appear to have the most success in terms of retention in treatment and low rates of relapse.

Programs that have been successful in rehabilitating women are the PROTO-TYPES program in Los Angeles (Brown 1991) and Women, Inc., in Dorchester, Massachusetts (Portis 1990). Both programs treat the whole woman, not just her drug use. They work daily with women who are also battered, often homeless, and have a multitude of problems. The programs' HIV prevention efforts have been built into this perspective and have necessarily expanded into the community as well, working with women in other institutions and in their own neighborhoods.

HIV prevention programs for women who are sexual partners of men who inject drugs have the same goals as all prevention programs. But the standard prevention messages have a higher potential for failure (Cohen 1991) because they are more likely to be seen by women as irrelevant. After all, the standard advice is to abstain, be monogamous, or use condoms. For women, this translates into: abstain and have no partner, hence no support, get your partner to be monogamous, or persuade him to use condoms. The first message denies the need for love and support, and the latter two contradict widespread cultural assumptions about a man's biological and sexual nature. Further, the last two contain the even less plausible assumption that it is possible for a woman to control a man's sexual behavior.

Efforts to increase condom promotion among women at risk have emphasized current condom use skills. What may be needed more is condom promotion strategies targeted to men and more female-controlled barrier methods. Intervention efforts that rely on women to introduce (male) condoms into a sexual situation are expecting women to assume new roles in an intensely emotional and private situation. In many cultural contexts, negative connotations include presumptions of infidelity and disease or of attempts to control a man's sexuality (Worth 1990). The range of reactions from male partners can include sexual rejection, domestic violence, and termination of the relationship. Clearly there is a strong need for prevention methods for women to use that are under their control.

One intervention program in Philadelphia, Blacks Educating Blacks About Sexual Health Issues (BEBASHI), has developed community efforts to address these issues within the black community (Hassan 1990). BEBASHI provides education at many levels, from private homes to schools and churches. As in the programs previously described, the leaders and staff members come from the community. Education and intervention are therefore conveyed by peers in a context that reflects understanding of the day-to-day issues faced by women at risk. Another program, Sister Love, began in Atlanta as a response to the AIDS epidemic in women in the black community there (Dixon 1990). It focuses on the home and family, providing safer sex parties that are also educational and support groups organized and run by peers. The groups encourage discussion of a wide range of issues in addition to HIV risk, with the intent to build social support and community social change.

With funding from the Community Research Demonstration Program of the National Institute on Drug Abuse, the Women's AIDS Risk Network (WARN) program was begun in several cities and Puerto Rico in 1989. WARN offers an extensive intervention program designed for women at risk for HIV infection through their own drug use or that of their sexual partners. Women who participate in the program are given individual and group support concerning drug use and health, family dynamics, negotiation of safer sexual relationships, and other issues related to their lives that affect risk for HIV infection (Slaughter 1990). A recent report of early findings from the program indicates that among women who injected drugs more than half have ceased their use; 35 percent have obtained treatment; and 42 percent have been able to reduce to some degree their risk of becoming infected from sexual partners (Weissman 1991; MMWR 1991).

As described in previous chapters, the major strategy in the United States to prevent vertical HIV transmission has been HIV antibody testing of women in prenatal and family planning clinics. The expectation is that knowing one's HIV status is important and will influence decision making about beginning or continuing a pregnancy. The evidence to date, however, indicates that the opposite is often true. Many women at risk are not eager to know their HIV status and may avoid programs that expect them to be tested because of fears of discovery of drug use or the likelihood that their babies will be taken from them. Further, knowledge of HIV status appears to have little effect on decisions about pregnancy (Holman et al. 1989). The profound meaning of childbearing to women of many cultures is more central to their decision making than are external factors like illness or economics (Weissman 1991). Interventions designed solely with the intent of influencing women's potential reproductive decisions are insufficient at best. Interventions designed to address the entire health and social context in which women function are more likely to have a positive impact.

AWARE, another community-based program in the Bay Area of San Francisco, began in 1984 with a health focus. The program's design involved women from high-risk backgrounds and lifestyles providing community education and support for behavior change in terms of women's health, particularly to reduce the risk of exposing oneself to HIV and other sexually transmitted diseases. Messages were personalized, nonjudgmental, and delivered on the streets. In addition, health screening, limited treatment, and referral service to health and drug treatment resources were brought to community locations by a team of outreach staff members, counselors, and health providers. The most direct measure of success is that AWARE has seen more than 2,000 women to date; only two have become HIV-infected since they joined the program (Cohen, Derish, and Dorfman in press).

Another example of how cultural and environmental factors affect prevention efforts is emerging from recent observations of the drug-using cultural pattern surrounding crack cocaine. The use of crack is prevalent among young adults in the inner city, and the lifestyle associated with crack use has a major impact on HIV- and STD-related risk behavior, including unsafe sexual behavior with many partners (Marx et al. 1991). This lifestyle has already been associated with epidemic increases in syphilis, and there is concern than HIV infection will increase concomitantly in areas of high crack use (Minkoff et al. 1990).

Comparison of prevention efforts that have reduced risk with efforts that have not leads to several conclusions that can guide the development of additional prevention efforts. First, some of the most expensive efforts, which are directed at general audiences via the mass media and nonspecific educational materials like brochures, fail to reach those who do not perceive themselves to be at risk. Most women still do not personalize HIV risk because they do not know anyone like themselves who has AIDS. Therefore, prevention efforts that are more personalized and that are delivered by plausible interpersonal efforts are most likely to be heard.

The most effective prevention programs are presented in community outreach efforts by women who are like those at risk and are delivered in ways and locations that are part of women's everyday lives.

The examples provided here show that successful programs can come from a variety of bases. What matters is that they are grounded in the communities of women at risk and that they address all of the issues related to HIV risk, not just the probability of transmission of the virus. An equally important characteristic of such programs is that peer staff also serve as credible role models, providing evidence that growth and change can happen (Dorfman, Derish, and Cohen 1992).

Finally, prevention messages that expect women to deny other more important or pressing daily realities and cause dissonant pressures are to be avoided. Often, women who know that they are at risk of HIV infection from a spouse still need to stay with that spouse for many reasons that outweigh the perceived distant or vague risk of acquiring HIV infection. Included in this contextual framework is the reality that, for most women, major decisions about their own health-related sexual behavior are influenced or controlled by men. It is men who wear or do not wear condoms, and the power to negotiate their use is not balanced. Unless prevention efforts to slow the spread of heterosexual transmission are aimed at men as well, existing prevention efforts will be limited in their effectiveness.

Recommendations for Policies and Programs

Women worldwide are at increasing risk of HIV infection and AIDS. As has been described throughout this book, women constitute the fastest growing group of people newly infected with HIV in the United States and throughout many parts of the globe. There is an urgent need for prevention policies and programs specifically for adolescent and adult women.

To develop appropriate interventions, there is a need for more social science research to better understand women's (and men's) risk behaviors, as well as the social, economic, and cultural context in which these behaviors take place. In particular, additional research is needed to identify women's opportunities and constraints for risk reduction and to develop appropriate programs and messages for women. It is essential that women's heterogeneity be recognized and that erroneous generalizations about women in the context of HIV and AIDS be avoided.

It is critical that all prevention programs be developed and implemented in a manner that takes into account gender differences. It is well recognized that women and men have a number of gender-specific biological and behavioral risk factors for HIV transmission, as well as unique opportunities and constraints for prevention. To be successful, programs and policies should address those gender-specific variables that are significant to HIV transmission and those that will enhance or constrain risk-reduction behaviors.

It is essential that prevention programs be evaluated and that their successes and failures be documented. Programs too often are designed and implemented without sufficient attention to how success will be defined and measured or how specific interventions will be evaluated. By incorporating evaluation plans, an ongoing program can be more readily and appropriately modified. Most important, successful programs can then be expanded or replicated to reach other women at risk.

Community-based groups and nongovernmental organizations play an essential and often unique role in HIV and AIDS prevention, complementary to that of government. Many community-based groups have initiated rapid and innovative responses to the pandemic. Their achievements often arise from their origins in, and access to, groups at risk of HIV infection, giving them a credibility with and understanding of the people they serve (Mercer 1991). Consequently, there is a critical need for increased financial and technical support to community-based organizations concerned with HIV and AIDS prevention and care for women.

Finally, there is an urgent need to develop products or technologies that women can use to protect themselves against HIV and AIDS (Stein 1990). In family planning, women are offered a variety of contraceptive choices that they can use without their partner's cooperation or consent. Female-controlled methods are likewise needed for HIV and AIDS prevention, particularly methods that will minimize negotiation as a precondition for use. There is a specific need to develop methods that will protect against HIV and AIDS but still allow conception. The development and testing of female-controlled methods should be of primary importance to increase women's options.

Constructively changing the milieu in which women and men become infected with HIV may be the most effective "cure" of all. To do so requires not only financial and scientific resources, but that most powerful and elusive element: human will.

Resources:
Service Organizations, Materials, and Further Reading

Ann Kurth and Laura J. Wittig

Sometimes I see women who are positive and still using drugs, adding a second disease to their first one. A lot of women don't want to accept help. They're going through changes, especially if they're taking chemicals. Maybe God put them in my life to help tell these women not to mess themselves up. They don't love themselves, is the thing. I do, and I want to live, so I do what's right. The help is there if you really want it. I have faith that one day that medicine will come. Till then, I have help: my doctor, my nurse-practitioner, my mother, my social worker. . . . I have lots of supportive people in my life. They give me what we all need, and that's lots of love. Unconditional love is all I need.
—Sylvia Cintron

While reviewing listings for resources that would reflect this book's purpose, it became evident that prevention and education efforts dominate the concerns of HIV service agencies and that, for the most part, sexual identities and gender are blended in many agencies' missions. This resource directory reflects an attempt to provide information about organizations working on the front line with women and HIV. Where this was not possible, organizations are listed that can provide information and referrals for direct services.

This listing is best used by reviewing the table of contents to determine the service area or geographical region of interest. The directory begins with a listing of national and international organizations that target specific populations and offer practical and technical assistance. Next, several national organizations are presented that highlight different areas of interest. Information is provided about agencies, projects, and materials based mostly in the United States. The regional section lists one or more resources for each state and the District of Columbia. A bibliography for further reading on women and HIV is included.

We do not list national, state, or local AIDS hot lines, or state or local departments of health; nor is there an exhaustive list of clinical service sites. Despite contacting every agency by phone prior to publication to validate the information contained for each entry, some changes will have inevitably occurred. This may also mean that new women's HIV service organizations have come into existence. Consider calling on the experience of some of these agencies in the development of women-specific projects in your area.

Resource Directory Contents

Populations

Adolescents

Safe Choices Project
Phone: (202) 783–7949
National Network of Runaway Youth Services
1319 F Street NW, No. 401
Washington, DC 20054

Safe Choices is a national initiative to provide HIV-prevention training materials and technical assistance to agencies that serve youth in high-risk situations. The program addresses the needs of women, particularly adolescents.

Culture-Specific Programs

Association for Drug Abuse, Prevention, and Treatment
Phone: (212) 289–1957
236 East 111th Street
New York, NY 10029

ADAPT is funded by the Centers for Disease Control to provide training materials and technical assistance to organizations interested in providing street-based outreach. The focus is on education, prevention, and referrals for HIV and substance abuse, especially for minority populations. The association provides support groups, some specifically for women, on a local level.

Blacks Educating Blacks About Sexual Health Issues
Phone: (215) 546–4140
1233 Locust Street, Suite 401
Philadelphia, PA 19107

BEBASHI provides education at many levels in the African-American community, from private homes to schools and churches. Leadership and staff members come from the community. The group provides direct client services—counseling, testing, case management—that are culture-specific, and it works with the client's entire family. It has a CDC grant to provide technical assistance in a five-state area for similar program development and is willing to provide information to programs outside its area.

Boston Women's AIDS Information Project
Phone: (617) 859–8689
464 Massachusetts Avenue
Boston, MA 02118

This multiracial and multicultural coalition targets women in the African-American, Hispanic, Haitian, and Cape Verdean communities. It focuses on prevention education and refers women to the appropriate resources for direct services.

Haitian Women's Program
Phone: (718) 783–0883
465 Dean Street
New York, NY 11217

This program is primarily prevention-focused, developing educational materials specific to the Haitian culture and training people from the Haitian community to teach others in the community about HIV prevention. It provides materials and information on their program model nationally.

IMANI and the Women's AIDS Project of the Kupona Network
Phone: (312) 536–3000
4611 South Ellis Avenue
Chicago, IL 60653

IMANI, an active advisory panel to the Women's AIDS Project, ensures that the Project networks efficiently with local, regional, and national service agencies working on AIDS with African-American women. Its members also advocate on behalf of HIV-positive African-American women and their families. The Kupona Network, a community-based organization in the national El Centro Human Services Women of Color AIDS Project Partnership, was established to develop effective models for preventing transmission of HIV among African-American and Haitian women and Latinas.

Native American Women's Health Education Resource Center
Phone: (605) 487–7072
Box 572
Lake Andes, SD 57357

This national forum for Native American women's issues provides AIDS awareness education to adult and teenage women and men, pre- and post-test HIV counseling, a nutrition program, and technical assistance to other groups and individuals.

SisterLove
Phone: (404) 753–7733
1237-R Abernathy Boulevard SW
Atlanta, GA 30310

SisterLove networks with local and regional women-focused service agencies to provide HIV and AIDS outreach to all women at risk, primarily those in the African-American community. Training includes education, support development, support groups, and safer-sex workshops.

Family Support

Mothers of AIDS Patients, Families, and Concerned Others
Phone: (310) 542–3019
Box 1763
Lomita, CA 90717-9998

This national organization connects family members who are affected by HIV and AIDS with others in the state who are or have been in the same situation.

National Hemophilia Foundation
Phone: (800) 424–2634
110 Greene Street, Room 303
New York, NY 10012

The foundation provides information and written materials on treatment and psychosocial issues, as well as a program for wives of hemophiliacs.

Health Care and Other Workers

American College of Obstetricians and Gynecologists, the Nurses Association of ACOG, and the Organization for Obstetric, Gynecologic and Neonatal Nurses
Phone: (202) 638–5577
Phone: (202) 863–2439
409 12th Street SW
Washington, DC 20024-2191

This professional organization specializes in the education of obstetric, gynecologic, and neonatal physicians and nurses. Members can order printed material pertaining to HIV for health care workers and patients. The group offers seminars on sexually transmitted diseases and HIV.

Association of Nurses in AIDS Care
Phone: (800) 962–4515
704 Stony Hill Road
Suite 106
Yardley, PA 19067

This group provides a network for its more than 2,300 U.S. and international members. It publishes the quarterly *Journal of the Association of Nurses in AIDS Care* and the quarterly newsletter *ANACDOTES* and hosts an annual conference.

Medical Expertise Retention Program
Phone: (415) 864–0408
273 Church Street
San Francisco, CA 94114

This program of the American Association of Physicians for Human Rights provides help for HIV-infected physicians and other health care workers, including counseling, policy updates, legal services, employment and retraining information, and advocacy.

National AIDS Minority Education Program
Phone: (202) 865–3720
Howard University
2139 Georgia Avenue, No. 3-B
Washington, DC 20001

This five-year CDC-funded program trains health care workers who work with the African-American community. It provides up-to-date information on experimental drugs, psychosocial issues, and epidemiology, and it maintains a speakers bureau of HIV-infected women and men.

National Family Planning and Reproductive Health Association
Phone: (202) 628–3535
122 C Street NW, Suite 380
Washington, DC 20001-2109

This national membership organization represents family planning providers and consumers. Its goal is to improve and expand the delivery of reproductive health care services nationwide. The agency has developed a set of medical protocols on AIDS for the family planning setting that covers such topics as infection control and staff and client education.

Physician Association for AIDS Care
Phone: (312) 222–1326
101 West Grand, Suite 200
Chicago, IL 60610

This group provides information on medical treatment and psychosocial issues via satellite, video, cable television, a monthly journal, and sponsorship of national and international conferences. It can provide some referrals to physicians who are treating patients with HIV.

Service Employees International
Phone: (202) 898–3386
Union AIDS Education Program
1313 L Street NW
Washington, DC 20005

Through this program, union members working in a health care setting receive education and training workshops on protecting themselves against HIV infection on and off the job. The union also makes available information on health and safety contract language negotiated by SEIU members to protect themselves from HIV and AIDS and to fight discrimination against workers who are infected with HIV; a manual on AIDS in the workplace; and research and assistance on other topics relating to AIDS.

International Women and HIV Organizations

Africa
Women and AIDS Support Network
Box 1554
Harare, Zimbabwe

The AIDS Support Organisation (TASO)
Plot 21 Kitante Road
Box 10443
Kampala, Uganda

Society for Women and AIDS in Africa
UTH, Department of Pathology and Microbiology
Box 50110
Lusaka, Zambia

Asia
South India AIDS Action Programme
65, Kamaraj Avenue
1st Street, Adyar, Madras-20
India

Europe
Positively Women
5 Sebastian Street
London ECIV 0HE
U.K.

International Community of Women Living with HIV/AIDS
Box 2338
London W8 4ZG
U.K.

North America
Positive Women's Network
1107 Seymour Street
Vancouver, British Columbia
Canada V6B 5S8

Pacific
Positive Women
76 Grafton Road
Auckland, New Zealand

Lesbian and Gay Issues

Lesbian AIDS Project of the Gay Men's Health Crisis
Phone: (212) 807–7517
129 West 20th Street
New York, NY 10011

GMHC distributes brochures on various subjects related to HIV and AIDS and produces a newsletter entitled *Treatment Issues*. Women-specific materials and projects include pamphlets and videos and the Lesbian AIDS Project.

National Center for Lesbian Rights
Phone: (415) 621–0674
1663 Mission Street, Fifth Floor
San Francisco, CA 94103

This nonprofit public interest law firm focuses on family law and employment discrimination. It serves as an information clearinghouse on legal cases and provides advice, counseling, and technical assistance to other attorneys working on cases in these two areas. Publication *AIDS and Child Custody* is available on request.

National Gay and Lesbian Task Force
Phone: (202) 332–6483
Policy Institute
1734 14th Street NW
Washington, DC 20009-4309

Institute focuses on activism, lobbying, advocacy, and referral. It assists states in organizing activism programs, provides public presentations, and lobbies on all aspects of HIV.

National Lesbian and Gay Health Foundation
Phone: (202) 797–3708
Box 65472
Washington, DC 20035

This group promotes community networking, organization, and action as it relates to the health care needs of lesbians, gay men, and people with AIDS. It publishes an annual directory of lesbian and gay health services and sponsors the annual Gay and Lesbian Health Conference.

Sex Workers

California Prostitutes Education Project
AIDS Research and Healthy Start
Phone: (510) 874–7850
620 20th Street
Oakland, CA 96412
Mailing address: Box 23855, Oakland, CA 94623-0055

CAL-PEP is a five-year CDC-funded research project to develop interventions that
empower women to negotiate safer sex. Services include education, information and
referrals, street-based outreach (includes distributing bleach kits and condoms), safer-sex
workshops, support groups, testing in a mobile unit for HIV and STDs, and vocation
rehabilitation for sex workers who leave the industry. Available publications include
Prostitutes Prevent AIDS: A Manual for Health Educators.

Come Off Your Old Tired Ethics (COYOTE)
Phone: (415) 474-3037
2269 Chestnut Street
Suite 452
San Francisco, CA 94123

Empower Thailand
Box 1065 Silom
Bangkok 10504
Thailand

Network for Sex Work Related HIV/AIDS Projects
4 Place Armand Carrol
75019 Paris
France

Red Thread
International Congress for Prostitutes' Rights
Box 12042 1100 AA Amsterdam
The Netherlands

Scarlet Alliance
Ground Floor
GK Ross House
Flinderslane
Melbourne 3000
Australia

Women and Prison

ACLU National Prison Project
AIDS in Prison Project
Phone: (202) 234–4830
1875 Connecticut Avenue NW, No. 410
Washington, DC 20009

This is a national resource clearinghouse for AIDS educators and activists on AIDS and prison issues. It also serves as a national legal referral agency for prisoners with HIV and AIDS.

AIDS Counseling and Education
Bedford Hills Correctional Facility
Phone: (914) 241–3100, extension 275
247 Harris Road
Bedford Hills, NY 10507

This group promotes peer counseling and education among prisoners, inmate and worker education, training of inmates to do peer counseling, and acts as a nationwide model for peer education at other prisons.

Areas of Interest

Education and Prevention

New Jersey Women and AIDS Network
Phone: (908) 846–4462
5 Elm Row, Suite 112
New Brunswick, NJ 08901

In this statewide organization, members of independent agencies and individuals come together to coordinate culturally sensitive, gender-specific prevention education initiatives, share information about problems faced by HIV-infected women, and work to advocate for appropriate legislation, public health policies, and resources for direct HIV services for women. It provides a quarterly newsletter, *NJWAN News;* educational presentations; a speakers bureau; and the Women and AIDS Clearinghouse, a database of literature.

Project AWARE
Phone: (415) 476–4091
3180 18th Street, No. 205
San Francisco, CA 94110

AWARE is a community-based participatory research and educational organization conducting epidemiological, behavioral, and clinical studies of lesbian, heterosexual, and bisexual women and HIV in the San Francisco Bay and Oakland area.

Women's AIDS Network
Phone: (415) 864–4376, extension 2007
San Francisco AIDS Foundation

Box 426182
San Francisco, CA 94142-6182

WAN is a citywide model for sharing information and coordinating advocacy. It provides education, prevention, and information referrals, with a focus on women with HIV who work or live in the San Francisco Bay Area. WAN facilitates monthly networking with other women's groups.

Research and Policy

AIDS Coalition to Unleash Power (ACT-UP)
Phone: (212) 564–2437
135 West 29th Street
New York, NY 10001

This nonpartisan, diverse group of individuals is united in anger and committed to direct action in ending the AIDS crisis. ACT-UP meets with government and health officials, researches and distributes the latest medical information, and conducts protests and demonstrations. Its publications include a weekly newsletter called *Treatment and Data;* information on how to start new ACT-UP groups; and an AIDS awareness brochure, among other publications.

American Foundation for AIDS Research
Phone: (212) 682–7440
733 Third Avenue, 12th Floor
New York, NY 10017

AmFar raises and distributes funding for scientific research, education, prevention, public policy, and clinical trials at community-based organizations. Through the National AIDS Clearinghouse it provides a free directory of clinical trials.

Center for Women's Policy Studies
Phone: (202) 872–1770
National Resource Center on Women and AIDS
2000 P Street NW, Suite 508
Washington, DC 20036

The center is instrumental in policy and legislation concerning women and AIDS. It coordinates and publishes *The Guide to Resources on Women and AIDS* and develops written materials, videos, and programs to help local groups meet the needs of women of color and low-income women confronting AIDS. Along with the National Women's Health Network, it chairs the Women and AIDS Coalition, in which 230 organizations and individuals provide input on HIV issues.

Feminist Institute
Phone: (301) 951–9040
Box 30563
Bethesda, MD 20814

This nonprofit research and advocacy organization provides educational and information services to people interested in feminist issues. It also researches psychosocial issues affecting women living with AIDS.

Office of AIDS Research
Phone: (301) 496–0357
National Institutes of Health
Building 1, Room 201
9000 Rockville Pike
Bethesda, MD 20892

This office coordinates National Institutes of Health policies and programs. It provides copies of *The Status on Women and AIDS Activities* (Congressional report, January 10, 1992), listing current institute biomedical research and future research priorities.

Sex Information and Education Council of the United States
Phone: (212) 819–9770
130 West 42nd Street, 25th Floor
New York, NY 10036

This national research library includes literature on women and AIDS. Its bimonthly newsletter, *SIECUS,* had a special issue focused on women and AIDS.

Treatment Information

AIDS Clinical Trials Information Service
Phone: (800) 874–2572
Spanish speakers available
TTY/TDD (English): (800) 243-7012
Box 6421
Rockville, MD 20850

ACTIS provides information on U.S. clinical trials and eligibility requirements, and on specific drugs (both experimental and federally approved).

AIDS Treatment News
Phone: (800) 873–2812
Box 411256
San Francisco, CA 94141

AIDS Treatment News is a bimonthly newsletter providing information on approved and unapproved AIDS treatments and on political issues, including those pertaining to women. ATN has a yearly subscription rate; it will also handle inquiries.

AIDS Treatment Registry
Phone: (212) 268–4196
Box 30234
New York, NY 10011-0102

Information, educational materials, and access to AIDS-related clinical drug trials are available through the AIDS Treatment Registry.

Notes from the Underground
Phone: (212) 255–0520
PWA Health Group

150 West 26th Street, Suite 201
New York, NY 10001

Notes from the Underground is a newsletter published six times a year that provides information on approved and unapproved AIDS treatments and on political issues, including those pertaining to women. It has a yearly subscription rate. It also will handle inquiries on drugs and drug prices.

Project Inform
Phone: (800) 822–7422
1965 Market Street, No. 220
San Francisco, CA 94103

Project Inform provides up-to-date treatment information and options to people with HIV or at risk for infection. It publishes *PI Perspective* three or four times a year and offers an introductory packet of treatment information.

Legal Issues

American Bar Association
AIDS Coordination Project
Phone: (202) 331–2248
1800 M Street NW
Washington, DC 20036

The association has developed a directory of legal resources for people with HIV or AIDS and a document *(The Legal Issues)* analyzing the impact of AIDS in fifteen areas of the law. The ABA also helps local bar associations and individual attorneys create their own legal referral programs.

American Bar Association
Immigration Law Project
Phone: (202) 331–2268
1800 M Street NW
Washington, DC 20036

The ABA offers educational materials for advocates and attorneys on discrimination against HIV-positive immigrants.

American Civil Liberties Union
AIDS Project
Phone: (212) 944–9800, extension 545
132 West 43rd Street
New York, NY 10036

The ACLU AIDS Project provides a directory of representatives and services available to those who are HIV-positive. It produces written materials pertaining to legal issues, problems, and policies that affect people with HIV. Test case litigation is taken on by affiliate offices in almost every state.

American Civil Liberties Union
Immigrants' Rights Project
Phone: (212) 944–9800, extension 715
132 West 43rd Street
New York, NY 10036

Provides backup, consultation, and referrals for attorneys and service providers assisting immigrants with HIV-related problems.

Lambda Legal Defense and Education Fund
Phone: (212) 995–8585
666 Broadway, 12th Floor
New York, NY 10012

The Fund provides test-case litigation for HIV-positive persons. It also provides this service for lesbian and gay legal rights issues.

National Lawyers Guild AIDS Network
Phone: (415) 824–8884
588 Capp Street
San Francisco, CA 94102

The group acts as a bridge between the legal community and AIDS service organizations, involving more than 700 attorneys and legal workers in over 300 AIDS organizations in 47 states, the District of Columbia, Puerto Rico, Canada, and Micronesia. It also provides a consultant service to attorneys, educational materials, and a legal and policy journal called *The Exchange*.

Regional HIV Organizations

Eastern United States

Bridgeport Women's and Men's Project
Phone: (203) 335–3634
135 Washington Avenue
Bridgeport, CT 06604

Services include case management, counseling, information and referrals, outpatient substance abuse aftercare program, and support services.

Yale–New Haven Hospital AIDS Care Program
Phone: (203) 785–5303
20 York Street
New Haven, CT 06504

Services include adult and pediatric AIDS outpatient clinics. The hospital is also an AIDS Clinical Trials Unit. Information, medical services, and referrals are provided.

District of Columbia Women's Council on AIDS Sister Care
Phone: (202) 544–8255
725 Eighth Street SE
Washington, DC 20003

Services include case management, child care for HIV-positive children and children of parents with AIDS, information and referrals, support groups, and support services.

Grandma's House
TERRIFIC, Inc.
Phone: (202) 462–8526, HIV program
(202) 234–4128, administration
1222 T Street NW
Washington, DC

Services include housing for children who have been abandoned, abused, neglected, prenatally drug-exposed, or are HIV-positive. This agency works to restore the family unit and offers assessment and referrals for drug rehabilitation, counseling, education, entitlement application, and support services. The adolescent program provides teen peer education on HIV and drugs; adolescents may participate in an internship to work with the younger children in the homes.

Impact—DC, Inc.
Phone: (202) 546–7228
300 I Street NE
Washington, DC 20002

Services include case management, information and referrals, legal services, nutritional assessment, counseling, support groups, and support services.

Pediatric AIDS/HIV Care Inc.
Phone: (202) 347–7707
1317 G Street NW
Washington, DC 20005

Services include child care for HIV-positive children, family support, information and referrals, and respite care.

Whitman-Walker Clinic
AIDS/Medical Services Programs
Phone: (202) 797–3500
TTY/TDD: (202) 797–3547
American Sign Language and Spanish speakers available
1407 S Street NW
Washington, DC 20009

Services include case management, clinical trials, direct health services and care, information and referrals, mental health services, substance abuse prevention and treatment, support groups, support services, and testing.

Delaware Lesbian and Gay Health Advocates AIDS Committee
Phone: (302) 652–6776
Hot line: (800) 422–0429 (in-state)
Spanish speakers available
800 West Street
Wilmington, DE 19801

Services include AA meetings, buddy program, information and statewide referrals, support groups, support services, and testing.

Health Education Resource Organization
Phone: (301) 685–1180
Hot line: (301) 945–2437
Hot line: (800) 638–6352 (outside of Baltimore)
101 West Read Street, No. 825
Baltimore, MD 21201

HERO services include advocacy, buddy support group, case management, counseling, information and referrals, support services.

Maine Department of Human Services, Bureau of Health
Office on AIDS
Phone: (207) 289–3747
Augusta, ME 04333

Services include statewide referrals to local resources for case management, counseling, information and referrals, support groups, and testing.

AIDS Action Committee
Phone: (617) 437–6200
131 Clarendon Street
Boston, MA 02116

Services include advocacy, case management, counseling, legal services, respite, support groups, support services. Group provides a free HIV/AIDS resource guide for women in the greater Boston area.

Women, Inc.
AIDS Department
Phone: (617) 442–6166
Spanish speakers available
244 Townsend Street
Dorchester, MA 02121

Services include advocacy, information and referrals, outreach to sex workers, support groups, support services, testing, and counseling.

AIDS Service Agency of Wake County
Phone: (919) 834–2437
324 South Harrington Street
Raleigh, NC 27603

Services include buddy program, education, family care home for individuals requiring care, information and referrals, support groups, and support services.

The AIDS Services Project
Phone: (919) 286–7475
Box 3203
Durham, NC 27715-3203

Services include buddy program, case management, emergency housing, information and referrals, support services.

Woman Reach
Phone: (704) 334–3614
Midtown Square
Suite 605, Gallery
Charlotte, NC 28204

Group provides information and one-on-one counseling to help HIV-positive women assess their needs, then provides referrals.

New Hampshire Division of Public Health Services
STD/HIV/AIDS Program
Phone: (603) 271–4576
Hot line: (800) 752–2437
(information tapes)
6 Hazen Drive
Health and Welfare Building
Concord, NH 03301

Services include case management, financial assistance for medications, information and referrals, statewide resource directory, and testing.

Hyacinth Foundation
Phone: (800) 433–0254
Spanish speakers available
103 Bayerd Street
New Brunswick, NJ 08901

Services include advocacy, counseling, legal services, information and referrals, support groups, support services, and testing.

The Family Place
United Hospital Medical Center/CHAP
Phone: (201) 481–0242
Spanish speakers available
15 South Ninth Street
Newark, NJ 07107

This group provides advocacy, case management, counseling, "family friends" emotional support, information and referrals, legal services, respite, substance abuse assessment, support groups, and support services. It also makes video and audio tapes of women with AIDS for their children.

University of Medicine and Dentistry of New Jersey
Medical School University Hospital
Women's HIV Clinic
Phone: (201) 456–4300
Spanish speakers available
150 Bergen Street
Newark, NJ 07103

Services include case management, clinical trials, counseling, direct health care and services, information and referrals, and testing. Full service care, including gynecological and obstetrical care, is available for women. Services are provided mostly to women with HIV but also to men and children.

AIDS Council of Northeastern New York
Phone: (518) 434–4686
Hot line: (518) 445–2437
Spanish speakers available
750 Broadway
Albany, NY 12207

Services include case management, education counseling, information and referrals, support groups, and support services.

Bronx-Lebanon Hospital Center
Infectious Disease Clinic
Phone: (212) 901–8940
Spanish speakers available
1309 Fulton Avenue
Bronx, NY 10456

Services include case management, counseling, crisis intervention, family treatment, and gynecological and medical treatment.

Caribbean Women's Health Association
Phone: (718) 826–2942
French, Haitian, Creole, and Spanish speakers available
2725 Church Avenue
Brooklyn, NY 11226-4104

Services include case management, counseling, legal services (immigration), information and referrals, and support groups to women and families of Caribbean origin.

Community Family Planning Council
Health Center and Executive Offices
Phone: (212) 447–1120
92–94 Ludlow Street
New York, NY 10002

Citywide clinics provide reproductive and primary health care to hundreds of thousands of low-income, minority, and homeless women and their families in New York. HIV and AIDS services include education, case management, counseling and testing, early intervention primary care, and outreach.

Community Health Network

Phone: (716) 244–9000

758 South Avenue

Rochester, NY 14620

Advocacy, case management, clinical trials, direct health care and services, support groups, support services, and testing are provided.

Montefiore Medical Center Women's Center

Phone: (212) 920–4280

Spanish speakers available

3320 Rochambeau Avenue

Bronx, NY 10467

Services include case management, counseling, information and referrals, legal services, recreational activities, substance abuse aftercare, support groups, and support services. Services are provided for women of African-American and Hispanic origin and their families.

New York City Department of Health
Pediatric Resource Unit

Phone: (718) 643–7630

111 Livingston Street

Brooklyn, NY 11201

Services include advocacy, case management with HIV-positive children and their biological parents or foster families, and assessment for day care, school, and social services. Unit provides families with training on HIV and information and referrals.

People with AIDS Coalition

Phone: (212) 532–0290

Hot line: (800) 828–3280

Spanish speakers available

31 West 26th Street

New York, NY 10010-1090

Services include education, information and referrals, and a support group. Mothers of children with AIDS operate the hot line. The group's *Newsline* newsletter is written by individuals with HIV/AIDS.

Women and AIDS Resource Network

Phone: (718) 596–6007

30 Third Avenue, Suite 212

Brooklyn, NY 11217

Services provided for women and their families include case management, counseling, crisis intervention, empowerment workshops for women, information and referrals, and safer sex counseling.

Elizabeth Blackwell Health Center for Women
HIV Testing and AIDS Counseling for Women Only
Phone: (215) 923–7577
1124 Walnut Street
Philadelphia, PA 19107

Services include abortion services, direct health care, gynecological care, and testing.

Family AIDS Center for Treatment and Support
Phone: (401) 461–6330
Creole and Spanish speakers available
239 Oxford Street
Providence, RI 02905

Services include advocacy, case management, child care for HIV-positive children, counseling, information and referrals, support groups, support services, transitional housing, and twenty-four-hour nursery.

Central Virginia AIDS Services and Education
Phone: (804) 359–4783
1627 Monument Avenue
Richmond, VA 23220

Services include advocacy, child care for HIV-positive children and for children of parents with AIDS, information and referrals, legal services, support groups, and support services.

Vermont Cares
Phone: (802) 863–2437
30 Elmwood Avenue
Burlington, VT 05401

Services include advocacy, case management, educational services, information and referrals, support groups, and support services.

West Virginia Department of Health and Human Resources
West Virginia AIDS Program
Phone: (304) 558–2950
Hot line: (800) 642–8244 (in-state)
1422 Washington Street E
Charleston, WV 25301

Services include case management, counseling, information and referrals, legal services, physician referrals, support groups, support services, and testing

Midwestern United States

Chicago Women's AIDS Project
Phone: (312) 271–2070
5249 North Kenmore
Chicago, IL 60640

Services include case management, counseling, information and referrals, safer-sex counseling, and support groups for HIV-positive women and their families.

Kupona Network
Phone: (312) 536–3000
Spanish speakers available
4611 South Ellis Avenue
Chicago, IL 60653

Services include case management, counseling, information and referrals, residential housing, support groups (includes family support groups for African-Americans), supportive care designed to meet the needs of African-Americans affected by HIV/AIDS. The Network can provide a free copy of the Greater Chicago Area HIV/AIDS Services Directory.

Women and Children HIV Program
Cook County Hospital
Phone: (312) 633–5080
Spanish speakers available
1835 West Harrison Street
CCSN# 912
Chicago, IL 60612

Services include case management, counseling, direct health care and services, information and referrals, substance abuse counseling, support groups, and support services.

HIV LifeCare Clinic
Methodist Hospital of Indiana, Inc.
Phone: (317) 929–2915
Medical Tower, Suite 105
1633 Capitol Avenue
Indianapolis, IN 46202

Services include case management, clinical trials, information and referrals, outpatient care and treatment, and support groups.

Broadlawns Primary Care
Phone: (515) 282–2427
Spanish speakers available
18th and Hickman Road
Des Moines, IA 50314-1597

Services include advocacy, case management, crisis intervention, direct health care and services, information and referrals, support groups, and testing.

Connect Care
Phone: (316) 265–9468
317 East 11th Street
Wichita, KS 67203

Services include case management, housing (group residence), support groups, and support services for women with HIV and their families.

Kansas Department of Health and Environment
Phone: (913) 232–3100
109 SW Ninth Street
Mills Building, Suite 605
Topeka, KS 66612-1271

Services include statewide information and referrals.

Detroit Medical Center
HIV/AIDS Program
Phone: (313) 745–1941
Harper Professional Building
4160 John R Street, Suite 730
Detroit, MI 48201

This program offers both HIV-positive and HIV-negative women comprehensive free treatment as part of CDC-funded HERS HIV Epidemiology Research Study. Women receive blood work, gynecological care, transportation, and lunch.

Michigan Department of Public Health
HIV/AIDS Prevention and Intervention Section
Phone: (517) 335–8371
Hot line: (800) 872–2437 (in-state)
3423 North Logan Street
Lansing, MI 48906

Services include statewide information and referrals. Office also can provide a single free copy of the state resource directory.

Simon House
Phone: (313) 863–1400
16260 Dexter
Detroit, MI 48221

Services include case management, counseling, hospice care for child with mother or guardian, information and referrals, support groups, support services, and transitional housing.

Minnesota AIDS Project
Phone: (612) 870–7773
Hot line: (800) 248–2437
Spanish speakers available
2025 Nicollet Avenue, No. 200
Minneapolis, MN 55044-2555

Services include statewide referral for services, advocacy, case management, legal services, supportive care, and transitional housing.

St. Louis Effort for AIDS
Phone: (314) 367–2382
Hot line: (314) 367–8400
French and Spanish speakers available
5622 Delmar Boulevard
Suite 104E
St. Louis, MO 63112

Services include case management, drop-in and activities center, information and referrals, support groups, and support services.

North Dakota State Department of Health and Consolidated Laboratories
Phone: (701) 224–2370
Judicial Wing, Second Floor
600 East Boulevard Avenue
Bismark, ND 58505-0200

Services include statewide information and referrals.

Nebraska AIDS Project
Phone: (402) 342–4233
Hot line: (800) 782–2437
3624 Leavenworth Street
Omaha, NE 68105

Services include buddy program, case management, counseling, education, information and referrals, and support services.

Columbus AIDS Task Force
Phone: (614) 466–4643
Hot line: (800) 332–2437
TTY/TDD: (800) 332–3889
American Sign Language available
1500 West Third Avenue, Suite 329
Columbus, OH 43266-0588

Services include buddy program, case management, counseling, education, information and referrals, legal services, support groups, and support services.

South Dakota Department of Health AIDS Program
Phone: (605) 773–3364
Hot line: (800) 592–1861
523 East Capitol
Pierre, SD 57501-3182

Services include statewide information and referrals.

Madison AIDS Support Network
Phone: (608) 238–6276
Hot line: (800) 486–6276
303 Lathrop Street
Madison, WI 53705

Services include case management, information and referrals, support groups, and support services.

The Milwaukee AIDS Project
Phone: (414) 273–1991
Hot line: (414) 273–2437
315 West Court Street
Milwaukee, WI 53212

Services include case management, counseling, information and referrals, legal services, library resource center, support groups, and support services.

Southern United States

Birmingham AIDS Outreach
Phone: (205) 322–4197
Box 550070
Birmingham, AL 35255

Services include buddy program, education, information and referrals, peer counseling, support groups, and support services.

Mobile AIDS Support Services
Phone: (205) 433–6277
Hot line: (205) 432–AIDS
107 North Ann
Mobile, AL 36604

Services include advocacy, buddy program, case management, counseling, education, information and referrals, support groups, and support services.

Arkansas AIDS Foundation
Phone: (501) 663–7833
5911 H Street
Little Rock, AR 72205

Services include case management, information and referrals, and testing.

Regional AIDS Interfaith Network
Phone: (501) 375–5908
509 South Scott Street
Little Rock, AR 72202

This group trains and coordinates care teams who provide services to allow the person with AIDS to remain at home.

Central Florida AIDS Unified Resources, Inc.
Phone: (407) 849–1452
TTY/TDD: (407) 843–3145
Spanish speakers available
1235 South Orange Avenue
Orlando, FL 32806

Services include counseling, information and referrals, peer counselors, support groups, and support services.

Health Crisis Network, Inc.
Phone: (305) 326–8833
Hotline: (305) 634–4636
Spanish speakers available
Box 42-1280
Miami, FL 33242-1280

Services include buddy program, information and referrals, licensed outpatient substance abuse program, support groups, and support services.

HRS Alachua Public Health Unit HIV Testing/Clinic
Phone: (904) 336–2415
Spanish speakers available
730 North Waldo Road
Gainesville, FL 32601

Services include case management, information and referrals, support groups, STD clinic, specialty clinic for those with low income, and testing services for adults.

HRS Broward County Public Health Unit
Phone: (305) 467–4532
Creole, French, Spanish, and Patou speakers available
Northwest Health Center
624 NW 15 Way
Fort Lauderdale, FL 33311

Services include counseling, dental care, early intervention program, home services (contracts with home care agencies), information and referrals, medical care, specialty clinic for those with low income.

Tampa AIDS Network
Florida Women's AIDS Resource Movement
Phone: (813) 978–8683
Hot line: (800) 359–9276
Spanish speakers available
11215 North Nebraska Avenue, Suite B3
Tampa, FL 33612

Services for HIV-positive women and their families include buddy program, case management, counseling, education, information and referrals, outreach, support groups, and support services.

AID Atlanta

Phone: (404) 872–0600
Hot line: (404) 876–9944
Spanish speakers available
1438 West Peachtree Street NW
Suite 100
Atlanta, GA 30309

Services include buddy program, case management (includes pediatric), direct health care and services, treatment center for alcohol or drug addiction, information and referrals, social support network, telephone support, testing, and transitional housing.

Emory AIDS Training Network

Phone: (404) 727–2929
735 Gatewood Road NE
Atlanta, GA 30322

Network provides *Key Contacts,* a free directory of HIV/AIDS services in Georgia.

AIDS Services Center

Phone: (502) 625–5490
810 Barret Avenue
Louisville, KY 40204

Services include AIDS library, community-based services, education, housing grants, information and referrals statewide, medication, residential facilities, support groups. Center provides free copy of the *AIDS Resources Directory* for southern Indiana and Kentucky.

Associated Catholic Charities
New Orleans AIDS Project

Phone: (504) 523–3755 (TAP and RAIN programs)
(504) 523–4320 (housing program)
1231 Prytania Street
New Orleans, LA 70130-4313

Through case management referrals, individuals with HIV/AIDS can obtain transportation (TAP); in-home care through care teams (RAIN); and low-income, independent living housing.

Central Louisiana AIDS Support Services

Phone: (318) 443–5216
Hot line: (800) 444–7993
824 16th Street
Alexandria, LA 71301-6809

Services include buddy program, care teams, case management, counseling, education, information and referral, support groups, support services, teen peer groups, and testing.

AIDS/HIV Prevention Program
Phone: (601) 960–7723
2324 North State Street
Jackson, MS 39202-1165

Services include statewide information and referrals and resource directory.

New Mexico AIDS Services
Phone: (505) 266–0911
Spanish speakers available
Services and Administration Office
4200 Silver SE, Suite D
Albuquerque, NM 87108

Services include buddy program, client services, education, emotional support, housing, support services, and testing.

New Mexico Association of People Living with AIDS
Phone: (505) 266–0342
Hot line: (800) 658–6717
126 Jackson NE
Albuquerque, NM 87108-1257

Services include advocacy, AIDS library, education, statewide database referrals, and support groups.

University of New Mexico Hospitals
Partners-in-Care Program
Phone: (505) 843–2111 (department of infectious disease)
Phone: (505) 843–2328 (department of clinical social work)
2211 Lomas Boulevard NE
Albuquerque, NM 87106

Services include counseling and direct health care and services for HIV/AIDS clients.

SHANTI—Tulsa
Phone: (918) 749–7898
Box 4318
Tulsa, OK 74159-0318

Services include buddy program, case management, counseling, education, support groups, and support services.

Palmetto AIDS Life Support Services of South Carolina, Inc.
Phone: (803) 779–7257
Hot line: (800) 723–7257 (in-state)
Box 12124
Columbia, SC 29211-2124

Services include buddy program, case management, counseling, education, information and referrals statewide, legal services, and support services.

Tennessee Department of Health
AIDS Program
Phone: (615) 741–7500
Hot line: (800) 525–2437
C2-221 Cordell Hull Building
Nashville, TN 37247-4947

Services include statewide referrals for clinical trials, counseling, legal services, medical care, medication assistance, support groups, and testing.

AIDS Foundation Houston
Phone: (713) 524–2437
Spanish speakers available
3202 West Leyen
Houston, TX 77027

Services include advocacy, case management, information and referrals, support groups, and support services.

AIDS Foundation of San Antonio
Phone: (512) 225–4715
818 East Grayson
San Antonio, TX 78208

Services include buddy program, case management, counseling, dental and health services, residential facility, support services, and testing. Services are only for the adult individual who is HIV-positive.

AIDS Interfaith Network, Inc., of North Texas
Phone: (214) 559–4899
2727 Oaklawn, Suite 108
Dallas, TX 75219

Services include home chores, information and referrals, pastoral counseling, respite care, support groups, weekend retreats.

AIDS Resource Center
Phone: (214) 521–5124
Hot line: (214) 559–2437
2701 Reagen Street
Dallas, TX 75219

Services include case management, counseling, information and referrals, pet pals, support groups, and support services.

Omega House, Inc.
Phone: (713) 523–7110
Hot line: (713) 523–1139
Spanish speakers available
2615 Waugh Drive
Houston, TX 77006

Services include counseling, direct health care and services, hospice care for adult individuals who are HIV-positive.

Open Arms, Inc.
Bryan's House
Phone: (214) 559–3946
Box 191402
Dallas, TX 75219

Services include child care for families affected by HIV, information and referrals, on-site day care, respite, support services.

Western United States

Alaskan AIDS Assistance Association
Phone: (907) 276–1400
Hot line: (800) 276–4880 (in-state)
7030 I Street, Suite 100
Anchorage, AK 99501

Services include buddy system, case management, counseling, drop-in center, education, support groups, support services. A free HIV resource manual is available.

Arizona AIDS Project
Phone: (602) 420–9396
Spanish speakers available
919 North First Street
Phoenix, AZ 85004-1902

Services include buddy program, case management, education, hospital visitation, information and referrals statewide, legal clinic, support groups (includes culture-specific), and support services.

Tucson AIDS Project
Phone: (602) 322–6226
Hot line: (602) 326–2437
151 South Tucson Boulevard, No. 252
Tucson, AZ 85716-5523

Services include advocacy, case management, education, information and referrals, support groups, and support services. A program for children of parents with AIDS called "Not Just the Facts" provides family assessment, counseling, training, and support.

AIDS Project Los Angeles
Phone: (213) 962–1600
Spanish speakers available
6721 Romaine Street
Hollywood, CA 90038

Services include advocacy, buddy program, case management, clinical trials, counseling (includes addictive behavior), dental clinic, education, information and referral, legal services, support groups, and support services.

AIDS Project of the East Bay
Women's Service Division
Phone: (510) 834–8181
Hot line: (800) 273–2057 (in-county)
Spanish speakers available
565 16th Street, Third Floor
Oakland, CA 94612

Services include advocacy, emotional and practical support volunteers, information and referrals, support groups, and support services geared toward the needs of HIV-positive women.

Inland AIDS Project
Phone: (714) 784–2437
Hot line: (800) 499–2437 (in-state)
Spanish speakers available
1240 Palmyrita Avenue
Riverside, CA 92501

Services include buddy program, case management, counseling, information and referrals, outreach, support groups (includes anger management and addiction recovery group), and support services.

Lyon-Martin Women's Health Services
Phone: (415) 565–7667
1748 Market Street
San Francisco, CA 94102

Services include case management, counseling, direct health care and services to African-American women.

Orange County Health Care Agency
Phone: (714) 834–7991
Spanish and Vietnamese speakers available
1725 West 17th Street
Santa Ana, CA 92706

Services include case management, information and referrals, medical clinic, outreach to sex workers and prisoners, substance abuse program, and testing.

Prototypes/Women and AIDS Risk Network
Phone: (310) 641–7795
5601 West Slauson Avenue, No. 200
Culver City, CA 90230

This group assists women at risk for AIDS through risk reduction, education, and behavior modification intervention programs. Specific targets are sex partners of male injection-drug users, adolescent prostitutes, and adult prostitutes. Information and referrals are provided for women who are HIV-positive.

San Francisco AIDS Foundation
Women and Children Services Program
Phone: (415) 864–5855
French, German, Filipino, and Spanish speakers available
Box 6182
San Francisco, CA 94101-6182

Services include case management, information and referrals, and support services.

San Francisco Women's Centers
Phone: (415) 431–1180
Spanish speakers available
Women's Buildings,
Women with HIV/AIDS Project
3543 18th Street
San Francisco, CA 94117

Several organizations with a focus on women (HIV-positive and negative) are housed in this building, such as those providing support groups, job listings, and lesbian and health coalitions

Santa Cruz AIDS Project
Phone: (408) 427–3900
TTY/TDD: (408) 426–1964
American Sign Language, French, Portuguese, and Spanish speakers available
911A Center Street
Santa Cruz, CA 95060

Services include advocacy, child care for HIV-positive children and children of parents with AIDS, counseling, information and referrals, support groups, and support services.

Shanti Project
Phone: (415) 777–2273
TTY/TDD: (415) 495–7495
Spanish speakers available
525 Howard Street
San Francisco, CA 94105

Services include child care for children with HIV and children of parents with AIDS, counseling, housing, information and referrals, recreational activities and free tickets, support for families and caregivers of people with AIDS, support groups, support services, van transportation to medical appointments, and volunteers for practical and emotional support. Certain services are available for the deaf.

Colorado AIDS Project
Phone: (303) 830–2437
Hot line: (800) 333–2437 (in-state)
Spanish speakers available
1576 Sherman Street
Denver, CO 80218-0529

Services include buddy program, case management, information and referrals statewide, legal services, outreach (education), support groups, and support services.

The Empowerment Program
Phone: (303) 863–7817
Spanish speakers available
1245 East Colfax Avenue, No. 404
Denver, CO 80218-2216

Services include case management, education, information and referrals, outreach (women prisoners, sex workers, the homeless, and injection-drug users), recreational activities, safer-sex counseling, sisters program (similar to a buddy program), support groups, and support services for HIV-positive women and their families.

Hawaii State Department of Health
STD/AIDS Prevention Branch Clinic
Phone: (808) 735–5303 (clinic)
(808) 733–9010 (services)
Hot line: (808) 922–1313
Chinese, Italian, Japanese, Korean, Llocano, Filipino, Samoan, Spanish, and Visayan speakers available
3627 Kilauea Avenue, No. 306
Honolulu, HI 96816

Services include clinical trials, direct health care and services, information and referrals statewide, support services, testing, and counseling.

Idaho Department of Health and Welfare
STD/AIDS Program
Phone: (208) 334–5937
450 West State Street
Boise, ID 83720

Services include statewide resource referral, information, and medication assistance.

Montana Department of Health and Environmental Services
AIDS Program
Phone: (406) 444–3565
Hot line: (800) 233–6668 (in-state)
Helena, MT 59260

Services include statewide information and referrals, free resource directory.

Nevada AIDS Foundation
Information and Referral Line
Phone: (702) 329–2437
1225 West Field Avenue, Suite 8
Reno, NV 89509

Services include buddy program, direct services, rent subsidy program, support program, support groups, and support services.

Cascade AIDS Project
Phone: (503) 223–5907
Hot line: (800) 777–2437 (in-state)
Cantonese and Spanish speakers available
620 SW Fifth, Suite 300
Portland, OR 97204

Services include advocacy, case management, informal telephone network that connects newly HIV-positive women and men with other HIV-positive women and men, information and referrals, legal services, support groups, and support services.

Utah AIDS Foundation
Phone: (801) 487–2323
Hot line: (800) 366–2437 (in-state)
450 South 900 East, Suite 105
Salt Lake City, UT 84102

Services include buddy program, case management, education, information and referrals statewide, peer support (visits clients in institutional settings), support groups, and support services.

Bailey and Boushay
Phone: (206) 322–5300
2720 East Madison
Seattle, WA 98112

Organization is primarily a residential, twenty-four-hour skilled care facility for adults with AIDS (requires Medicaid, Medicare, a third-party insurer, or private pay). It also offers an adult day health program that includes a support group for family and partners.

Seattle-King County Department of Public Health
Northwest Family Center
Phone: (206) 720–4300
Spanish speakers available
1001 Broadway Avenue, No. 210
Seattle, WA 98122

Services include advocacy, child care for HIV-positive children, clinical trials, direct health care and services, public resource center on women, children, families and HIV, substance abuse counseling, and support services.

State of Wyoming Department of Health
Division of Prevention Medicine
Wyoming HIV/AIDS Program
Phone: (307) 777–5800
Hot line: (800) 327–3577 (in-state)
Spanish speakers available
2001 Capitol Avenue
Hathaway Building, No. 475
Cheyenne, WY 82002

Services include statewide referrals for case management, child care, clinical trials, counseling, direct health care and services, substance abuse prevention and treatment, support groups, support services, and testing.

Informational Resources

Telephone Hot Lines—National

National Aids Hotline
Phone: (800) 342–2437
(919) 361–8430 (administration)
(800) 344–7432 (Spanish speakers available)
(800) 243–7889 (TTY, English only)
American Social Health Association
Box 13827
Research Triangle Park, NC 27709

Hotline, funded by the CDC, is available seven days a week, twenty-four hours a day. It provides a computerized list of names and phone numbers of organizations across the country, including HIV counseling and testing centers, drug treatment services, general AIDS information, hot lines in each state, and teen and runaway services.

Native American AIDS Hotline
Phone: (800) 283–2437

Services include counseling, information, and referral.

Pediatric and Pregnancy AIDS Hot Line
Phone: (212) 430–3333
(212) 430–2940 (administration)
Albert Einstein College of Medicine
1300 Morris Park Avenue
Bronx, NY 10461

Hot line can answer HIV questions concerning pediatrics, pregnancy, and counseling.

Teens TAP and AIDS Hotline
Phone: (800) 234–8336

Services include counseling, information, and referral.

U.S. Centers for Disease Control and Prevention
Phone: (404) 639–3311
(404) 639–2957 (statistics)
1600 Clifton Road NE
Atlanta, GA 30333

National AIDS Clearing House
Phone: (800) 458–5231
Box 6003
Rockville, MD 20850

Hot line provides everything that has been printed by the CDC (e.g., Universal Precautions, Directory of Clinical Trials).

Women and AIDS Periodicals and Publications

The Positive Woman
Phone: (202) 898–0372
Box 34372
Washington, DC 20043-4372

This is a private, nonprofit, volunteer organization dedicated to the empowerment of HIV-infected women. It produces a bimonthly newsletter, *The Positive Woman,* that includes information on traditional medical practices and holistic approaches to well-being. A telephone hot line is available for HIV-positive women to talk with other HIV-positive women.

Womyns Braille Press
Phone: (612) 872–4352
Box 8475
Minneapolis, MN 55408

This group produces audiotapes and braille books for the blind on feminism, sexuality, lesbianism, writings by women of color, radical feminist theory, writings on violence against women, and women's health issues, including AIDS.

Women Organizing to Respond to Life-Threatening Diseases
Phone: (510) 658–6930
Box 11535
Oakland, CA 94611

This organization produces a monthly newsletter by, for, and about women with HIV and those affected by HIV/AIDS. A quarterly newsletter in Spanish entitled *Mujer imagen de vida* (Woman, symbol of life) is also available. Both newsletters provide personal testimonies, treatment information, general education, letters, and announcements of conferences and support groups.

Women and AIDS Videos

"AIDS Is About Secrets"
HIV Center
722 West 168th Street
New York, NY 10032

This thirty-seven-minute video tells the story of four African-American women whose male partners are IV-drug users. It is based on real-life stories.

"AIDS: Me and My Baby"
HIV Center
722 West 168th Street
New York, NY 10032

This twenty-two-minute video illustrates the issues around HIV infection and pregnancy with a series of dramatized vignettes.

"A Promise Kept"
McNabb & Connolly
60 Briarwood Avenue
Port Credit, Ontario
Canada L5G 3N6

This forty-six-minute documentary is about a woman who stays with her spouse through his death from AIDS.

"Vida"
Aidsfilms/Select Media
74 Varick Street, Suite 305
New York, NY 10013

This eighteen-minute story of a young Hispanic woman is aimed at AIDS prevention among urban U.S. teenagers.

"My Body's My Business"
Cultural Research and Communication, Inc.
2600 Tenth Street
Berkeley, CA 94710

This sixteen-minute documentary features prostitutes and ex-prostitutes with the CAL-PEP project who speak frankly about staying safe on the streets with their dates, as well as at home with their boyfriends.

The Orphan Generation
Small World Productions
Teaching Aids at Low Cost
Box 49, St. Albans
Hertfordshire, AL 4AX
U.K.

This forty-minute video focuses on the struggle of one Ugandan village to cope with the deepening orphan crisis.

Further Reading on Women and AIDS

Anthologies and Women's Stories

Kaleeba, N., with S. Ray and B. Wilmore. 1992. *We miss you all. Noerine Kaleeba: AIDS in the family.* Harare, Zimbabwe: Women and AIDS Support Network.

O'Sullivan, S., and K. Thompson, eds. 1992. *Positively women—Living with AIDS.* London: Sheba Feminist Press.

Rieder, I., and P. Ruppelt, eds. 1988. *AIDS: The women*. Pittsburgh: Cleis Press.

Rudd, A., and D. Taylor, eds. 1992. *Positive women—Voices of women living with AIDS*. Toronto: Second Story Press.

Women's Health Resource Collective. 1992. *Positive women—Women with HIV/AIDS speak out*. Victoria, Australia: WHRC.

Clinical and Psychosocial Care Issues

Cohen, F., and J. Durham., eds. 1993. *Women, children, and HIV/AIDS*. New York: Springer.

Dorn, N., S. Henderson, and N. South, eds. 1992. *AIDS: Women, drugs, and social care*. London: Falmer Press.

Schinazi, R., and A. Nahmias, eds. 1988. *AIDS in children, adolescents, and heterosexual adults: An interdisciplinary approach to prevention*. New York: Elsevier.

Squire, C., ed. 1993. *Women and AIDS: Psychological perspectives*. Newbury Park, Calif.: Sage.

General Audience

ACT-UP/NY Women and AIDS Book Group. 1990. *Women, AIDS, and activism*. Edison, N.J.: South End Press.

Corea, G. 1992. *The invisible epidemic: The story of women and AIDS*. New York: HarperCollins.

Norwood, C. 1987. *Advice for life: A woman's guide to AIDS risks and prevention*. New York: Pantheon.

Patton, C., and J. Kelly. 1987. *Making it: A woman's guide to sex in the age of AIDS*. Ithaca, N.Y.: Firebrand Books.

Richardson, D. 1988. *Women and AIDS*. New York: Methuen.

International Impact

Radelet, M. 1991. *Triple jeopardy*. London: PANOS Institute.

Legal Periodicals and Publications

ABA policy and report on AIDS. 1990. Washington, D.C.: American Bar Association.

AIDS law and litigation reporter. Frederick, Md.: University Publishing Group.

AIDS policy and law. Washington, D.C.: Buraff Publications.

Albert, P., R. Eisenberg, D. Hansell, and J. Marcus, eds. 1991. *National Lawyers Guild AIDS practice manual*, 3rd ed. Washington, D.C.: National Lawyers Guild.

Goodwin, S., ed. *AIDS reference guide: A sourcebook for planners and decision makers*. Washington, D.C.: Atlantic Information Services.

LaGamma, D., A. Herb, N. Dubler, and M. Pinott. 1993. *Legal services for a parent with AIDS.* Bronx, N.Y.: Montefiore Medical Center.

Rennert, S. 1989. *AIDS and persons with developmental disabilities: Legal perspective.* Washington, D.C.: American Bar Association.

Rubenfeld, A., ed. 1991. *AIDS benchbook.* Reno, Nev.: National Judicial College.

Zavos, M., ed. 1991. *Directory of legal resources for people with AIDS and HIV.* Washington, D.C.: American Bar Association.

Prenatal Testing and Counseling

Faden, R., G. Geller, and M. Powers, eds. 1991. *AIDS, women, and the next generation.* New York: Oxford University Press.

Melice, F., ed. 1992. *AIDS and human reproduction* (Proceedings of the First International Symposium on AIDS and Reproduction, Genoa, December 12–15, 1990). Basel: Karger.

Sherr, L. 1991. *HIV and AIDS in mothers and babies: A guide to counseling.* London: Blackwell.

Resource Listings

Berer, M. 1993. *Women and HIV/AIDS.* London: Pandora Press.

Center for Women Policy Studies. 1991. *The guide to resources on women and AIDS,* 2nd ed. Washington, D.C.: CWPS.

Hammrich, H., and J. M. Dunn. 1992. *National directory of AIDS care,* 3rd ed. Albuquerque, N.M.: National Directory of AIDS Care (Richards Publishing).

National AIDS Information Clearinghouse. December 1990. *Educational materials for women on HIV/AIDS.* Washington, D.C.: NAIC.

NOVA Research Company. September 1991. *Women, AIDS, and drug use,* rev. ed. Rockville, Md.: NIDA.

Watstein, A., and R. A. Laurich. 1991 *AIDS and women: A sourcebook.* Phoenix, Ariz.: Onyx.

References

ACLU. *See* American Civil Liberties Union.

ACSF Investigators. 1992. AIDS and sexual behavior in France. *Nature* 360: 407–409.

ACTIS. *See* AIDS Clinical Trial Information Service.

Adam, B. D. 1992. Sociology and people living with AIDS. In *The social context of AIDS*, ed. J. Huber and B. Schneider. Newbury Park, Calif.: Sage.

AIDS Clinical Trial Information Service (ACTIS). 1992a. Demographic summary by OI protocol from beginning to January 10, 1992. Rockville, Md.: ACTIS. Phone: (800) 874–2572.

———. 1992b. Demographic summary of ACTG study entries by protocol from beginning to January 17, 1992. Rockville, Md.: ACTIS. Telephone (800) 874–2572.

AIDS Epidemiology Program. 1991. AIDS surveillance quarterly update, December 1991. Albany: State University of New York.

AIDS policy and law. 1991. Women with HIV gets jail term for felony solicitation charge. October 16, 1991: 2.

AIDS Policy Center. 1992. Intergovernmental Health Policy Project, George Washington University.

AIDS Reference Guide. 1990. Washington, D.C.: Atlantic Information Services.

Albert, P., R. Eisenberg, D. Hansell, and J. K. Marcus (eds.). 1991. *AIDS practice manual: Personal and estate planning,* 3rd ed., sec. 4.3: 4–7. Washington, D.C.: National Lawyer's Guild.

Alden, J. S., G. M. Salole, and J. Williamson. 1991. Managing Uganda's orphan crisis. Unpublished report. Washington, D.C.: Technologies for Primary Care, Pritec Project.

Allen, J., and V. Setlow. 1991. Heterosexual transmission of HIV: A view of the future. *Journal of the American Medical Association* 266: 1695–96.

Allen, M. 1990. Primary care of women infected with the human immunodeficiency virus. *Obstetrics and Gynecology Clinics of North America* 17(3): 557–69.

Allen, M., and C. Marte. 1992. HIV infection in women: Presentations and protocols. *Hospital Practice,* March 15, 113–20.

Allen, S., C. Lindan, A. Serufilira, P. Van de Perre, A. C. Rundle, F. Nsengumuremyi, M. Carael, J. Schwalbe, and S. Hulley. 1991. Human immunodeficiency virus infection in urban Rwanda: Demographic and behavioral correlates in a representative sample of child-bearing women. *Journal of the American Medical Association* 266(12): 1657–63.

AMA. *See* American Medical Association.

Amaro, H., L. Fried, H. Cabral. 1990. Violence during pregnancy and substance abuse. *American Journal of Public Health* 80: 5.

American Academy of Neurology AIDS Task Force. 1989. Human immunodeficiency virus infection and the nervous system. *Neurology* 39: 119–22.

American Academy of Pediatrics, Task Force on Pediatric AIDS. 1989. Infants and children with acquired immunodeficiency syndrome: Placement in adoption and foster care. *Pediatrics* 83: 609–12.

American Civil Liberties Union (ACLU). 1991. *In re: Jane Doe.* AIDS Project Docket. October.

American College of Obstetricians and Gynecologists (ACOG). 1987. Prevention of human immunodeficiency virus infection and acquired immunodeficiency syndrome. ACOG Committee Statement. Washington, D.C.: ACOG.

American Medical Association (AMA), Council on Ethical and Judicial Affairs. 1991. Gender disparities in clinical decision making. *Journal of the American Medical Association* 266: 559–62.

American Medical Association Physician Guidelines. 1991. *HIV Early Care.* Chicago: AMA.

Anastos, K. 1992. Epidemiology of HIV infection in women. *HIV/AIDS Clinical Insight* 2(3): 2–7.

Anastos, K. et al. 1991. Hypertension in women: What is really known? The Women's Caucus, Working Group on Women's Health of the Society of General Medicine. *Annals of Internal Medicine* 115: 287–93.

Anastos, K., R. Denenberg, L. Solomon, and S. Rein. 1992. Relationship of CD4 cell counts to cervical cytologic abnormalities and gynecologic infections in 150 HIV-infected women. Paper presented at the Eighth International Conference on AIDS. Amsterdam, July 19–24.

Anastos, K., and S. M. Palleja. 1991. Caring for women at risk of HIV infection. *Journal of General Internal Medicine* 6 (Suppl.): S40-S46.

Anderson, D. J., T. R. O'Brien, J. A. Politch, A. Martinez, G. R. Seage III, N. Padian, C. R. Horsburgh, Jr., and K. H. Mayer. 1992. Effects of disease stage and zidovudine therapy on the detection of human immunodeficiency virus type 1 in semen. *Journal of the American Medical Association* 267(20): 2769–74.

Ankrah, E. M. 1991. AIDS and the social side of health. *Social Science and Medicine* 32(9): 967–80.

Aral, S. O., and K. K. Holmes. 1991. Sexually transmitted diseases in the AIDS era. *Scientific American* 264(2): 62–69.

Archibald, D. W., D. J. Witt, D. E. Craven, M. W. Vogt, M. S. Hirsch, and M. Essex. 1987. Antibodies to human immunodeficiency virus in cervical secretions from women at risk for AIDS. *Journal of Infectious Diseases* 156(1): 240–41.

Arno, P. 1992. *Insurance coverage: New models, new challenges.* Paper presented at the Fifth National AIDS Update Conference. San Francisco, October 9.

Arpadi, S., and W. B. Caspe. 1991. HIV testing. *Journal of Pediatrics* 119(1), part 2: S8–S13.

Arras, J. D. 1990. AIDS and reproductive decisions: Having children in fear and trembling. *Milbank Quarterly* 68(3):353–82.

Associated Press. 1992a. Curbing prostitution on demand side. *New York Times,* April 20, B8.

Associated Press. 1992b. Survey of victims shows increase in violent crime. *New York Times,* B12.

Atkinson, J. H., I. Grant, C. J. Kennedy, D. D. Richman, S. A. Spector, and J. A. Mc-Cutchan. 1988. Prevalence of psychiatric disorders among men infected with human immunodeficiency virus. *Archives of General Psychiatry* 45: 859–64.

Auer, L. 1992. Pap testing and cervical disease: Implications for women with HIV. *PI Perspective Project Inform* 12 (April): 6–8.

Auger, I., P. Thomas, V. De Gruttola, et al. 1988. Incubation periods of pediatric AIDS patients. *Nature* 336: 575–77.

Austin, H., W. C. Louv, and W. J. Alexander. 1984. A case control study of spermicides and gonorrhea. *Journal of the American Medical Association* 251: 2822.

Aybouya, Y. L., A. Beaumel, S. Lucas, A. Dago-Akribi, G. Coulibaly, M. N'Dhatz, J. B. Konan, A. Yapi, and K. M. de Cock. 1992. Pneumocystis carinii pneumonia: An uncommon cause of death in African patients with acquired immunodeficiency syndrome. *American Review of Respiratory Diseases* 145: 617–20.

Ayd, F. J. 1988. Psychopharmacotherapy for HIV-infected, AIDS-related complex (ARC), and AIDS patients. *International Drug Therapy Newsletter* 23: 25–28.

Bader, E. 1990. Pregnant drug users face jail. *New Directions for Women* 19(2). Englewood, N.J.: New Directions for Women.

Baer, J. W. 1989. Study of 60 patients with AIDS or AIDS-related complex requiring psychiatric hospitalization. *American Journal of Psychiatry* 146: 1285–88.

Baker, D. A., C. Hameed, N. Tejani, P. Milch, J. Thomas, A. G. Monheit, and R. J. Dattwyler. 1985. Lymphocytic subsets in women on low-dose oral contraceptives. *Contraception* 32(4): 377–82.

Barbacci, M., R. Chaisson, J. Anderson, and J. Horn. 1989. Knowledge of HIV serostatus and pregnancy decisions. Paper presented at the Fifth International Conference on AIDS. Montreal, June 4–9.

Barbacci, M., J. T. Repke, and R. Chaisson. 1991. Routine prenatal screening for HIV infection. *Lancet* 337: 709–11.

Barnett, T., P. Blaikie, and C. Obbo. 1990. Community coping mechanisms in the face of exceptional demographic change. Final Report to the Overseas Development Administration. London: ODA.

Barrett, J. E., J. A. Barrett, T. E. Oxman, and P. D. Gerber. 1988. The prevalence of psychiatric disorders in a primary care practice. *Archives of General Psychiatry* 45: 1100–1106.

Barringer, F. 1992. New census data reveal redistribution of poverty. *New York Times,* May 29, A14.

Bassett, M., and M. Mhloyi. 1991. Women and AIDS in Zimbabwe: The making of an epidemic. *International Journal of Health Services* 21(1): 127–30.

Bateson, M. C. 1990. *Composing a life.* New York: Plume.

Bayer, R. 1990. AIDS and the future of reproductive freedom. *Milbank Quarterly* 68 (Suppl. 2): 179–204.

———. 1991. AIDS and the future of reproductive freedom. In *A disease of society: Cultural and institutional responses to AIDS*, ed. D. Nelkin, D. P. Willis, and S. V. Parris. New York: Cambridge University Press.

Bayer, R., C. Levine, and S. M. Wolf. 1986. HIV antibody screening: An ethical framework for evaluating proposed programs. *Journal of the American Medical Association* 256: 1768–74.

Bayer, R., L. H. Lumey, and L. Wan. 1990. The American and Dutch responses to unlinked anonymous HIV seroprevalence studies: An international comparison. *AIDS* 4: 4283–90.

Becker, T. M., K. M. Stone, and E. R. Alexander. 1987. Genital human papillomavirus. *Obstetrics and Gynecology Clinics of North America* 14(2): 389–96.

Beckett, A. 1990. The neurobiology of human immunodeficiency virus infection. In *American Psychiatric Press review of psychiatry,* ed. A. Tasman, S. M. Goldfinger, and C. A. Kaufmann, vol. 19, 593–613. Washington, D.C.: American Psychiatric Press.

Beckett, A., P. Summergrad, T. Manschreck, H. Vitagliano, M. Henderson, M. L. Buttolph, and M. Jenike. 1987. Symptomatic HIV infection of the CNS in a patient without clinical evidence of immune deficiency. *American Journal of Psychiatry* 144: 1342–44.

BEMFAM and AIDSCOM. 1992. Criacao de programa de apoio visando o incentivo ao uso do condon. Final Quantitative Research Report. Rio de Janeiro: AIDSCOM, May.

Benson, C., B. Sha, P. Urbanski, J. Pottage, and H. Kessler. 1992. Women with HIV disease: Clinical progression and survival in a cohort followed at a university medical center. Presented at the Eighth International Conference on AIDS. Amsterdam, July 19–24.

Benson, D. J. D., and C. Maier. 1990. Challenges facing women with HIV. *Focus: A Guide to Research and Counseling* 6(1): 1–2.

Benton, E. 1990. The constitutionality of pregnancy clauses in living will statutes. *Vanderbilt Law Review* 43: 1821.

Beresford, L. 1991. Cracking the big case. *TCM,* July 1991, 50–58.

Berkelman, R., P. Fleming, S. Chu, and D. Hanson. 1991. Women and AIDS: The increasing role of heterosexual transmission in the United States. Abstract presented at the Seventh International Conference on AIDS. Florence, June 16–21.

Berkely, S., W. Naamara, S. Okware, R. Downing, J. Konde-Lule, M. Wawer, M. Musagaara, and S. Musgrave. 1990. AIDS and HIV infection in Uganda: Are more women infected than men? *AIDS* 4: 1237–47.

Berkely, S., S. Okware, and W. Naamara. 1989. Surveillance for AIDS in Uganda. *AIDS* 3: 79–85.

Berkman, L. F. 1984. Assessing the physical health effects of social networks and social support. *Annual Review of Public Health* 5: 413–32.

Berkman, L. F., and L. Breslow. 1983. Social networks and mortality risk. In *Health and Ways of Living: The Alameda County Study,* ed. L. F. Berkman and L. Breslow. New York: Oxford University Press.

Berkman, L. F., and S. L. Syme. 1989. Social networks, host resistance, and mortality: A nine-year follow-up study of Alameda County residents. *American Journal of Epidemiology* 109(2): 186–204.

Berkowitz, K., and A. LaSala. 1990. Risk factors associated with the increasing prevalence of pneumonia during pregnancy. *American Journal of Obstetrics and Gynecology* 163: 981–85.

Bernstein, G., V. A. Clark, A. H. Coulsen, R. Frezieres, L. H. Kilzer, R. M. Nakamura, and T. Walsh. 1986. Use-effectiveness study of cervical caps: Final report. Washington, D.C.: National Institute of Child Health and Human Development (contract N01-HD-1-2804).

Bertrand, J. T., M. Bakutuvwidi, D. Balowa, and L. N. Kinavwidi. 1989. Connaissances du SIDA et comportement sexuel dans 10 sites au Zaire. Working paper, Tulane University.

Boue, F., J. C. Pons, L. Keros, V. Chambrin, E. Papiernik, R. Henrion, and J. F. Delfraissey. 1990. Risks for HIV-1 perinatal transmission vary with the mother's stage of HIV infection. Paper presented at the Sixth International Conference on AIDS. San Francisco, June 20–24.

Brandt, A. 1986. Historical analogies to the AIDS epidemic. In *AIDS and patient management: Legal, ethical and social issues,* ed. M. Witt. Washington, D.C.: National Health Publishing.

Bray, M. A., B. Soltes, L. Clarke, H. Minkoff, M. P. Sierra, and F. I. Reyes. 1991. Human immunodeficiency virus-1 infection in an infertile population. *Fertility and Sterility* 56(1): 16–19.

Brew, B. J., J. J. Sidtis, C. K. Petito, and R. W. Price. 1988. The neurologic complications of AIDS and human immunodeficiency virus infection. In *Advances in contemporary neurology,* ed. F. Plum, 1–49. Philadelphia: F. A. Davis.

Brew, B. J., J. J. Sidtis, M. Rosenblum, and R. W. Price. 1988. AIDS dementia complex. *Journal of the Royal College of Physicians of London* 22: 140–44.

Bridge, T. P. 1988. AIDS and HIV CNS disease: A neuropsychiatric disorder. In *Psychological, neuropsychiatric, and substance abuse aspects of AIDS,* ed. T. P. Bridge, 1–12. New York: Raven Press.

Brinton, L. A. 1991. Oral contraceptives and cervical neoplasia. *Contraception* 43(6): 581–95.

Broadhead, W. E., B. H. Kaplan, S. A. James, E. H. Wagner, V. J. Schoenbach, R. Grimson, et. al. 1983. The epidemiologic evidence for a relationship between social support and health. *American Journal of Epidemiology* 117 (5).

Brody, J. 1992. Vitamin C deficiency and sperm cells. *New York Times,* February 12, B7.

Bronx-Lebanon Hospital Center. 1992. HIV preventive care flow sheet. Courtesy of K. Anastos and R. Denenberg.

Brookmeyer, R. 1991. Reconstruction and future trends of the AIDS epidemic. *Science* 253: 37–42.

Brouwers, P., A. L. Belman, and L. G. Epstein. 1991. Central nervous system involvement: Manifestations and evaluation. In *Pediatric Aids: The challenge of HIV infection in infants, children, and adolescents,* ed. P. A. Pizzo and C. M. Wilfert, 318–35. Baltimore: Williams and Wilkins.

Brown, G. R., and J. R. Rundell. 1990. Prospective study of psychiatric morbidity in HIV-seropositive women without AIDS. *General Hospital Psychiatry* 12: 30–35.

Brown, P. 1992. HIV-2: Slower, still deadly. *WorldAIDS* 22: 10.

Brown, V. 1991. The Prototypes Program. Paper presented at the Annual Meeting of the American Psychological Association. San Francisco, August 1991.

Brown, Z. A., and D. H. Watts. 1990. Antiviral therapy in pregnancy. *Clinical Obstetrics and Gynecology* 33: 276–89.

Brunetti, A., G. Berg, R. Yarchoan, A. Wichman, J. Grafman, P. Pizo, R. D. Finn, R. M. Cohen, S. Broder, G. DiChiro, and S. M. Larson. 1988. PET-FDG studies in patients with AIDS-related dementia: Effect of treatment with azidothymidine. *Journal of Nuclear Medicine* 29: 852.

Brunetti, A., A. Soricelli, L. Mansi, and M. Salvatore. 1991. Functional brain imaging in AIDS-related dementia: A review. In *Biomedical and social developments in AIDS and associated tumors,* ed. G. Giraldo, M. Salvatore, M. Piazza, D. Zarrilli, and E. Beth-Giraldo, 227–34. Basel: Karger.

Burke, D. S., J. F. Brundage, M. Goldenbaum, L. T. Gardner, M. Peterson, R. Vistine, and R. Redfield. 1990. Human immunodeficiency virus in teenagers: Seroprevalence among applicants for U.S. military service. *Journal of the American Medical Association* 263: 2074–77.

Butler, C., J. Hittelman, and S. Hauger. 1991. Approach to neurodevelopmental and neurologic complications in pediatric HIV infection. *Journal of Pediatrics* 119(1), Part 2: S41-S46.

Calderone, M. 1989. Fetuses' rights not to be born. *New York Times,* September 16.

Campbell, C. A. 1990. Women and AIDS. *Social Science and Medicine* 30: 407–15.

Cancellieri, F. R., J. Fine, S. Holman, A. Sunderland, S. Landesman, and B. Bihari. 1988. Psychological reactions to human immunodeficiency virus infection in drug-using pregnant women. In *AIDS in children, adolescents, and heterosexual adults,* ed. R. F. Schinaze and A. J. Nahmias, 207–9. New York: Elsevier.

Carael, M., P. H. Van de Perre, P. H. Lepage, S. Allen, F. Nsengumuremy, C. van Goethem, M. Ntahorutaba, D. Nzaramba, and N. Clumeck. 1988. Human immunodeficiency virus transmission among heterosexual couples in Central Africa. *AIDS* 2(3): 201–5.

Carey, M. A., R. Jenkins, G. Brown, L. Temoshok, and J. Pace. 1991. Gender differences in psychosocial functioning in early-stage HIV patients. Paper presented at the Seventh International Conference on AIDS. Florence, June 16–21.

Carovano, K. 1991. More than mothers or whores: Redefining the AIDS prevention needs of women. *International Journal of Health Services* 21(1): 131–42.

Carpenter, C. C. J., K. H. Mayer, A. Fisher, M. B. Desai, and L. Durand. 1989. Natural history of acquired immunodeficiency syndrome in women in Rhode Island. *American Journal of Medicine* 86: 771–75.

Carpenter, C. C. J., K. H. Mayer, M. D. Stein, B. D. Leibman, A. Fisher, and T. C. Fiore. 1991. Human immunodeficiency virus infection in North American women: Experience with 200 cases and a review of the literature. *Medicine* 70: 307–25.

Carr, G. S., and G. Gee. 1986. AIDS and AIDS-related conditions: Screening for populations at risk. *Nurse Practitioner* 11(10): 25–26, 29, 32–34.

Caussy, D., J. J. Goedert, J. Palefsky, J. Gonzales, C. S. Rabkin, R. A. DiGioia, W. C. Sanchez, R. J. Grossman, G. Colclough, S. Z. Wiktor, et al. 1990. Interaction of human immunodeficiency and papilloma viruses: Association with anal epithelial abnormality in homosexual men. *International Journal of Cancer* 46: 214–19.

CCCM (Communications Consortium Media Center). 1992. *1991–1992 women of color reproductive health poll.* Washington, D.C.: CCCM–National Council of Negro Women.

Centers for Disease Control. 1981. Pneumocystis pneumonia—Los Angeles. *Morbidity and Mortality Weekly Report* 30: 250–52.

———. 1982. *Morbidity and Mortality Weekly Report* 31: 507–8.

———. 1983. *HIV/AIDS Surveillance Report,* December.

———. 1985. Recommendations for assisting in the prevention of perinatal transmission of human T-lymphotrophic virus type 3/lymphadenopathy-associated virus and acquired immunodeficiency syndrome. *Morbidity and Mortality Weekly Report* 34: 721–32.

———. 1986. Classification for human T-lymphotropic virus type 3/lymphadenopathy-associated virus infections. *Morbidity and Mortality Weekly Report* 35: 334.

———. 1987. *Morbidity and Mortality Weekly Report* 36 (Suppl. 1).

———. 1988a. Update: Universal precautions for prevention of transmission of human immunodeficiency virus, hepatitis B virus, and other bloodborne pathogens in health-care settings. *Morbidity and Mortality Weekly Report* 37: 377–82, 387–88.

———. 1988b. Semen banking, organ and tissue transplantation, and HIV antibody testing. *Morbidity and Mortality Weekly Report* 37: 57–58, 63.

References

————. 1989a. Tuberculosis and human immunodeficiency virus infection: Recommendations of the Advisory Committee for the Elimination of Tuberculosis. *Morbidity and Mortality Weekly Report* 38: 243–50.

————. 1989b. Guidelines for prophylaxis against Pneumocystis carinii pneumonia for persons infected with human immunodeficiency virus. *Morbidity and Mortality Weekly Report* 38: S-5.

————. 1989c. *HIV/AIDS Surveillance Report*. July.

————. 1990a. Risk for cervical disease in HIV-infected women—New York City. *Morbidity and Mortality Weekly Report* 39(47): 846–49.

————. 1990b. HIV-1 infection and artificial insemination with processed semen. *Morbidity and Mortality Weekly Report* 39(15): 249–56.

————. 1991a. *HIV/AIDS Surveillance Report,* September.

————. 1991b. Purified protein derivative (PPD)-tuberculin anergy and HIV infection: Guidelines for anergy testing and management of anergic persons at risk of tuberculosis. *Morbidity and Mortality Weekly Report* 40 (RR-5), 27–33.

————. 1991c. Recommendations for preventing transmission of human immunodeficiency virus and hepatitis B virus to patients during exposure-prone invasive procedures. *Morbidity and Mortality Weekly Report* 40 (No. RR-8): 1–9.

————. 1991d. Guidelines for prophylaxis against Pneumocystis carinii pneumonia for children infected with human immunodeficiency virus. *Morbidity and Mortality Weekly Report* 40, RR-2.

————. 1992. 1993 revised classifaction system for HIV infection and expanded surveillance case definition for AIDS among adolescents and adults. *Morbidity and Mortality Weekly Report* 41, RR-17, i–19.

————. 1993. *HIV/AIDS Surveillance Year-End Edition.* Atlanta: CDC, February.

Chaisson, M. A., R. L. Stoneburner, and S. C. Joseph. 1990. Human immunodeficiency virus transmission through artificial insemination. *Journal of Acquired Immune Deficiency Syndromes* 3: 69–72.

Chaisson, M. A., D. Hildebrandt, W. Ewing, R. Stoneburner, and K. Castro. 1991. Similar risk of HIV infection through heterosexual transmission for men and women at a New York City sexually transmitted disease clinic. Paper presented at the Seventh International Conference on AIDS. Florence, June 16–21.

Chaisson, R., and P. Volberding. 1990. Clinical manifestations of HIV infection. In *Mandell's principles and practices of infectious diseases,* 1059–91. New York: Churchill Livingstone.

Charney, P., and C. Morgan. 1992. Do treatment recommendations reported in the research literature consider differences between women and men? Written communication, August 10, on subset analysis of data from *Clinical Research* 40(2): 554A.

Chavkin, W. 1989. Testimony presented April 27 to the U.S. House of Representatives Select Committee on Children, Youth, and Families. Washington, D.C.

————. 1990. Drug addiction and pregnancy: Policy crossroads. *American Journal of Public Health* 80: 483–87.

Chemical & Engineering News. 1993. Prominent AIDS researcher paints bleak outlook. March 1, pp. 29–30.

Chene, G., P. Morlat, D. Commenges, F. Dabis, R. Salamon, and the Groupe d'Epidém-
iologie Clinique du SIDA en Aquitaine. 1991. Low hemoglobin level is associated with
shorter survival in symptomatic HIV-infected patients: A prospective cohort study,
Bordeaux, France, 1985–1990. Paper presented at the Seventh International Conference on AIDS. Florence, June 16–21.

Chin, J. 1990. Current and future dimensions of the HIV/AIDS pandemic in women and
children. *Lancet* 336: 221–24.

———. 1991. The increasing impact of the HIV/AIDS pandemic on women and children.
Paper presented at the Annual Meeting of the American Public Health Association.
Atlanta, November 12.

Chin, J., and J. M. Mann. 1988. The global patterns and prevalence of AIDS and HIV
infection. *AIDS* 2 (Suppl. 1): S247–S252.

Chiodo, F., G. Marinacci, P. Costigliola, E. Ricchi, and V. Colangeli. 1990. Risk factors in
the heterosexual transmission of HIV. Presented at the Sixth International Conference on
AIDS. San Francisco, June 20–24.

Christie, K. A., J. D. Burke, D. A. Regier, D. S. Rae, J. F. Boyd, and B. Z. Locke. 1988.
Epidemiologic evidence for early onset of mental disorders and higher risk of drug abuse
in young adults. *American Journal of Psychiatry* 145: 971–75.

Chu, S. Y., J. W. Buehler, and R. L. Berkelman. 1990. Impact of the human immunodeficiency virus epidemic on mortality in women of reproductive age, United States. *Journal of the American Medical Association* 264: 225–29.

Chu, S. Y., J. W. Buehler, P. L. Fleming, and R. L. Berkelman. 1990. Epidemiology of
reported cases of AIDS in lesbians, United States, 1980–89. *American Journal of Public
Health* 80: 11, 1380–1.

Cicourel, A. V. 1983. Hearing is not believing: Language and the structure of belief in
medical communication. In *The social organization of doctor-patient communication,*
ed. S. Fisher and A. Todd. Washington: Center for Applied Linguistics.

Ciesielski, C., P. Fleming, R. Berkelman, and Centers for Disease Control. 1991. Changing
trends in AIDS indicator diseases in the United States. Paper presented at the Seventh
International Conference on AIDS. Florence, June 16–21.

Clark, B. 1988. Case management: An overview. In *The AIDS manual: A guide for health
care administrators,* ed. J. A. DeHovitz and T. J. Altimont, 257–74. Baltimore: National Health Publishing.

Clark, R., J. Dumestre, C. Pindaro, W. Brandon, and T. Wisniewski. 1992. Gynecologic
findings in HIV+ women in New Orleans. Paper presented at the Eighth International
Conference on AIDS. Amsterdam, July 19–24.

Cleary, P., D. Mechanic, and J. R. Greenley. 1982. Sex differences in medical care utilization: An empirical investigation. *Journal of Health and Social Behavior* 23: 106–18.

Coates, T. J., D. C. DesJarlais, H. G. Miller, L. E. Moses, C. F. Turner, and D. Worth. 1990.
The AIDS epidemic in the the second decade. In *AIDS: The second decade,* ed. H. G.
Miller, C. F. Turner, L. E. Moses. Washington, D.C.: National Academy Press.

Cohen, D. 1992. To increase condom use, target men. *AIDSline* (Spring): 1–2.

Cohen, J., and C. Wofsy. 1989. Association for Women's AIDS Research and Education
(AWARE) fact sheet. San Francisco: Project AWARE.

References

Cohen, J. B. 1990. Epidemiology of HIV infection in women: A crosscutting view. Plenary address at the National Conference on Women and HIV Infection. Washington, D.C., December 14.

———. 1991. Why woman partners of drug users will continue to be at high risk for HIV infection. *Journal of Addictive Diseases* 10(4): 99–110.

Cohen, J. B., P. A. Derish, and L. E. Dorfman. In press. AWARE: A community-based research and peer intervention program for women. In *Community-based research, prevention, and services,* ed. J. Van Vugt. New York: Praeger.

Cohen, P. T. 1990. Safe sex, safer sex, and prevention of HIV infection. In *The AIDS knowledge base,* ed. M. A. Sande and P. A. Volberding. Waltham, Mass.: Medical Publishing Group.

Cole, R., and S. Cooper. 1991. Lesbian exclusion from HIV/AIDS education: Ten years of low-risk identity and high-risk behavior. *SIECUS Report* December 1990–January 1991.

Coleman, E. 1987. Child physical and sexual abuse among chemically dependent individuals. *Journal of Chemically Dependent Treatment* 1: 27–37.

Communications Consortium Media Center. *See* CCCM.

Connecticut Department of Health Services. 1991. AIDS in Connecticut: Annual surveillance report. December 31.

Connell, E. B. 1989. Barrier contraceptives. *Clinical Obstetrics and Gynecology* 32(2): 377–86.

Contraceptive Technology Update. 1992. HIV-infected women may need special attention. 13(3): 41–56.

Cooper, E. B. 1992. Women and the criminalization of HIV. *Health/PAC Bullentin* (Winter).

Costello, C. G. 1982. Social factors associated with depression: A retrospective community study. *Psychological Medicine* 12: 329–39.

Cotton, D., J. Feinberg, and D. Finkelstein. 1991. Participation of women in a multicenter HIV clinical trials program in the United States. Presented at the Seventh International Conference on AIDS. Florence, June 16–21.

Covino, J., and W. McCormack. 1990. Vulvar ulcer of unknown etiology in a human immunodeficiency virus-infected woman: Response to treatment with zidovudine. *American Journal of Obstetrics and Gynecology* 163: 116–18.

Creagh, T., M. Thompson, A. Morris, ARCA Spectrum of Disease Working Groups, and B. Whyte. 1992. Gender differences in the spectrum of HIV disease. Paper presented at the Eighth International Conference on AIDS. Amsterdam, July 19–24.

Currier, J. S., C. Spino, and D. J. Cotton. 1992. Women and power: The impact of accrual rates of women on the ability to detect gender differences in toxicity rates and response to therapy in clinical trials. Presented at the Eighth International Conference on AIDS. Amsterdam, July 19–24.

D'Adesky, A., J. Eigo, R. Lederer, M. Milano, D. Kirschenbaum, and I. Long. 1990. *Access to AIDS clinical trials and experimental drugs in New York state: History, assessment of performance, patient access and demographics, and comprehensive recommendations.* Albany: New York State Department of Health.

Dalton, H. L., and S. Burris. 1987. *AIDS and the law.* New Haven: Yale University Press.

Dattel, B. J. 1990. Substance abuse in pregnancy. *Seminars in Perinatology* 14: 179–87.

Dattel, B. J., N. Padian, M. Shannon, J. Miller, W. R. Cronbleholme, and R. L. Sweet. 1991. HIV serostatus and risk unrelated to pregnancy planning or contraceptive use. Paper presented at the Seventh International Conference on AIDS. Florence, June 16–21.

Dear, M. J. 1976. Abandoned housing. In *Urban policy making and metropolitan development,* ed. J. Adams, 30. Cambridge: Balanger.

De Ferrari, E. 1989. Counseling women regarding high-risk behaviors associated with HIV infection. *Journal of Nurse-Midwifery* 34(5): 276–80.

de Jung, T., S. Holman, A. Fairchild Carrino, S. Caplan-Cotenoff, D. de Leon. 1993. HIV-related discrimination in abortion clinics, New York City, U.S.A.: 1988–1992. Paper presented at the Ninth International Conference on AIDS. Berlin, June 7–11.

de la Vega, Ernesto. 1990. Considerations for reaching the Latino populations with sexuality and HIV/AIDS information and education. *SIECUS Report* 18(3), February–March: 1–8.

Denenberg, R. 1991. Pregnancy and HIV. *Treatment Issues* 5: 6–10. (Published by Gay Men's Health Crisis, New York).

———. 1992. Gynecological care manual for HIV-positive women in primary care settings. Bronx-Lebanon Hospital, N.Y. Photocopy.

DesJarlais, D. C., S. R. Friedman, D. M. Novick, J. L. Sotheran, T. F. Yankovitz, Sr., D. Mildvan, J. Weber, M. J. Kreek, and R. Maslansky. 1989. HIV-1 infection among intravenous-drug users in Manhattan, New York City, from 1977 through 1987. *Journal of the American Medical Association* 261: 1008–12.

De Vincenzi, I., R. Ahrelle-Park, and European Study Group on Heterosexual Transmission of HIV. 1990. Heterosexual transmission of HIV: Follow-up of a European cohort of couples. Presented at the Sixth International Conference on AIDS. San Francisco, June 20–24.

Dew, M. A., M. V. Ragni, and P. Nimorwicz. 1990. Infection with human immunodeficiency virus and vulnerability to psychiatric distress. *Archives of General Psychiatry* 47: 737–44.

Diaz, A. L., R. Settlage, M. Barrett, and A. Kovacs. 1990. Mother-child HIV disease: A model for collaborative care. *Clinical Issues in Perinatal and Women's Health Nursing: AIDS in Women* 1(1): 60–66.

Dilley, J. W., and M. Forstein. 1990. Psychosocial aspects of HIV epidemic. In *American Psychiatric Press Review of Psychiatry,* ed. A. Tasman, S. M. Goldfinger, and C. A. Kaufmann, vol. 19, 635–55. Washington, D.C.: American Psychiatric Press.

Diric, M., and G. Lindmark. 1992. The risk of medical complications after female circumcision. *East African Medical Journal* 69: 477–78.

Dixon, D. A. 1990. The Sister Love Women and AIDS Project: Communicating issues and strategies. Presented at the National Conference on Women and HIV Infection. Washington, D.C., December 14.

Dixon-Mueller, R., and J. Wasserheit. 1991. *The culture of silence: Reproduction tract infections among women of the developing world.* Washington, D.C.: International Women's Health Coalition.

References

Dondero, T. J., M. Pappaioanou, and J. Curran. 1988. Monitoring the levels and trends of HIV infection: The Public Health Service's HIV surveillance program. *Public Health Reports* 103(3): 213–20.

Dorfman, L. E., P. A. Derish, and J. B. Cohen. 1992. Hey girlfriend: An evaluation of AIDS prevention among women in the sex industry. *Health Education Quarterly* 19: 25–40.

Dorrucci, M., and the Italian Seroconversion Study. 1992. Age accelerates the progression from HIV-seroconversion to AIDS in women. Paper presented at the Eighth International Conference on AIDS. Amsterdam, July 19–24.

Dupont, B., 1990. Fungal infections and AIDS. In *Chemotherapy of fungal diseases,* ed. J. F. Ryley. Chicago: Springer.

Dyke, M. 1990. A matter of life and death: Pregnancy clauses in living will statutes. *Boston University Law Review* 70: 867.

Ekholm, S., and J. H. Simon. 1988. Magnetic resonance imaging and the acquired immunodeficiency syndrome dementia complex. *Acta Radiologica* 29: 227–30.

Elford, J., and P. Summers. 1991. Research into HIV and AIDS between 1981 and 1990: The epidemic curve. *AIDS* 5: 1515–19.

Elias, C., and L. Heise. 1993. *The development of microbicides: A new method of HIV prevention for women.* NY: Population Council.

Ellerbrock, T. V., T. J. Bush, M. G. Chamberland, and M. J. Oxtoby. 1991. Epidemiology of women with AIDS in the United States, 1981 through 1990: A comparison with heterosexual men with AIDS. *Journal of the American Medical Association* 265(22): 2971–75.

Ellerbrock, T. V., and M. F. Rogers. 1990. Epidemiology of human immunodeficiency virus infection in women in the United States. *Obstetrics and Gynecology Clinics of North America* 17(3): 523–44.

Endeley, G. 1984. Traditional practices affecting the health of women and children in Africa. In *Report on a seminar on traditional practices affecting the health of women and children in Africa,* 185–189. Senegal.

European Study Group. 1989. Risk factors for male to female transmission of HIV. *British Medical Journal* 298(6671): 411–15.

Faden, R., G. Geller, and M. Powers. 1992. *AIDS, women and the next generation.* New York: Oxford University Press.

Faden, R. R., J. Chwalow, K. Quaid, G. A. Chase, C. Lopes, C. O. Leonard, and N. A. Holtzman. 1987. Prenatal screening and pregnant women's attitudes toward the abortion of defective fetuses. *American Journal of Public Health* 77(3): 288–90.

Faich, G., K. Pearson, D. Fleming, S. Sobel, and C. Amello. 1986. Toxic shock syndrome and the vaginal contraceptive sponge. *Journal of the American Medical Association* 255(2): 216–18.

Falloon, J. 1992. Current therapy for HIV infection and its infectious complications. A practical summary for primary care physicians. *Postgraduate Medicine* 91(8): 115–32.

Farizo, K. M., J. W. Buehler, M. E. Chamberland, B. M. Whyte, E. S. Fruelicher, S. G. Hopkins, C. M. Reed, E. D. Mokotoff, D. L. Cohn, S. Troxler, A. F. Phelps, and R. L. Berkelman. 1992. Spectrum of disease in persons with human immunodeficiency virus

Feingold, A. R., S. H. Vermund, R. D. Burk, K. F. Kelley, L. K. Schrager, K. Schreiber, G. Munk, G. H. Friedland, R. S. Klein. 1990. Cervical cytologic abnormalities and papilloma virus in women infected with human immunodeficiency virus. *Journal of Acquired Immune Deficiency Syndrome* 3: 896–903.

Fenton, T. W. 1988. Psychiatric aspects of HIV infection: Implications for the U.K. *Journal of the Royal College of Physicians of London* 22: 145–48.

Fernandez, F., F. Adams, J. K. Levy, V. F. Holmes, M. Neidhart, and P. W. A. Mansell. 1988. Cognitive impairment due to AIDS-related complex and its response to psychostimulants. *Psychosomatics* 29: 38–46.

Fernandez, F., V. F. Holmes, J. K. Levy, and P. Ruiz. 1989. Consultation-liaison psychiatry and HIV-related disorders. *Hospital and Community Psychiatry* 40: 146–53.

Fernandez, F., and J. K. Levy. 1990. Psychiatric diagnosis and pharmacotherapy of patients with HIV infection. In *American Psychiatric Press Review of Psychiatry,* ed. A. Tasman, S. M. Goldfinger, and C. A. Kaufmann, vol. 19, 614–30. Washington, D.C.: American Psychiatric Press.

Fernandez, F., J. K. Levy, and P. W. A. Mansell. 1990. Management of delirium in terminally ill AIDS patients. *International Journal of Psychiatry Medicine* 19: 165–72.

Finnegan, W. 1990. Out there, I and II. *New Yorker,* September 10 and 17.

Fischl, M. A., G. M. Dickinson, G. B. Scott, N. Klimas, M. A. Fletcher, and W. Parks. 1987. Evaluation of heterosexual partners, children, and household contacts of adults with AIDS. *Journal of the American Medical Association* 257(5): 640–44.

Fischl, M. A., D. D. Richman, M. H. Grieco, M. S. Gottlieb, P. A. Volberding, O. L. Laskin, J. M. Leedom, J. E. Groopman, D. Mildvan, R. T. Schooley, G. G. Jackson, D. T. Durack, D. King, AZT Collaborative Working Group. 1987. The efficacy of azidothymidine (AZT) in the treatment of patients with AIDS and AIDS-related complex: A double-blind, placebo-controlled trial. *New England Journal of Medicine* 317: 185–91.

Flaskerud J. H., and C. E. Rush. 1989. AIDS and traditional health beliefs and practices of black women. *Nursing Research* 38(4): 210–15.

Fleming, P., C. Ciesielski, and R. Berkelman. 1991. Sex-specific differences in the prevalence of reported AIDS-indicative diagnoses, United States, 1988-1989. Paper presented at the Seventh International Conference on AIDS. Florence, June 16–21.

Franke, K. M. 1989. HIV-related discrimination in abortion clinics in New York City. City of New York Commission on Human Rights, AIDS Discrimination Division. June.

Freedman, L. 1991. Women, health, and third world debt: A critique of the public health response in economic crisis. Unpublished paper, Development Law and Policy Program, Columbia University.

Friedland, G. H., B. Saltzman, J. Vileno, K. Freeman, L. K. Schrager, and R. S. Klein. 1991. Survival differences in patients with AIDS. *Journal of Acquired Immunodeficiency Syndrome* 4: 144–53.

Fruchter, R., M. Maiman, E. Serur, and S. Cuthill. 1992. Cervical intraepithelial neoplasia in HIV-infected women. Paper presented at the Eighth International Conference on AIDS. Amsterdam, July 19–24.

References

Fullilove, M. T., E. A. Lown, and R. E. Fullilove. 1992. Crack 'hos and skeezers: Traumatic experiences of women crack users. *Journal of Sex Research* 29(2): 275–87.

Gail, M. H., P. S. Rosenberg, and J. J. Goedert. 1990. Therapy may explain recent deficits in AIDS incidence. *Journal of Acquired Immune Deficiency Syndrome* 3: 296–306.

Gallagher, J. 1987. Prenatal invasions and interventions: What's wrong with fetal rights. *Harvard Women's Law Journal* 9: 47.

———. Fetus as patient. 1988. *Reproductive laws for the 1990s.* Clifton, N.J.: Humana.

Garris, I., E. Rodriguez, A. De Moya, et al. 1991. Heterosexual predominance in the Dominican Republic. *Journal of Acquired Immunodeficiency Syndrome* 4: 1173–1175.

Genero, N., J. B. Miller, J. Surrey, and L. Baldwin. 1992. Measuring perceived mutuality in close relationships: Validation of mutual psychological development questionnaire. *Journal of Family Psychology* 6: 36–48.

Genero, N., J. Surrey, A. Arons, and D. Angiloillo. 1990. Toward prevention of depression in mothers of young children. Symposium presented at the Annual Meeting of New England Psychological Association, Worcester, Mass.

Gillespie, S. 1989. Potential impact of AIDS on farming systems: A case study from Rwanda. *Land Use Policy* (October): 301–12.

Global Programme on AIDS, World Health Organization. 1989. Unlinked anonymous screening for the public health surveillance of HIV infections: Proposed international guidelines. Geneva. June.

Goedert, J. J., M. E. Eyster, R. J. Biggar, and W. A. Blattner. 1987. Heterosexual transmission of human immunodeficiency virus: Association with severe depletion of T-helper lymphocytes in men with hemophilia. *AIDS Research and Human Retroviruses* 3(4): 355–61.

Goedert, J. J., H. Mendez, J. E. Drummon, M. Robert-Guroff, H. Minkoff, S. Holman, R. Stevens, A. Rubinstein, W. A. Blattner, A. Willoughby, and S. Landesman. 1989. Mother-to-infant transmission of human immunodeficiency virus type 1: Association with prematurity or low anti-gp120. *Lancet* 2: 1351–54.

Gollub, E., M. Rosenberg, and J. Michael. 1992. Methods women can use that may prevent sexually transmitted disease including sexually acquired HIV. Submitted to the *American Journal of Public Health.*

Gollub, E. L., and I. Sivin. 1989. The Prentif cervical cap and Pap smear results: A critical appraisal. *Contraception* 40(3): 343–49.

Gonsalves, G., and M. Harrington. 1992. *AIDS research at the NIH: A critical review.* New York: Treatment Action Group. Monograph available at the Eighth International Conference on AIDS. Amsterdam, July 1992.

Gorna, R. 1992. Everything you always wanted to know about oral sex . . . but you won't find it here. Conference newspaper at Eighth International Conference on AIDS. Amsterdam, July 21.

Goroll, A. H. et al. 1987. *Primary care medicine,* 2d ed. Philadelphia: J. B. Lippincott.

Gottlieb, M. S., R. Schroff, H. M. Schanker, J. D. Weisman, P. T. Fan, R. A. Wolf, and A. Saxon. 1981. Pneumocystis carinii pneumonia and mucosal candidiasis in previously healthy homosexual men: Evidence of a new acquired cellular immunodeficiency. *New England Journal of Medicine* 305: 1425–31.

Gove, W. R., and M. Hughes. 1979. Possible causes of apparent sex differences in physical health: An empirical investigation. *American Sociological Review* 44: 126–46.

Grant, I., J. H. Atkinson, J. R. Hesselink, C. J. Kennedy, D. D. Richman, S. A. Spector, and J. A. McCutchan. 1987. Evidence for early central nervous system involvement in the acquired immunodeficiency syndrome and other human immunodeficiency virus infections. *Annals of Internal Medicine* 107: 828–36.

Grant, I., J. H. Atkinson, J. R. Hesselink, C. J. Kennedy, D. D. Richman, S. A. Spector, and J. A. McCutchan. 1988. Human immunodeficiency virus-associated neuro-behavioural disorder. *Journal of the Royal College of Physicians of London* 22: 149–57.

Grant, I., S. Carter, K. Anastos, and J. Ernst. 1991. Gender differences in AIDS defining illnesses. Paper presented at the Eighth International Conference on AIDS. Florence, June 16–21.

Gray, F., R. Gherardi, and F. Scaravilli. 1988. The neuropathology of the acquired immune deficiency syndrome (AIDS): A review. *Brain* 111: 245–66.

Greene, W. 1991. The molecular biology of human immunodeficiency virus type 1 infection. *New England Journal of Medicine* 324: 308.

Gross, J. 1989. Grandmothers bear a burden sired by drugs. *New York Times,* April 7.

Guimaraes, C., K. Carovano, S. Middlestadt, V. Vital, and E. Ferraz. 1991. Can we talk? Paper presented at the USAID AIDS Prevention Conference. Washington, D.C., November.

Guinan, M. 1992. HIV, heterosexual transmission, and women. *Journal of the American Medical Association* 268(4): 520–21.

Guinan, M. E., and A. Hardy. 1987. Epidemiology of AIDS in women in the United States, 1981 through 1986. *Journal of the American Medical Association* 257(17): 2039–42.

Gwinn, M., M. Pappaioanou, J. R. George, H. Hannon, S. C. Wasser, M. A. Redus, R. Hague, R. A., J. Y. Q. Mok, L. MacCallum, S. Burns, and P. L. Yap. 1991. Do maternal factors influence the risk of HIV infection? Paper presented at the Seventh International Conference on AIDS, Florence, June 16–21.

Halpert, R., R. G. Fruchter, A. Sedlis, K. Butt, J. G. Boyce, and F. H. Sillman. 1986. Human papillomavirus and lower genital neoplasia in renal transplant patients. *Obstetrics and Gynecology* 68: 251–58.

Hamburg, D. A. 1982. Human society, family, social support and health. In *Health and behavior: Frontiers of research in the biobehavioral sciences,* ed. D. A. Hamburg, G. R. Elliott, and D. L. Parron. Washington, D.C.: National Academy Press.

Hampton, J. 1991. *Meeting AIDS with compassion: AIDS care and prevention in Agomanya, Ghana.* Strategies for Hope Series No. 4. London: Actionaid.

Haseltine, W. 1992. Testimony presented December 15 to the U.S. Senate, Washington, D.C.

Hassan, R. L. 1990. BEBASHI: Blacks educating blacks about sexual health issues. Presented at the National Conference on Women and HIV Infection. Washington, D.C., December 13.

Hassig, S. 1989. Contraceptive utilization and reproductive desires in a group of HIV-positive women in Kinshasa. Paper presented at the Fifth International Conference on AIDS. Montreal, June 7.

Hatcher, R. A., F. Stewart, J. Trussell, D. Kowal, F. Guest, G. K. Stewart, and W. Cates.1992. *Contraceptive Technology, 1990–1992,* 15th rev. ed. New York: Irvington Publishers.

Hausermann, J., and R. Danziger. 1991. Women and AIDS: A human rights perspective. Paper presented at the Seventh International Conference on AIDS. Florence, June 16–21.

Heagarty, M. C., and E. J. Abrams. 1992. Caring for HIV-infected women and children. *New England Journal of Medicine* 326(13): 887–88.

Heise, L. 1992. Violence against women: The missing agenda. In *Women's health: A global perspective,* ed. M. A. Koblinsky, J. Timyan, and J. Gay. Boulder, Colo.: Westview Press.

Helquist, M., and S. Middlestadt. 1991. *National AIDS/HIV KABP survey: St. Vincent and the Grenadines* and *St. Lucia: Preliminary report of comparative data.* Washington, D.C.: AIDSCOM. March.

Hicks, D. R., L. S. Martin, J. P. Getchell, J. L. Heath, D. P. Francis, J. S. McDougal, J. W. Curran, and B. Voeller. 1985. Inactivation of HTLV-III/LAV-infected cultures of normal lymphocytes by nonoxynol-9 in vitro. *Lancet* 2: 1422–23.

Hilton, E., et al. 1992. Ingestion of yogurt containing lactobacillus acidophilus as prophylaxis for candidal vaginitis. *Annals of Internal Medicine* 116: 353–57.

Hoegsberg, B., O. Abulafia, A. Sedlis, J. Feldman, D. DesJarlais, S. Landesman, and H. Minkoff. 1990. Sexually transmitted diseases and human immunodeficiency virus infection among women with pelvic inflammatory disease. *American Journal of Obstetrics and Gynecology* 163(4): 1135–38.

Hoegsberg, B., T. Dotson, O. Abulatia, et al. 1989. Social, sexual, and drug use profile of HIV-positive and HIV-negative women with PID. Paper presented at the Fifth International Conference on AIDS. Montreal, June.

Hoff, G., F. Grady, A. Willoughby, A. C. Novello, L. R. Peterson, T. J. Dondero, and J. W. Curran. 1991. Prevalence of HIV infection in childbearing women in the United States. *Journal of the American Medical Association* 265(13): 1704–8.

Holman, S., M. Berthaud, A. Sunderland, G. Moroso, F. Cancellieri, H. Mendez, E. Beller, and A. Marcel. 1989. Women infected with human immunodeficiency virus: Counseling and testing during pregnancy. *Seminars in Perinatology* 13(1): 7–15.

Holmberg, S. D., C. R. Horsburgh, Jr., J. W. Ward, and H. W. Jaffe. 1989. AIDS commentary: Biologic factors in the sexual transmission of human immunodeficiency virus. *Journal of Infectious Diseases* 160(1): 116–25.

Holmes, K. K. 1991. The changing epidemiology of HIV transmission. *Hospital Practice* 15: 89–110.

Holmes, K. K., and J. Kreiss. 1988. Heterosexual transmission of human immunodeficiency virus: Overview of a neglected aspect of the AIDS epidemic. *Journal of Acquired Immune Deficiency Syndromes* 1(6): 602–10.

Holtzman, D. M., D. A. Kaku, and Y. T. So. 1989. New-onset seizures associated withhuman immunodeficiency virus infection: Causation and clinical features in 100 cases. *American Journal of Medicine* 87:173–77.

Horsburgh, C. R., D. Hanson, S. A. Fann, J. A. Havlik, and S. E. Thomson. 1991. Predictors of survival in HIV infection including CD4+ cell count, AIDS defining condition and therapy but not sex, age, race, or risk activity. Paper presented at the Seventh International Conference on AIDS. Florence, June 16–21.

House, J. S., C. Robins, H. L. Metzner. 1982. The association of social relationships and activities with mortality: Prospective evidence from the Tecumseh community health study. *American Journal of Epidemiology* 116: 123–40.

Hutchison, M., and A. Kurth. 1990. *HIV and reproductive decision-making.* Master's thesis, Yale University.

Hutchison, M., and A. Kurth. 1991. 'I need to know that I have a choice': a study of women, HIV, and reproductive decision-making. *AIDS Patient Care* (February): 17–25.

Ickovics, J. 1991. *Medical utilization of HIV-positive women affiliated with Yale-New Haven Hospital (preliminary analysis).* New Haven: Yale Department of Psychology.

Ickovics, J., and J. Rodin. 1992. Women and AIDS in the United States: Epidemiology, natural history, and mediating mechanisms. *Health Psychology* 11(1): 1–16.

Imam, N. C., C. J. Carpenter, K. H. Mayer, A. Fisher, M. Stein, and S. B. Danforth. 1990. Hierarchical pattern of mucosal candida infections in HIV seropositive women. *American Journal of Medicine* 89: 142–46.

Institute of Medicine, National Academy of Sciences. 1988. *Confronting AIDS: Update 1988.* Washington, D.C.: National Academy Press.

Institute of Medicine. 1991. *HIV Screening of Pregnant Women and Newborns,* ed. L. M. Hardy. Washington: National Academy Press.

Instone, S. L., and A. Fraser. 1991. Maternal-child HIV infection: A model for family-focused care. *Nurse Practitioner Forum* 2(2): 108–12.

International Center for Research on Women. 1989. *Strengthening women: Health research priorities for women in developing countries.* Washington, D.C.: ICRW.

———. January 1992. The women and AIDS research program. *ICRW Information Bulletin.* Washington, D.C.: ICRW.

International Gay and Lesbian Human Rights Commission. 1992. AIDS and human rights abuses in Burma. Press release, Eighth International Conference on AIDS. Amsterdam, July 19–24.

Jacobson, J. L. 1991. Women's reproductive health: The silent emergency. Worldwatch Paper 102. Washington, D.C.: Worldwatch Institute.

Jaffe, L. R., M. Seehaus, C. Wagner, and B. Leadbeater. 1988. Anal intercourse and knowledge of acquired immunodeficiency syndrome among minority-group female adolescents. *Journal of Pediatrics* 112(6): 1005–7.

James, M. E. 1988. HIV seropositivity diagnosed during pregnancy: Psychosocial characterization of patients and their adaptation. *General Hospital Psychiatry* 10: 309–16.

Jason, J., B. L. Evatt, and Hemophilia-AIDS Collaborative Study Group. 1990. Pregnancies in human immunodeficiency virus-infected sex partners of hemophilic men. *American Journal of the Diseases of Children* 144: 485–90.

Jemmott, L. S., and J. B. Jemmott III. 1991. Applying the theory of reasoned action to AIDS risk behavior: Condom use among black women. *Nursing Research* 40(4): 228–34.

References

Johns, D. R., M. Tierney, and D. Felsenstein. 1987. Alteration in the natural history of neurosyphilis by concurrent infection with the human immunodeficiency virus. *New England Journal of Medicine* 316: 1569–72.

Johnson, A. M., J. Wadsworth, K. Wellings, S. Bradshaw, and J. Field. Sexual lifestyles and HIV risk. *Nature* 360: 410–12.

Johnstone F. D., R. P. Brettle, L. R. MacCallum, J. Mok, J. F. Peutherer, S. Burns. 1990. Women's knowledge of their HIV antibody state: Its effect on their decision whether to continue the pregnancy. *British Medical Journal* 300: 23–24.

Judson, F. N., J. M. Ehret, G. F. Bodin, M. J. Levin, and C. A. M. Reitmeijer. 1989. In vitro evaluations of condoms with and without nonoxynol-9 as physical and chemical barriers against chlamydia trachomatis, herpes simplex virus type 2, and human immunodeficiency virus. *Sexually Transmitted Diseases* 16(2): 51–56.

Kaplan, M. H., B. Farber, W. H. Hall, C. Mallow, C. O'Keefe, and R. G. Harper. 1989. Pregnancy arising in HIV-infected women while being repetitively counseled about "safe sex." Paper presented at the Fifth International Conference on AIDS. Montreal, June 4–9.

Karan, L. D. 1989. AIDS prevention and chemical dependence treatment needs of women and their children. *Journal of Psychoactive Drugs* 21(4): 395–99.

Kaslow, R. A., J. P. Phair, H. B. Friedman, D. Lyter, R. E. Solomon, J. Dudley, B. F. Polk, and W. Blackwelder. 1987. Infection with the human immunodeficiency virus: Clinical manifestations and their relationship to immune deficiency. *Annals of Internal Medicine* 107: 474–80.

Keeling, R. P. 1993. HIV disease: Current concepts. *Journal of Counseling and Development* 71: 261–74.

Kegeles, S. M., N. E. Adler, and C. E. Irwin. 1988. Sexually active adolescents and condoms: Changes over one year in behaviors, attitudes, and use. *American Journal of Public Health* 78(4): 460–61.

Kent, J. 1990. Michigan State Department of Health. Personal communication, telephone, December 1990.

Kessler, L. G., P. D. Cleary, and J. D. Burke. 1985. Psychiatric disorders in primary care. *Archives of General Psychiatry* 42: 583–87.

Kieburtz, K. D., L. Ketonen, A. E. Zettelmaier, D. Kido, E. D. Caine, and J. H. Simon. 1990. Magnetic resonance imaging findings in HIV cognitive impairment. *Archives of Neurology* 47: 643–45.

Kirschstein, R. L. 1991. Research on women's health. *American Journal of Public Health* 81(3): 291–93.

Kizer, K. W., M. Green, C. I. Perkins, G. Doebbert, and M. J. Hughes. 1988. Letter: AIDS and suicide in California. *Journal of the American Medical Association* 260: 1881.

Klein, R., A. Adachi, I. Fleming, G. Y. F. Ho, and R. Burk. 1992. A prospective study of genital neoplasia and human papillomavirus in HIV-infected women. Paper presented at the Eighth International Conference on AIDS. Amsterdam, July 19–24.

Kline, M. W., and W. T. Shearer. 1991. Serious bacterial complications of HIV infection in infants and children. *The AIDS Reader* 1: 82–86.

Koff, W. C., and D. F. Hoth. 1988. Development and testing of AIDS vaccines. *Science* 241: 426–32.

Koonin, L. M., T. V. Ellerbrock, H. K. Atrash, M. F. Rogers, J. C. Smith, C. J. R. Hogue, M. A. Harris, W. Chavkin, A. L. Parker, and G. J. Halpin. 1989. Pregnancy-associated deaths due to AIDS in the United States. *Journal of the American Medical Association* 261: 1306–9.

Koop, C. E. 1986. Surgeon general's report on acquired immune deficiency syndrome. *Journal of the American Medical Association* 256(20): 2784–89.

Kraus, E. M., D. B. Brettler, A. D. Forsberg, and J. L. Sullivan. 1991. Pregnancy in a cohort of long-term partners of human immunodeficiency virus-seropositive hemophiliacs. *Obstetrics and Gynecology* 78 (5, part 1): 735–38.

Kreiss, J., E. Ngugi, K. Holmes, J. Ndinya-Achola, P. Waiyaki, P. Roberts, I. Rumenjo, J. Kimata, T. Fleming, A. Anzala, D. Holton, and F. Plummer. Efficacy of nonoxynol-9 contraceptive sponge use in preventing heterosexual acquisition of HIV in Nairobi prostitutes. *Journal of the American Medical Association* 268(4): 477–82.

Kübler-Ross, E. 1969. *On Death and Dying*. New York: Macmillan.

Kuni, C. C., F. S. Rhame, M. J. Meier, M. C. Foehse, R. B. Loewenson, B. C. P. Lee, R. J. Boudreau, and R. P. duChret. 1991. Quantitative I-123-IMP brain SPECT and neuro-psychological testing in AIDS dementia. *Clinical Nuclear Medicine* 16: 174–77.

Kurth, A., and M. Hutchison. 1990. Reproductive health policy and HIV: Where do women fit in? *Pediatric AIDS and HIV Infection: Fetus to Adolescent* 1(6): 121–33.

Ladner, J. 1971. *Tomorrow's tomorrow: The black woman*. Garden City, N.Y.: Anchor Doubleday.

Laga, M., J. P. Icenogle, R. Marsella, A. T. N. Nzila, R. W. Ryder, S. H. Vermund, W. L. Heyward, A. Nelson, and W. C. Reeves. 1991. Genital papillomavirus infection and cervical dysplasia—Opportunistic complications of HIV infection. *International Journal of Cancer* 50: 45–48.

Lagakos, S., A. F. Margaret, D. S. Stein, L. Lim, and P. Volberding. 1991. Effects of zidovudine therapy in minority and other subpopulations with early HIV infection. *Journal of the American Medical Association* 266: 2709–12.

Lambert, J. S., M. Seidlin, R. C. Reichman, C. S. Plank, M. Laverty, G. D. Norse, C. Knupp, C. McLaren, C. Pettinelli, F. T. Valentine, and R. Dolin. 1990. Dideoxy-yinosine Knupp, C. McLaren, C. Pettinelli, F. T. Valentine, and R. Dolin. 1990. Dideoxyinosine (ddI) in patients with the acquired immunodeficiency syndrome or AIDS-related complex. *New England Journal of Medicine* 322: 1333–40.

Langhoff, E., E. F. Terwilliger, M. C. Poznansky, H. Bos, K. H. Kalland, and W. A. Haseltine. 1991. Prolific HIV-1 growth in human dendritic cells. Paper presented at the Seventh International Conference on AIDS. Florence, June.

Lapointe, N., J. Michaud, D. Pekovic, J. P. Chausseau, and J. M. Dupuy. 1985. Transplacental transmission of HTLV-III virus. *New England Journal of Medicine* 312: 1325–26.

Lazzarin, A., A. Saracco, M. Musicco, and A. Nicolosi (Italian Study Group on HIV Heterosexual Transmission). 1991. Man-to-woman sexual transmission of the human immunodeficiency virus: Risk factors related to sexual behavior, man's infectiousness, and woman's susceptibility. *Archives of Internal Medicine* 151(12): 2411–16.

Leary, W. E. 1992. U.S. panel backs approval of first condom for women. *New York Times,* February 1.

Lebowohl, M., and P. Contard. 1990. Interferon and condylomata acuminata. *International Journal of Dermatology* 29: 699–705.

Lemp, G. F., S. Payne, D. Neal, T. Temelso, and G. W. Rutherford. 1990. Survival trends for patients with AIDS. *Journal of the American Medical Association* 263: 402–6.

Lemp, G. F., A. M. Hirozawa, J. B. Cohen, P. A. Derish, K. C. McKinney, and S. R. Hernandez. 1992. Survival for women and men with AIDS. *Journal of Infectious Diseases* 166: 74–79.

Lepage, P., P. Van de Perre, M. Carael, F. Nsengumuremyi, J. Nkurunziza, J. P. Butzler, and S. Sprecher. 1987. Letter: Postnatal transmission of HIV from mother to child. *Lancet* 2(8555): 400.

Lerner, G. 1972. *Black women in white America: A documentary history.* New York: Pantheon. (For discussion of the matriarchal tradition, see pp. 624–26.)

Levine, C., and N. N. Dubler. 1990. Uncertain risks and bitter realities: The reproductive choices of HIV-infected women. *Milbank Quarterly* 68(3): 321–51.

Lifshiz, A. 1986. Inmunodeficiencia adquirida en un sujeto de bajo riesgo: Primera mujer en Mexico (Acquired immune deficiency in a low-risk subject: The first woman in Mexico). In *Revista Medica.* Mexico City: Instituto Mexicano de Seguro Social.

Lifson, A. R. 1988. Do alternative modes for transmission of human immunodeficiency virus exist? A review. *Journal of the American Medical Association* 259: 1353–56.

Lindan, C., S. Allen, M. Careal, F. Nsengumuremyi, P. Van de Perre, A. Serufilira, J. Tice, D. Black, T. Coates, and S. Hulley. 1991. Knowledge, attitudes, and perceived risk of AIDS among urban Rwandan women: Relationship to HIV infection and behavior change. *AIDS* 5: 993–1002.

Long, I. 1993 Women's access to government-sponsored AIDS/HIV clinical trials: Status report, critique, and recommendations. New York: ACT-UP, 1–15.

Los Angeles Times. 1986. Woman accused of contributing to baby's demise during pregnancy. October 1, Metro sec., col. 4.

Louv, W. C., A. Harland, W. J. Alexander, S. Stagno, and J. Cheeks. 1988. A clinical trial of nonoxynol-9 for preventing gonococcal and chlamydial infections. *Journal of Infectious Diseases* 158: 518–23.

Lucas, S. B. 1990. Missing infections in AIDS. *Trans. R. Society for Tropical Medicine and Hygiene* 84 (Suppl. 1): 34–38.

Lundberg, G. D. 1989. The 1988 Bethesda system for reporting cervical/vaginal cytological diagnosis. *Journal of the American Medical Association* 262: 931–34.

McArthur J. C., P. S. Becker, J. E. Parisi, B. Trapp, O. A. Selnes, D. R. Cornblath, J. Balakrishnan, J. W. Griffin, and D. Price. 1989. Neuropathological changes in early HIV-1 dementia. *Annals of Neurology* 26: 681–84.

McCusker, J., A. M. Stoddard, J. G. Zapka, M. Zorn, and K. H. Mayer. 1989. Predictors of AIDS-preventive behavior among homosexually active men: A longitudinal study. *AIDS* 3(7): 443–48.

MacDonald, M. G., H. M. Ginzburg, and J. C. Bolan. 1991. HIV infection and pregnancy: Epidemiology and clinical management. *Journal of AIDS* 4(2): 100–108.

McGovern, T. 1992. The CDC surveillance definition. Roundtable presentation at the Eighth International Conference on AIDS. Amsterdam, July 19–24.

McMahon, K. M. 1988. The integration of HIV testing and counseling into nursing practice. *Nursing Clinics of North America* 23(4): 803–21.

Maiman, M. 1991. Human immunodeficiency virus infection and cervical neoplasia. *Journal of NIH Research* 3: 81–83.

Maiman, M., R. G. Fruchter, E. Serur, and J. Boyce. 1988. Prevalence of human immunodeficiency virus in a colposcopy clinic. *Journal of the American Medical Association* 260(15): 2214–15.

Maiman, M., R. G. Fruchter, E. Serur, J. C. Remy, G.Feur, and J. Boyce. 1990. Human immunodeficiency virus infection and cervical neoplasia. *Gynecologic Oncology* 38: 377–82.

Maiman, M., N. Tarricone, J. Vieira, J. Suarez, E. Serur, and J. G. Boyce. 1991. Colposcopic evaluation of human immunodeficiency virus seropositive women. *Obstetrics and Gynecology* 78: 84–88.

Maldonado, M. 1990. Latinas and HIV/AIDS. *SIECUS Report* 19(2): 11–15.

Malele, M., T. Manoka, M. Kivuvu, M. Tuliza, B. Edidi, F. Behets, W. L. Heyward, P. Piot, and M. Laga. 1991. The impacts of HIV infection on the incidence of STD in high-risk women. Paper presented at the Seventh International Conference on AIDS. Florence, June 16–21.

Malkovsky, M., A. Newell, and A. G. Dagleish. 1988. Inactivation of HIV by nonoxynol-9. *Lancet* 1: 645.

Mann, J., D. J. M. Tarantola, and T. W. Netter, eds. 1992. *AIDS in the world, 1992.* Cambridge: Harvard University Press.

Marotta, R., and S. Perry. 1989. Early neuropsychological dysfunction caused by human immunodeficiency virus. *Journal of Neuropsychiatry and Clinical Neurosciences* 1: 225–33.

Marte, C. 1989. *Community Health Project gynecology protocol.* New York: Community Health Project.

Marte, C., et al. 1989. Need for gynecologic protocols in AIDS primary care clinics. Presented at Fifth International Conference on AIDS, Montreal, June 4–9.

Marte, C., and M. Allen. 1991. HIV-related gynecologic condition: Overlooked complications. *Focus: A guide to AIDS research and counseling* 7 (1): 1–4.

Marx, R., S. O. Aral, R. T. Rolfs, C. E. Sterk, and J. G. Kahn. 1991. Crack, sex and STDs. *Sexually Transmitted Diseases* 18(2): 92–101.

Marzuk, P. M., H. Tierney, K. Tardiff, E. M. Gross, E. B. Morgan, M.-A. Hsu, and J. J. Mann. 1988. Increased risk of suicide in persons with AIDS. *Journal of the American Medical Association.* 259: 1333–37.

Mason, J., J. Preisinger, R. Sperling, V. Walther, J. Berrier, and V. Evans. 1991. Incorporating HIV education and counseling into routine prenatal care: A program model. *AIDS Education and Prevention* 3: 118–23.

Masur, H., M. A. Michelis, J. B. Greene, I. Onorato, R. A. VandeStouwe, R. S. Holzman, G. Wormser, L. Brettman, M. Lange, H. W. Murray, and S. Cunningham-Rundles. 1981. An outbreak of community-acquired Pneumocystis carinii pneumonia: Initial manifestation of cellular immune dysfunction. *New England Journal of Medicine* 305: 1431–38.

Masur, H., M. A. Michelis, G. Wormser, S. Lewin, J. Gold, M. L. Tapper, J. Giron, C. W. Lerner, D. Armstrong, U. Setia, J. A. Sender, R. S. Siebken, P. Nicholas, Z. Arlen, S. Maayan, J. A. Ernst, F. P. Siegal, and S. Cunningham-Rundles. 1982. Opportunistic infections in previously healthy women. *Annals of Internal Medicine* 97: 533–39.

Mathur-Wagh, U., N. Roche, J. Stein, R. Newman, I. Wilets, J. Weber, S. Middleton, M. Mack, and D. DeCarlo. Gynecological findings in an HIV positive outpatient population. Paper presented at the Eighth International Conference on AIDS. Amsterdam, July 19–24.

Maury, W., B. J. Potts, and A. B. Rabson. 1989. HIV-1 infection of first-trimester and term human placental tissue: A possible mode of maternal-fetal transmission. *Journal of Infectious Disease* 160: 583–88.

Mayer, K. H., S. Zeirler, L. Feingold, D. Laufer, and C. Carpenter. 1991. Gender specific differences in morbidity among HIV positive adults. Paper presented at the Seventh International Conference on AIDS. Florence, June 16–21.

Mays, V. M., and S. D. Cochran. 1988. Issues in the perception of AIDS risk and risk reduction activities by black and Hispanic/Latina women. *American Psychologist* 43(11): 949–57.

Mechanic, D. 1976. Sex, illness, and illness behavior and the use of health services. *Human Stress* 2: 2–49.

Medina, D. 1987. Latino culture and sex education. *SIECUS Report* 1: 1–4.

Meirik, O., and T. M. Farley. 1990. Oral contraceptives and HIV transmission. In *Heterosexual transmission of AIDS,* ed. N.J. Alexander, H. L. Gabelnick, and J. M. Spieler, 247–54. New York: Wiley-Liss.

Melnick, S., R. Sherer, D. Hillman, E. Rodriguez, C. Lackman, L. Capps, J. Korvick, S. H. Vermund, M. Carolyn, and L. Deyton. 1992. Gender, HIV-related clinical events, and mortality: Preliminary observational data from the Community Programs for Clinical Research on AIDS (CPCRA). Paper presented at the Eighth International Conference on AIDS. Amsterdam, July 19–24.

Mendez, H. 1991. Ambulatory care of HIV-seropositive infants and children. Journal of Pediatrics 119(1, part 2: S14–S20.

Mendez, H., and J. E. Jule. 1990. Care of the infant born exposed to human immunodeficiency virus. *Obstetrical and Gynecological Clinics of North America* 17(3): 637–49.

Menendez, B. S., E. Drucker, S. H. Vermund, R. Rivera-Castaño, R. R. Perez-Agosto, F. J. Parga, and S. Blum. 1990. AIDS mortality among Puerto Ricans and other Hispanics in New York City. *Journal of Acquired Immune Deficiency Syndrome* 3: 644–48.

Mercer, M. A., L. Liskin, and S. J. Scott. 1991. The role of nongovernmental organizations in the global response to AIDS. *AIDS Care* 3(3): 265–70.

MFY Legal Services. 1992. Memorandum on Social Security's proposed HIV disability standards. MFY Legal Services, HIV Project. January.

Michaels, D., and C. Levine. 1992. Projections of the number of motherless youth orphaned by AIDS in the United States. Presentation at the Eighth International Conference on AIDS. Amsterdam, July 19–24.

Miller, D., and M. Riccio. 1990. Nonorganic psychiatric and psychosocial syndromes associated with HIV-1 infection and disease. *AIDS* 4: 381–88.

Miller, J. B. 1988. Connection, disconnections, and violations. Work in progress no. 33. Wellesley, Mass.: Stone Center Working Paper Series.

Minkoff, H. L. 1991. Gynecologic care of HIV-infected women. *Contemporary OB/GYN* 35(9): 46–60.

Minkoff, H. L., and L. Feinkind. 1989. Management of pregnancies of HIV-infected women. *Clinical Obstetrics and Gynecology* 32: 467–76.

Minkoff, H. L., M. S. McCalla, I. Delke, R. Stevens, M. Salwen, and J. Feldman. 1990. The relationship of cocaine use to syphilis and human immunodeficiency virus infection among inner-city parturient women. *American Journal of Obstetrics and Gynecology* 163: 521–26.

Minkoff, H. L., and J. D. Moreno. 1990. Drug prophylaxis for human-immunodeficiency-virus-infected pregnant women: Ethical considerations. *American Journal of Obstetrics and Gynecology* 163(4): 1111–14.

Minkoff, H. L., and J. A. DeHovitz. 1991a. Care of women infected with the human immunodeficiency virus. *Journal of the American Medical Association* 266: 2253–58.

Minkoff, H. L., and J. A. DeHovitz. 1991b. HIV infection in women. *AIDS Clinical Care* 3(5): 33–35.

Minuk, G. Y., C. E. Bohme, T. J. Bowen, D. I. Hoar, S. Cassol, M. J. Gill, and H. C. Clark. 1987. Efficacy of commercial condoms in the prevention of hepatitis B virus infection. *Gastroenterology* 93: 710–14.

Mitchell, J. L. 1988. Women, AIDS, and public policy. *AIDS and Public Policy Journal* 3(2): 50–52.

Mitchell, J. L., and G. Brown. 1990. Physiological effects of cocaine, heroin, and methadone. In *Women: Alcohol and other drugs,* ed. R. Engs, 53–60. Dubuque, Iowa: Kendall/Hunt.

Mitchell, J. L., and M. Heagarty. 1991. Special considerations for minorities. In *Pediatric AIDS: The challenge of HIV infection in infants, children, and adolescents,* ed. P. A. Pizzo and C. M. Wilfert, 704–13. Baltimore: Williams and Wilkins.

Mitchell, J. L., J. Tucker, P. O. Loftman, and S. B. Williams. 1992. HIV and women: Current controversies and clinical relevance. *Journal of Women's Health* 1: 35–39.

Modan, B., R. Goldschmidt, E. Rubenstein, A. Vonsover, M. Zinn, R. Golan, A. Chetrit, and T. Gottlieb-Stematzky. Prevalence of HIV antibodies in transsexual and female prostitutes. *American Journal of Public Health* 82(4): 590–91.

Moore, R. D., J. Hidalgo, B. W. Sugland, and R. Chaisson. 1991. Zidovudine and the natural history of the acquired immunodeficiency syndrome. *New England Journal of Medicine* 324: 1412–16.

Moss, A. R., P. Bacchetti, D. Osmond, W. Krampf, R. E. Chaisson, D. Stites, J. Wilber, J. P. Allain, and J. Carlson. 1988. Seropositivity for HIV and the development of AIDS or AIDS related conditions: Three-year follow-up of the San Francisco General Hospital Cohort. *British Medical Journal* 296: 45–50.

Moss, G. B., D. Clemetson, L. D. Costa, F. A. Plummer, J. O. Ndinya-Achola, M. Reilly, K. K. Holmes, P. Piot, G. M. Maitha, S. L. Hillier, et al. 1991. Association of cervical ectopy with heterosexual transmission of human immunodeficiency virus: Results of a study of couples in Nairobi, Kenya. *Journal of Infectious Diseases* 164(3): 588–91.

Moss, G. B., and J. K. Kreiss. 1990. The interrelationship between human immunodeficiency virus infection and other sexually transmitted diseases. *Medical Clinics of North America* 74: 1647–60.

Moytl, M., B. Saltzman, M. Levi, J. C. McKitrick, H. H. Friedland, and R. S. Klein. 1990. The recovery of Mycobacterium avium complex and Mycobacterium tuberculosis from blood specimens of AIDS using the nonradiometric BACTEC NR 660 medium. *American Journal of Clinical Pathology* 94: 84–86.

Mukoyogo, M. C., and G. Williams. 1991. *AIDS orphans: A community perspective from Tanzania*. London: Actionaid.

Mundy, D. C., R. F. Schinazi, A. R. Gerber, A. J. Nahmias, and H. W. Randall. 1987. Letter: Human immunodeficiency virus isolated from amniotic fluid. *Lancet* 2: 459–60.

Muñoz, A., L. K. Schrager, I. Speizer, H. Bacellar, S. H. Vermund, R. Detels, A. J. Saah, C. Rinaldo, D. Seminara, and J. P. Phair. 1993. Trends and explanatory factors for the incidence of initial AIDS-defining outcomes in the Multicenter AIDS Cohort Study: 1984–1991. *American Journal of Epidemiology* 137: 423–38.

Musher, D. M., R. J. Hamill, and R. E. Baugh. 1990. Review: Effect of human immunodeficiency virus infection on the course of syphilis and on the response to treatment. *Annals of Internal Medicine* 113: 872–81.

Myers, J. K., M. M. Weissman, G. L. Tischler, C. E. Holzer III, P. J. Leaf, H. Orvaschel, J. C. Anthony, J. H. Boyd, J. D. Burke, M. Kramer, and R. Stoltzman. 1984. Six-month prevalence of psychiatric disorders in three communities (1980 to 1982). *Archives of General Psychiatry* 41: 959–67.

Nabarro, D., and C. McConnel. 1989. The impact of AIDS on socioeconomic development. *AIDS* 3(1): 826–28.

Nadler, J. P. 1992. HIV in your practice. *Emergency Medicine,* May 15, 133–153.

Nanda, D., and H. L. Minkoff. 1989. HIV in pregnancy-transmission and immune effects. *Clinical Obstetrics and Gynecology* 32: 456–66.

National Association of People with AIDS. 1992. Letter to the Commissioner, Social Security Administration. Washington, D.C.: NAPWA. February 18.

National Cancer Institute. 1989. The Bethesda system for reporting cervical/vaginal cytologic diagnoses. Developed at the NCI Workshop in Bethesda, Md., March 16.

National Institute of Allergy and Infectious Diseases (NIAID). 1990. Conference on state-of-the-art AZT therapy for early HIV infection: Executive summary. Bethesda, Md.

National Institute of Allergy and Infectious Diseases (NIAID) and Centers for Disease Control (CDC). 1991. U.S. Public Health Service National Conference: Women and HIV infection. *Clinical Courier* 9(6): 1–8.

National Institute on Drug Abuse (NIDA). 1992. Summary of research priorities from a five-year research planning meeting. Bethesda, Md., January 23–24, 1992.

National Institutes of Health. 1990. NIH/ADAMHA policy concerning inclusion of women in study populations. *NIH Guide* 19(31) August 24: 18–19.

National Institutes of Health. 1990. NIH/ADAMHA policy concerning inclusion of minorities in study populations. *NIH Guide* 19(35), September 28.

Navia, B. A., E. S. Cho, C. K. Petito, and R. W. Price. 1986. The AIDS dementia complex: II. Neuropathology. *Annals of Neurology* 19: 525–35.

Navia, B. A., B. D. Jordan, and R. W. Price. 1986. The AIDS dementia complex: I. Clinical features. *Annals of Neurology* 19: 517–24.

Negrini, B. P., M. H. Schiffman, R. J. Kurman, W. Barnes, L. Lannom, K. Malley, L. A. Brinton, G. Delgado, S. Jones, J. C. Tchabo, and W. D. Lancaster. 1990. Oral contraceptive use, human papillomavirus infection, and risk of early cytological abnormalities of the cervix. *Cancer Research* 50(15): 4670–75.

New York City Commission on Human Rights. 1990. HIV-related discrimination by reproductive health care providers in New York City. Law Enforcement Bureau, AIDS Discrimination Division.

New York City Department of Health. 1989. *Summary of vital statistics, 1988*. New York: Bureau of Health Statistics and Analysis.

———. 1991. *AIDS Surveillance Report*. December.

New York State Department of Health. 1989. Press release, *DOH News*. June 15.

———. 1991. *AIDS Surveillance Quarterly Update*. September.

———. 1992. *AIDS Surveillance Quarterly Update*. Cases reported through December 31, 1992.

New York State Department of Health, AIDS Institute. 1992. *Women and children with HIV infection in New York State: 1990–92 AIDS Institute program review.* January.

Newell, J. L. 1992. Risk factors for vertical transmission of HIV-1 infection. European Collaborative Study. Presented at the Eighth International Conference on AIDS. Amsterdam, July 19–24.

NIAID/NIH. 1991. *AIDS agenda,* ed. M. Warren. Rockville, Md.: NIAID/NIH.

Nicolau, D. P., and T. E. West. 1990. Treatment of severe recurrent aphthous stomatitis in patients with AIDS. *DICP, The Annals of Pharmacotherapy* 24: 1054–56.

Nicolosi, A., and Italian Partners Study. 1990. Different susceptibility of women and men to heterosexual transmission of HIV. Presented at Sixth International Conference on AIDS. San Francisco, June 21.

Niruthisard, S., R. Roddy, and S. Chutirongse. 1991. The effects of frequent nonoxynol-9 use on the vaginal and cervical mucosa. *Sexually Transmitted Diseases* 18(3): 176–79.

Nolan, K. 1989. Ethical issues in caring for pregnant women and newborns at risk for human immunodeficiency virus infection. *Seminars in Perinatology,* 13(1): 55–65.

Novell, M. K., G. I. Benrubi, and R. J. Thompson. 1984. Investigation of microtrauma after sexual intercourse. *Journal of Reproductive Medicine* 29: 269–71.

Novello, A. 1990. Excerpt from speech on women and HIV. *Journal of the American Medical Association* 265: 1805.

Novello, A. C., and J. R. Allen. 1991. Report of the U.S. Public Health Service panel on women, infants, and children with HIV infection and AIDS. Washington, D.C.: U.S. Public Health Service.

Novick L. F., D. M. Glebatis, R. L. Stricof, P. A. MacCubbin, L. Lessner, and D. S. Berns. 1991. Newborn seroprevalence study: Methods and results. *American Journal of Public Health* 81 (Suppl.): 15–21.

References

Obbo, C. 1991. HIV transmission: Men are the solution. A Ugandan perspective. Paper presented at AAAS Conference on Consequences of HIV in Eastern Africa, 14–19. Washington, D.C., February 14–19.

O'Dowd, M. A., and F. P. McKegney. 1990. AIDS patients compared with others seen in psychiatric consultation. *General Hospital Psychiatry* 12: 50–55.

O'Farrell, N., I. Windsor, and P. Becker. 1991. HIV-1 infection among heterosexual attenders at a sexually transmitted diseases clinic in Durban. *South African Medical Journal* 80: 17–20.

O'Grady, S. M., and K. E. Frasier. 1992. Recognizing and managing mycobacterial diseases in clients with AIDS. *Nurse Practitioner* 17(7): 41–45.

Olsen, W. L., F. M. Longo, C. M. Mills, and D. Norman. 1988. White matter disease in AIDS: Findings at MR imaging. *Radiology* 169: 445–48.

OPRR Reports of the NIH/PHS/HHS. Code of Federal Regulations: 45 CRF 46 (reprinted July 31, 1989).

Ostrow, D., I. Grant, and H. Atkinson. 1988. Assessment and management of the AIDS patient with neuropsychiatric disturbances. *Journal of Clinical Psychiatry* 49 (5, Suppl.): 14–22.

Padian, N. 1991. AIDSFILE 5(3): 2. Padian, N. S., S. C. Shiboski, and M. P. Jewel. 1991. Female-to-male transmission of human immunodeficiency virus. *Journal of the American Medical Association* 266(12): 1664–1667.

Padian, N., L. Marquis, D. P. Francis, R. E. Anderson, G. W. Rutherford, P. M. O'Malley, and W. Winklestein, Jr. 1987. Male-to-female transmission of human immunodeficiency virus. *Journal of the American Medical Association* 158(6): 788–90.

Padian, N., S. C. Shiboski, and N. P. Jewell. 1990. The effect of number of exposures on the risk of heterosexual HIV transmission. *Journal of Infectious Diseases* 161: 883–87.

Padian, N., J. Wiley, and W. Winkelstein. 1987. Male-to-female transmission of human immunodeficiency virus: Current results, infectivity rates, and San Francisco population seroprevalence estimates. Papers of the Third International Conference on AIDS. Washington, D.C., June 1–5.

PAHO/WHO. 1991. AIDS surveillance in the Americas: Health situation and trend assessment program. Press release, February 28, 1991.

Palefsky, J. M., J. Gonzales, R. M. Greenbelt, D. K. Ahn, and H. Hollander. 1990. Anal intraepithelial neoplasia and anal papillomavirus infection among homosexual males with group 4 HIV disease. *Journal of the American Medical Association* 263: 2911–16.

Panos Institute. 1990. *Triple jeopardy: Women and AIDS*. London: Panos Dossier.

Pappaioanou, M., T. J. Dondero, Jr., L. R. Petersen, I. M. Onorato, C. D. Sanchez, J. W. Curran. 1990. The family of HIV seroprevalence surveys: Objectives, methods, and uses of sentinel surveillance for HIV in the United States. *Public Health Reports* 105(2): 113–19.

Pelton, S. I, and J. O. Klein. 1991. Bacterial diseases in infants and children with infections due to human immunodeficiency virus. In *Pediatric AIDS: The challenge of HIV infection in infants, children, and adolescents*, ed. P. A. Pizzo and C. M. Wilfert, 199–208. Baltimore: Williams and Wilkins.

Pepin, J., et al. 1989. The interaction of HIV infection and other sexually transmitted diseases: An opportunity for intervention. *AIDS* 3: 3–9.

Perry, S., and R. R. Marotta. 1987. AIDS dementia: A review of the literature. *Alzheimer Disease and Associated Disorders* 1: 221–35.

Perry, S. W. 1990. Organic mental disorders caused by HIV: Update on early diagnosis and treatment. *American Journal of Psychiatry* 147: 696–710.

Peterson, E. P., N. J. Alexander, and K. S. Moghissi. 1988. A.I.D. and AIDS—too close for comfort. *Fertility and Sterility* 49(2): 209–11.

Pinn, V. 1992. Women's health research: Prescribing change and addressing issues. *Journal of the American Medical Association* 268(14): 1921–22.

Pivnick, A., M. Mulvihill, A. Jacobsen, M. A. Hsu, K. Eric, E. Drucker. 1991. Reproductive decisions among HIV-infected drug-using women: The importance of mother-child coresidence. *Medical Anthropology Quarterly* 5(2NS): 153–69.

Pizzo, P. A., and C. Wilfert. 1991. Treatment considerations for children with HIV infection. In *Pediatric AIDS: The challenge of HIV infection in infants, children, and adolescents,* ed. P. A. Pizzo and C. M. Wilfert, 478–94. Baltimore: Williams and Wilkins.

Plummer, F. A., J. N. Simonsen, D. W. Cameron, J. O. Ndinya-Achola, J. K. Kreiss, M. N. Gakinya, P. Waiyaki, M. Cheang, P. Piot, A. R. Ronald, and E. Ngugi. 1991. Cofactors in male-female sexual transmission of human immunodeficiency virus type-1. *Journal of Infectious Diseases* 163: 233–39.

Pohl, P., G. Vogl, H. Fill, H. Rossler, R. Zangerle, and F. Gerstenbrand. 1988. Single photon emission computed tomography in AIDS dementia complex. *Journal of Nuclear Medicine* 29: 1382–86.

Polk, B., R. Fox, R. Brookmeyer, S. Kanchanaraksa, R. Kaslow, B. Visscher, U. Rinaldo, and J. Phair. 1987. Predictors of the acquired immunodeficiency syndrome developing in a cohort of seropositive homosexual men. *New England Journal of Medicine* 316: 616.

Pond, S. M., M. J. Kreek, T. G. Tong, J. Raghunath, N. L. Benowitz. 1985. Altered methadone pharmacokinetics in methadone-maintained pregnant women. *Journal of Pharmacology and Experimental Therapy* 233: 1–6.

Portis, K. 1990. Women Inc.: A residential rehabilitation program for women in Dorchester, Mass. Presented at the National Conference on Women and HIV Infection. Washington, D.C., December.

Post, M. J. D., J. R. Berger, and R. M. Quencer. 1991. Asymptomatic and neurologically symptomatic HIV-seropositive individuals: Prospective evaluation with cranial MR imaging. *Radiology* 178: 131–39.

Preble, E. A. 1990. Impact of HIV/AIDS on African children. *Social Science and Medicine* 31(6): 671–80.

Price, R. W., B. Brew, J. Sidtis, M. Rosenblum, A. C. Scheck, and P. Cleary. 1988. The brain in AIDS: Central nervous system HIV-1 infection and AIDS dementia complex. *Science* 239: 586–92.

Price W., T. Merigan, T. Peterman, et al. 1989. Condom usage reported by female sexual partners of asymptomatic HIV seropositive hemophiliac men. Paper presented at the Fifth International Conference on AIDS. Montreal, June.

Provencher, D., et al. 1988. HIV status and positive Papanicolaou screening: Identification of a high-risk population. *Gynecologic Oncology* 31: 184–88.

Quick, P., M. Rees-Newton, I. Mackie, and J. Gilmour. 1991. Characteristics of women and men with HIV disease: A comparison of psychosocial issues. Paper presented at the Seventh International Conference on AIDS. Florence, June 16–21.

Quinn, T. C., R. L. Kline, N. Halsey, et al. 1991. Early diagnosis of perinatal HIV infection by detection of viral-specific IgA antibodies. *Journal of the American Medical Association* 266(24): 3439–42.

Rapp, R. 1987. Counseling women at risk: Models, myths, ambiguities. Talk presented at the Hastings Center, New York. December 1.

Reed, B. G. 1987. Developing women-sensitive drug dependence treatment services: Why so difficult? *Journal of Psychoactive Drugs* 19(2): 151–64.

Regan, D. O., S. M. Ehrlich, and L. P. Finnegan. 1987. Infants of drug addicts at risk for child abuse, neglect, and placement in foster care. *Neurotoxicology and Teratology* 9: 315–19.

Regier, D. A., J. H. Boyd, J. D. Burke, D. S. Rae, J. K. Myers, M. Karamer, L. N. Robins, L. K. George, M. Karno, and B. Z. Locke. 1988. One-month prevalence of mental disorders in the United States. *Archives of General Psychiatry* 45: 977–86.

Regier, D. A., M. E. Farmer, D. S. Rae, B. Z. Locke, S. J. Keith, L. L. Judd, and F. K. Goodwin. 1990. Comorbidity of mental disorders with alcohol and other drug abuse. *Journal of the American Medical Association* 264: 2511–18.

Rehmet, S., S. Staszewski, I. Von Wangenheim, L. Bergmann, E. B. Helm, H. W. Doerr, and W. Stille. 1990. HIV transmission rates and cofactors in heterosexual couples. Presented at Sixth International Conférence on AIDS. San Francisco, June 21.

Rekhart, M. L. 1988. HIV transmission by artificial insemination. Paper presented at the Fourth International Conference on AIDS. Stockholm, June.

Rhoads, J., C. Wright, R. Redfield, and D. Burke. 1987. Chronic vaginal candidiasis in women with human immunodeficiency virus infection. *Journal of the American Medical Association* 257: 3105–7.

Ricci, J. M., R. M. Fojaco, and M. J. O'Sullivan. 1989. Congenital syphilis: The University of Miami/Jackson Memorial Medical Center experience, 1986–1988. *Obstetrics and Gynecology* 74: 687–93.

Richwald, G., S. Greenland, M. M. Gerber, R. Potik, L. Kersey, and M. A. Comas. 1989. Effectiveness of the cavity-rim cervical cap: Results of a large clinical study. *Obstetrics and Gynecology* 74(2): 143–48.

Robins, L. N., J. E. Helzer, M. M. Weissman, H. Orvaschel, E. Gruenberg, J. D. Burke, and D. A. Regier. 1984. Lifetime prevalence of specific psychiatric disorders in three sites. *Archives of General Psychiatry* 41: 949–58.

Rodriguez, E. M., E. A. de Moya, E. Guerrero, E. R. Monterroso, T. C. Quinn, E. Paello, B. Thorington, P. D. Glasner, F. Zacharias, and S. H. Vermund. In press. HIV-1 and HTLV-1 in sexually transmitted disease clinics in the Dominican Republic. *Journal of Acquired Immune Deficiency Syndromes* 8(3): 313–18.

Rodriguez, E. M., L. Macy, S. Melnick, M. Caryln, G. Collins, and L. Deyton. 1991. Demographic and clinical characteristics of women enrolled in the Community Programs for Clinical Research on Aids. Paper presented at the Seventh International Conference on AIDS. Florence, June 16–21.

Rodriguez, E. M., S. Melnick, J. Korvick, R. Sherer, D. Lackman, D. Hillman, M. Carlyn, L. Capps, and L. Deyton. 1992. Gender and HIV-related therapy: Preliminary findings of the Observational Data Base of the Community Programs for Clinical Research on AIDS. Presented at the Eighth International Conference on AIDS, Amsterdam, July.

Rolfs, R. T., and A. K. Nakashima. 1990. Epidemiology of primary and secondary syphilis in the United States, 1981 through 1989. *Journal of the American Medical Association* 264: 1432–37.

Rosenberg, P. S., M. H. Gail, L. K. Schrager, S. H. Vermund, T. Creagh-Kirk, E. B. Andrews, W. Winkelstein, Jr., M. Marmor, D. C. DesJarlais, R. J. Biggar, and J. J. Goedert. 1991. National AIDS incidence trends and the extent of zidovudine therapy in selected demographic and transmission groups. *Journal of Acquired Immune Deficiency Syndrome* 4: 392–401.

Rosenblum, L., W. Darrow, J. Witte, J. Cohen, J. French, P. S. Gill, J. Potterat, K. Sikes, R. Reich, and S. Hadler. 1992. Sexual practices in the transmission of hepatitis B virus and prevalence of hepatitis delta virus infection in female prostitutes in the United States. *Journal of the American Medical Association* 267(18): 2477–81.

Rothenberg, R., M. Woelfel, R. Stoneburner, J. Milberg, R. Parker, and B. Truman. 1987. Survival with the acquired immunodeficiency syndrome: Experience with 5,833 cases in New York City. *New England Journal of Medicine* 317: 1297–1302.

Rottenberg, D. A., J. R. Moeller, S. C. Strother, J. J. Sidtis, B. A. Navia, V. Dhawan, J. Z. Ginos, and R. W. Price. 1987. The metabolic pathology of the AIDS dementia complex. *Annals of Neurology* 22: 700–706.

Rubinow, D. R., R. T. Joffe, P. Brouwers, K. Squillace, H. C. Lane, and A. F. Mirsky. 1988. Neuropsychiatric impairment in patients with AIDS. In *Psychological, neuropsychiatric, and substance abuse aspects of AIDS,* ed. T. P. Bridge, 111–15. New York: Raven Press.

Rubinstein, A., T. Calvelli, K. J. Reagan, and E. I. Devash. 1990. Antibodies to the gp120 principal neutralizing domain of the HIV-MN strain (gp120-MN-PND) as predictors of maternal-fetal transmission. Paper presented at the Sixth International Conference on AIDS. San Francisco, June.

Rundell, J. R., K. M. Kyle, G. R. Brown, and J. L. Thomason. 1992. Risk factors for suicide attempts in a human immunodeficiency virus screening program. *Psychosomatics* 33: 24–27.

Rutabanzibwe-Ngaiza, J., K. Heggenbougen, and G. Walt. 1985. *Women and health: A review of parts of sub-Saharan Africa, with a selected annotated bibliography.* London: Evaluation and Planning Centre for Health, London School of Hygiene and Tropical Medicine.

Rwandan HIV Seroprevalence Study Group. 1989. National community-based serologic survey of HIV 1 and other human retrovirus infections in a central African country. *Lancet* 1: 941–43.

Ryder, R. W., T. Mazila, E. Baende, U. Kabagabo, F. Behets, V. Batter, E. Paquot, E. Binyinggo, and W. L. Hayward. 1991. Evidence from Zaire that breastfeeding by HIV-1-seropositive mothers is not a major route for perinatal HIV-1 transmission but does decrease morbidity. *AIDS* 5: 709–14.

Ryndes, T. 1989. The coalition model of case management for care of HIV-infected persons. *Quality Review Bulletin* 15(1): 4–8.

Safrin, S., B. J. Dattel, I. L. Hauer, and R. I. L. Sweet. 1990. Seroprevalence and epidemiologic correlates of human immunodeficiency virus infection in women with acute pelvic inflammatory disease. *Obstetrics and Gynecology* 75: 666–70.

St. Louis, M. E., et al. 1991. Human immunodeficiency virus infection in disadvantaged adolescents. *Journal of the American Medical Association* 266: 2387.

Santangelo, J., and J. Schnack. 1991. Primary care intervention and management for adults with early HIV infection. *Nurse Practitioner* 16(6): 9–15.

Schafer, A., W. Friedmann, M. Mielke, B. Schwartlander, and M. A. Koch. 1991. The increased frequency of cervical dysplasia-neoplasia in women infected with the human immunodeficiency virus. *American Journal of Obstetrics and Gynecology* 164: 593–98.

Schecter, M. T., K. J. Craib, T. N. Le, B. Willoughby. 1989. Progression to AIDS and predictors of AIDS in seroprevalent and seroincident cohorts of homosexual men. *AIDS* 3(6): 347–53.

Schielke, E., K. Tatsch, H. W. Pfister, C. Trenkwalder, G. Leinsinger, C. M. Kirsch, A. Matuschke, and K. M. Einhaupl. 1990. Reduced cerebral blood flow in early stages of human immunodeficiency virus infection. *Archives of Neurology* 47: 1342–45.

Schietinger, H. 1990. Observations from Malawi, April through May.

———. 1992a. Observations from Rwanda, March 1 to April 15.

———. 1992b. Project to train volunteers to teach families to care for people with chronic illness including AIDS at home: Evaluation report. Kigali: Rwanda Red Cross.

Schilling, R. F., N. Ei-Bassel, S. P. Schinke, K. Gordon, and S. Nichols. 1991. Building skills of recovering women drug users to reduce heterosexual AIDS transmission. *Public Health Reports* 106(3): 297- 304.

Schilling, R. F., S. P. Schinke, S. E. Nichols, L. H. Zayas, S. O. Miller, M. O. Orlandi, and G. J. Botvin. 1989. Developing strategies for AIDS prevention research with black and Hispanic drug users. *Public Health Reports* 104(1): 2–11.

Schmid, G. P. 1990. Approach to the patient with genital ulcer disease. *Medical Clinics of North America* 74: 1559–72.

Schmitt, F. A., J. W. Bigley, R. McKinnis, P. E. Logue, R. W. Evans, J. L. Drucker, and the AZT Collaborative Working Group. 1988. Neuropsychological outcome of zidovudine treatment of patients with AIDS and AIDS-related complex. *New England Journal of Medicine* 319: 1573–78.

Schrager, L. K., G. H. Friedland, D. Maud, K. Schreiber, A. Adachi, D. J. Pizzuti, L. G. Koss, and R. S. Klein. 1989. Cervical and vaginal squamous cell-abnormalities in women infected with human immunodeficiency virus. *Journal of Acquired Immune Deficiency Syndrome* 2: 571–575.

Schuman, P., R. Kauffman, L. R. Crane, and D. Philpot. 1990. Pharmacokinetics of zidovudine during pregnancy. Paper presented at the Sixth International Conference on AIDS. San Francisco, June.

Scott, G. B., and C. Hutto. 1991. Prognosis in pediatric HIV infection. In *Pediatric AIDS: The challenge of HIV infection in infants, children, and adolescents,* ed. P. A. Pizzo and C. M. Wilfert, 187–98. Baltimore: Williams and Wilkins.

Scura, K. W., and B. Whipple. 1990. Older adults as an HIV-positive risk group. *Journal of Gerontological Nursing* 16: 6–10.

Seitz V., L. Rosenbaum, and N. Apfel. 1985. Effects of family support intervention: A ten year follow-up. *Child Development* 56: 376–91.

Selwyn, P. A., R. J. Carter, E. E. Schoenbaum, V. J. Robertson, R. S. Klein, M. F. Rogers. 1989b. Knowledge of HIV antibody status and decisions to continue or terminate pregnancy among intravenous drug users. *Journal of the American Medical Association* 261: 3567–71.

Selwyn, P. A., E. E. Schoenbaum, K. Davenny, V. J. Roberston, A. R. Feingold, J. F. Shulman, M. M. Mayers, R. S. Klein, G. H. Friedland, and M. F. Rogers. 1989a. Prospective study of human immunodeficiency virus infection and pregnancy outcomes in intravenous drug users. *Journal of the American Medical Association* 261: 1289–94.

Septimus, A. 1989. Psychosocial aspects of caring for families of infants infected with HIV. *Seminars in Perinatology* 13: 49–54.

Serrano, Y. 1990. The Puerto Rican intravenous-drug user. In *AIDS and intravenous drug use: Future directions for community-based prevention research,* NIDA research monograph no. 93, 24–34, ed. C. G. Leukefeld, R. J. Battjes, and Z. Amsel. Washington, D.C.: U.S. Department of Health, Education and Welfare.

Sillman, F. H., and A. Sedlis. 1987. Anogenital papillomavirus infection and neoplasia in immunodeficient women. *Obstetrics and Gynecology Clinics of North America* 14(2): 537–57.

Simon, L. L. 1989. Report of the Connecticut Commission on Children, General Assembly, Hartford.

Simonsen, J., B. Cameron B, M. Gakina M, M. N. Gakinya, J. O. Ndinya-Achola, L. J. da Costa, et al. 1988. Human immunodeficiency virus among men with sexually transmitted diseases: Experiences from the center in Africa. *New England Journal of Medicine* 319: 274–78.

Simpson B. J. 1991. Pediatric AIDS in the context of kinship foster care in Connecticut. Master's thesis, University of Connecticut.

Slaughter, R. 1990. HIV education and prevention strategies for women: The WARN Project. Presented at the National Conference on Women and HIV Infection. Washington, D.C., December.

Smith, E., V. Hasseltvedt, and M. Bottinger. 1991. Trends in the AIDS epidemic among Scandanavian women: A status by 30.9.1990. Presented at the Seventh International Conference on AIDS. Florence, June 16–21.

Smith, J. R., G. E. Forster, V. S. Kitchen, Y. S. Hooi et al. 1991. Infertility management in HIV-positive couples: A dilemma. *British Medical Journal* 302(6790): 1447–50.

Smith, P. F., J. Mikl, K. Kelley, and D. Putnam. 1992. Impact of the Centers for Disease Control proposed 1992 AIDS case definition on AIDS cases reported in New York State exclusive on New York City. Paper presented at the Eighth International Conference on AIDS. Amsterdam, July 19–24.

Sobel, J. D. 1990. Therapeutic considerations in fungal vaginitis. In *Chemotherapy of fungal diseases,* ed. J. F. Ryley. Chicago: Springer.

Society for Women and AIDS in Africa (SWAA). 1991. SWAA: Report on Third International Conference on women and AIDS in Africa. Yaonde, Cameroon, November 19–22.

Solomon, L., and R. Denenberg. 1992. Bronx-Lebanon Hospital Center. Personal communication, telephone, January 8.

Solomon, M. S., and W. DeJong. 1989. Preventing AIDS and other STDs through condom promotion: A patient education intervention. *American Journal of Public Health* 78(4): 460–61.

Sonsel, G. E. 1989. Case management in a community-based agency. *Quality Review Bulletin* 15(1): 31–36.

Sontag, S. 1988. *AIDS and its metaphors.* New York: Farrar, Straus, and Giroux.

Soyka, L. F., and J. M. Joffe. 1980. Male-mediated drug effects on offspring. In *Drug and Chemical Risks to the Fetus and Newborn,* ed. R. H. Schwartz and S. J. Yaffe. New York: Alan R. Liss.

Sperling, R. S., P. Stratton, and the Obstetric-Gynecologic Working Group of the AIDS Clinical Trials Group of the NIAID. 1992a. Treatment options for human immunodeficiency virus-infected pregnant women. *Obstetrics and Gynecology* 79: 443–48.

Sperling, R. S., P. Stratton, M. J. O'Sullivan, et al. 1992b. A survey of zidovudine use in pregnant women with human immunodeficiency virus infection. *New England Journal of Medicine* 326: 857–61.

Speroff, L, R. H. Glass, and N. G. Kase. 1989. Amenorrhea. In *Clinical gynecologic endocrinology and infertility,* 4th ed. Baltimore: Williams and Wilkins.

Spino, C. 1992. Statistical and Data Anaylsis Center, Boston, of the ACTG data base gender analysis through May 1992. Personal communication, letter.

Spitzer, P. G., and N. J. Weiner. 1989. Transmission of HIV infection from a woman to a man by oral sex. *New England Journal of Medicine* 320: 251.

Spurrett, B., D. S. Jones, and G. Stewart. 1988. Cervical dysplasia and HIV infection. *Lancet* 1: 237–39.

Squires, S. 1989. Leprosy's legacy. *Washington Post,* April 25, Health sec., 13–17.

Stack, C. B. 1974. *All our kin,* 62–120. New York: Harper and Row.

Stamm, W., H. Hammersfield, and A. Rompalo. 1988. The association between genital ulcer disease and acquisition of HIV infection in homosexual men. *Journal of the American Medical Association* 260: 1429–33.

Staugaart, S. Anderson, and F. Staugard. 1986. *Traditional medicine in Botswana: Traditional midwives,* 23. Gaborone, Botswana: Ipelegeng.

Stein, D. S., J. A. Korvick, and S. H. Vermund. 1992. CD4+ lymphocyte cell enumeration for prediction of clinical course of human immunodeficiency virus disease: A review. *Journal of Infectious Diseases* 165: 352–63.

Stein, M. D., J. Piette, V. Mor, T. Wachtel, J. Felishman, K. Mayer, and C. Carpenter. 1991. Differences in zidovudine among symptomatic HIV-infected persons. *Journal of General Internal Medicine* 6: 35–40.

Stein, Z. A. 1990. HIV Prevention: The need for methods women can use. *American Journal of Public Health* 80: 460–62.

Stevens, C. E., P. E. Taylor, E. A. Zong, J. M. Morrison, E. J. Harley, S. Rodriguez de Cordoba, C. Bacino, R. C.Y. Ting, A. J. Bodner, M. G. Sarngadharan, R. C. Gallo, and P. Rubinstein. 1986. Human T-cell lymphotropic virus-3 infection in a cohort of homosexual men in New York City. *Journal of the American Medical Association* 255: 2167–72.

Stewart, G. J., J. P. P. Tyler, A. L. Cunningham, J. A. Barr, G. L. Driscoll, J. Gold, and B. J. Lamont. 1985. Transmission of human T-cell lymphotropic virus type 3 by artificial insemination by donor. *Lancet* September 14: 581–84.

Stone, K., and H. Peterson. 1992. Spermicides, HIV, and the vaginal sponge. *Journal of the American Medical Association* 268(4): 521–23.

Stoneburner, A., M. A. Chaisson, I. B.Weisfuse, and P. A. Thomas. 1990. The epidemic of AIDS and HIV-1 infection among heterosexuals in New York City. *AIDS* 4(2): 99–106.

Sunderland, A. 1990. Influence of human immunodeficiency virus infection on reproductive decisions. *Obstetrics and Gynecology Clinics of North America* 17(3): 585–94.

Sunderland, A., G. Moroso, M. Berthaud, S. Holman, S. Landesman, H. Minkoff, F. Cancellieri, and H. Mendez. 1988. Influence of HIV infection on pregnancy decisions. Paper presented at the Fourth International Conference on AIDS, Stockholm, June.

Swigar, M. E., M. B. Bowers, and S. Fleck. 1976. Grieving and unplanned pregnancy. *Psychiatry* 39: 72–80.

Szabo, S., L. H. Miller, H. S. Sacks, A. C. Gurtman, D. N. Rose, R. A. Kee, T. W. Cheung, and S. E. Cohen. 1992. Gender differences in the natural history of HIV infection. Paper presented at the Eighth International Conference on AIDS. Amsterdam, July 19–24.

Temmerman, M., S. Moses, D. Kiragu, S. Fusallah, I. A. Wamola, and P. Piot. 1990. Impact of single session postpartum counselling of HIV infected women on their subsequent reproductive behavior. *AIDS Care* 2(3): 247–52.

Thiesen, R. J. 1984. *Agro-economic factors relating to the health and academic achievement of rural school children.* Salisbury [Harare], Zimbabwe: Tribal Areas of Rhodesia Research Foundation.

Thompson, E., and M. Thompson. 1976. *Homeboy came to Orange: A story of people's power.* Newark: Bridgebuilder Press.

Thompson, M., B. Whyte, A. Morris, D. Rimland, and S. Thompson. 1991. Gender differences in the spectrum of HIV disease in Atlanta. Paper presented at the Seventh International Conference on AIDS. Florence, June 16–21.

Tillmann, M., and B. Wigdahl. 1991. Neuropathogenesis of human immunodeficiency virus infection. *Seminars in the Neurosciences* 3: 131–39.

Tracy, C. E., and H. C. Williams. 1991. Social consequences of substance abuse among pregnant and parenting women. *Pediatric Annals* 20: 548–53.

Tross, S., and D. A. Hirsch. 1988. Psychological distress and neuropsychological complications of HIV infection and AIDS. *American Psychologist* 43: 929–34.

Tross, S., R. W. Price, B. Navia, H. T. Thaler, J. Gold, D. A. Hirsch, and J. J. Sidtis. 1988. Neuropsychological characteristics of the AIDS dementia complex: A preliminary report. *AIDS* 2: 81–88.

Trussell, J., R. A. Hatcher, W. Cates, Jr., F. H. Stewart, and K. Kost. 1990. Contraceptive failure in the United States: An update. *Studies in Family Planning* 21(1): 51–54.

Tuomala, R. 1990. Human immunodeficiency virus education and screening of prenatal patients. *Obstetrics and Gynecology Clinics of North America* 17(3): 571–83.

Turner, B. J., L. E. Markson, L. McKee, and T. Fanning. 1991. Survival patterns of women and men with AIDS: Impact of health care use prior to AIDS. Paper presented at the Seventh International Conference on AIDS. Florence, June 16–21.

Ulin, P. 1992. African women and AIDS: Negotiating behavior change. *Social Science and Medicine* 34(1): 63–73.

UNICEF. 1990. *Children and AIDS: An impending calamity.* New York: UNICEF.

United Nations. 1992. *AIDS: International response to a global threat.* Geneva: U.N. Dept. of Public Information.

Valenti, W. M. 1992. Early intervention in the management of HIV. Rochester, N.Y.: Community Health Network.

Van de Perre, P., D. Jacobs, and S. Sprecher-Goldberger. 1987. The latex condom, an efficient barrier against sexual transmission of AIDS-related virus. *Journal of AIDS* 1: 49–52.

Varney, H. 1987. *Nurse-Midwifery,* 2d ed. Boston: Blackwell Scientific.

Verdegem, T. D., F. R. Sattler, and C. T. Boylen. 1988. Increased fatality from Pneumocystis carinii pneumonia in women with AIDS. Poster presented at the Fourth International Conference on AIDS. Stockholm, June.

Vermund, S. H., M. A. Galbraith, S. C. Ebner, A. R. Sheon, and R. A. Kaslow. 1992. Human immunodeficiency virus/acquired immunodeficiency syndrome in pregnant women. *Annals of Epidemiology* 2(6) 773–803.

Vermund, S. H., and K. F. Kelley. 1990. Human papillomavirus in women: Methodologic issues and the role of immunosuppression. In *Reproductive and perinatal epidemiology,* ed. M. Kiely, 143–68. Boca Raton, Fla.: CRC Press.

Vermund, S. H., K. F. Kelley, R. D. Burk, A. R. Feingold, K. Schreiber, G. Munk, L. K. Schrager, and R. S. Klein. 1990. Risk of human papillomavirus and cervical squamous intraepithelial lesions highest among women with advanced HIV disease. Paper presented at the Sixth International Conference on AIDS. San Francisco, June 20–24.

Vermund, S. H., K. F. Kelley, R. S. Klein, A. R. Feingold, K. K. Schreiber, G. Munk, and R. D. Burk. 1991b. High risk of human papillomavirus infection and cervical squamous intraepithelial lesions among women with symptomatic human immunodeficiency virus infection. *American Journal of Obstetrics and Gynecology* 165: 392–400.

Vermund, S. H., A. R. Sheon, M. A. Gailbraith, S. C. Ebner, and R. D. Fischer. 1991a. Transmission of the human immunodeficiency virus. In *AIDS Research Reviews,* ed. C. Koff, F. Wong-Staal, and R. C. Kennedy, vol. 1, 81–136. New York: Marcel Dekker.

Vessey, M. P., K. McPherson, M. Lawless, and D. Yeates. 1983. Neoplasia of the cervix uteri and contraception: A possible adverse effect of the pill. *Lancet* 2: 930–34.

Voeller, B. 1991. AIDS and heterosexual anal intercourse. *Archives of Sexual Behavior* 20(3): 233–76.

Vogt, M. W., D. E. Craven, D. F. Crawford, D. J. Witt, R. Byington, R. T. Schooley, and M. S. Hirsch. 1986. Isolation of HTLV-3/LAV from cervical secretions of women at risk for AIDS. *Lancet* 1: 525–27.

Wagnild, G., and H. M. Young. 1990. Resilience among older women. *Image* 22: 252–55.

Wallace, D., and R. Wallace. 1990. The burning down of New York City: Its causes and its impacts. *Anthropos* 12: 256–72.

Wallace, R. 1988. A synergism of plagues: "Planned shrinkage," contagious housing destruction, and AIDS in the Bronx. *Environmental Research* 47: 1–33.

———. 1990. Urban desertification, public health, and public order: "Planned shrinkage," violent death, substance abuse and AIDS in the Bronx. *Social Science and Medicine* 31(7): 801–13.

Wallace, R., M. Thompson, R. Thompson, and P. Gould. 1992. The U.S. urban crisis and diffusion of HIV into affluent heterosexual populations. Article under review.

Warne, P. A., A. Ehrhardt, D. Schecter, J. Williams, and J. Gorman. 1991. Menstrual abnormalities in HIV+ and HIV- women with a history of intravenous drug use. Paper presented at the Seventh International Conference on AIDS. Florence, June.

Weil, M. 1985. Key components in providing efficient and effective services. In *Case management in human service practice,* ed. M. Weil and J. Karls, 29–71. San Francisco: Jossey-Bass.

Weinstein, M. 1991. *Add AIDS to the list: AIDS prevention in the black community.* San Francisco: San Francisco State University.

Weisman, M. F., P. B. Slobetz, M. Meritz, and P. Howard. 1976. Clinical depression among narcotic addicts maintained on methadone in the community. *American Journal of Psychiatry* 133: 1434–38.

Weissman, G. 1991. Working with pregnant women at high risk for HIV infection: Outreach and intervention. *Bulletin of the New York Academy of Medicine* 67: 291–300.

Weissman, G. 1991. Women at risk: Experience from a national prevention research program. Presented at the Annual Meeting of the American Psychological Association. Boston, August.

Weissman, G. 1992. *Morbidity and Mortality Weekly Report.* January.

West, H. M. 1988. Factors impacting on the pediatric AIDS population. Master's thesis, Yale University School of Nursing.

WHO. See World Health Organization.

Whyte, B., C. Swanson, and D. Cooper. 1989. Survival of patients with the acquired immunodeficiency syndrome in Australia. *Medical Journal of Australia* 150: 358–62.

Wilhelm, K., and G. Parker. 1989. Is sex necessarily a risk factor to depression? *Psychological Medicine* 19: 401–13.

Wilkins, H. A. 1992. HIV infection in Africa. *Nature* 356: 393–94.

Williams, A. 1990. Reproductive concerns of women at risk for HIV infection. *Journal of Nurse-Midwifery* 35(5): 292–98.

———. 1992. The epidemiology, clinical manifestations, and health-maintenance needs of women infected with HIV. *Nurse Practitioner* 17: 27–44.

References

Winkelstein, W., Jr., D. Lyman, N. Padian, R. Grant, M. Samuel, J. A. Wiley, R. E. Anderson, W. Lang, J. Riggs, and J. A. Levy. 1987. Sexual practices and risk of infection by the human immunodeficiency virus: The San Francisco Men's Health Study. *Journal of the American Medical Association* 257: 321–25.

Wiznia, A., C. Bueti, C. Douglas, T. Cabat, and A. Rubinstein. 1989. Factors influencing maternal decision-making regarding pregnancy outcome in HIV infected women. Paper presented at the Fifth International Conference on AIDS. Montreal, June.

Wiznia, A., and S. W. Nicholas. 1990. Organ system involvement in HIV-infected children. *Pediatric Annals* 19: 475–81.

Wofsy, C. B. 1987. Human immunodeficiency virus infection in women. *Journal of the American Medical Association* 257(15): 2075–76.

Wofsy, C. B., L. B. Hauer, B. A. Michaelis, J. B. Cohen, N. S. Padian, L. A. Evans, and J. A. Levy. 1986. Isolation of AIDS-associated retrovirus from genital secretions of women with antibodies to the virus. *Lancet* 1: 527–29.

Wofsy, C. B., N. S. Padian, J. B. Cohen, R. Greenblat, R. Coleman, and J. A. Korvick. 1992. Management of HIV disease in women. In *AIDS Clinical Review 1992,* ed. P. Volberding and M. A. Jacobson, 301–28. New York: Marcel Dekker.

World Health Organization (WHO). 1990. *Report of the second consultation on the neuropsychiatric aspects of HIV-1 infection.* Geneva: WHO.

———. 1991. *Review of six HIV/AIDS home care programmes in Uganda and Zambia.* Geneva: WHO GPA/IDS/HCS/91.3.

———. 1992a. *Global Programme on AIDS:. The current global situation of the HIV/AIDS pandemic.* Geneva: WHO.

———. 1992b. *Current and future dimensions of the HIV/AIDS pandemic.: A capsule summary.* Geneva: WHO (WHO/GPA/RES/SFI/92.1).

———. 1992c. AIDS prevention does work. Press release WHO/44, June 22.

Worth, D. 1990. Women at high risk of HIV infection. In *Behavioral Aspects of AIDS,* ed. D. G. Ostrow, 101–19. New York: Plenum.

Worth, D. 1990. Minority women and AIDS: Culture, race, and gender. In *Culture and AIDS,* ed. D. Feldman. New York: Praeger, 111–35.

Worth, D., and R. Rodriguez. 1987. Latina women and AIDS. *SIECUS Report* January–February: 6–7.

Wyatt, G. E. 1988. Ethnic and cultural differences in women's sexual behavior. In NIMH/NIDA Workshop on Women and AIDS: Promoting Healthy Behaviors. Volume of background papers for workshop in Bethesda, Md., Sept. 27–29. Rockville, Md.: National Institute of Mental Health.

Yale-New Haven Hospital. 1992. Demographic data from the Pediatric AIDS Care Program, obtained May 15 by research nurse B. Joyce Simpson.

Yarchoan, R., H. Mitsuya, R. V. Thomas, J. M. Pluda, N. R. Hartman, C.-P. Perno, K. S. Marczyk, J.-P. Allain, D. G. Johns, and S. Broder. 1989. In vivo activity against HIV and favorable toxicity profile of 2',3'-dideoxyinosine. *Science* 245: 412–15.

Yazigi, R. A., R. R. Odem, and K. L. Polakoski. 1991. Demonstration of specific binding of cocaine to human spermatozoa. *Journal of the American Medical Association* 266(14): 1956–59.

Ybarra, S. 1991. Women and AIDS: Implications for counseling. *Journal of Counseling and Development* 69: 285–87.

Young, M., E. Marx, I. Rafi, M. Doherty, and P. Pierce. 1992. Characteristics of HIV disease in an urban cohort of women in Washington, D.C. Paper presented at the Eighth International Conference on AIDS. Amsterdam, July 19–24.

Zarembka, A., and K. Franke. 1991. Women and AIDS, part two: Controlling HIV-positive women or meeting their needs. *The Exchange* NLG AIDS Network, San Francisco: 4.

Zwi, A. B., and A. J. R. Cabral. 1991. Identifying "high risk" situations for preventing AIDS. *British Medical Journal* 303: 1597–99.

Contributors

Kathyrn Anastos, MD, is a primary-care internist at Bronx-Lebanon Hospital Center, New York. She is medical director of the Bronx Morrisania Ambulatory Care Unit and director of HIV Primary Care Services.

Kathryn Carovano, MA, was a senior program officer for the Center for Communication Programs of Johns Hopkins University and a member of the technical advisory group for the Women and AIDS Program of the International Center for Research on Women.

Judith Cohen, MA, MPH, PhD, cofounded the Association for Women's AIDS Research and Education in 1984. She is program director for AWARE and a research epidemiologist at the University of California, San Francisco.

Risa Denenberg, FNP, is a nurse-practitioner and nurse-colposcopist in the HIV and gynecology clinics at Bronx-Lebanon Hospital Center, New York, and a primary-care scholar in HIV and substance abuse at Montefiore Medical Center, New York.

Ilene Fennoy, MD, is assistant clinical professor of pediatrics at Columbia University and associate attending and associate director of the department of pediatrics at Harlem Hospital Center, New York.

Mindy Thompson Fullilove, MD, is associate professor of clinical psychiatry and public health at Columbia University.

Helen Gasch, MPH, is a doctoral candidate in sociomedical sciences at Columbia University School of Public Health and director of the obstetrical initiative, New York Department of Health's AIDS Institute.

Susan Holman, RNC, MS, is a certified adult nurse-practitioner involved in AIDS-related research at SUNY Health Science Center, Brooklyn, New York. She is visiting assistant clinical professor at SUNY-HSC Brooklyn College of Nursing and consultant to the New York State Department of Health AIDS Institute.

Margaret Hutchison, MSN, CNM, is a certified nurse-midwife at the San Francisco General Hospital/University of San Francisco Nurse Midwifery Service and Education Program.

Joyce A. Korvick, MD, is associated with the Division of AIDS at the National Institute of Allergy and Infectious Diseases, National Institutes of Health.

Ann Kurth, MPH, MSN, CNM, is director of clinical data and research, Division of Acquired Diseases, Indiana State Department of Health.

Carol Levine, MA, is executive director of the Orphan Project: The HIV Epidemic and New York City's Children. She is author of *Taking Sides: Controversial Issues in Biomedical Ethics* (Dushkin, 4th ed., 1991).

Patricia Loftman, MS, CNM, is director of Midwifery Service at Harlem Hospital Center, New York, and instructor in clinical nursing at Columbia University.

Iris L. Long, PhD, is a certified professional chemist who has worked as the scientific adviser to AIDS Coalition to Unleash Power (ACT-UP) and as a consultant to the AIDS Institute of New York.

Jonathan Mann, MD, MPH, is François-Xavier Bagnoud Professor of Health and Human Rights; professor of epidemiology and international health, Harvard School of Public Health; and director of the International AIDS Center, Harvard AIDS Institute.

Janet L. Mitchell, MD, MPH, is chief of perinatology at Harlem Hospital Center, New York City, and assistant professor in obstetrics and gynecology at Columbia University.

Kathy M. Sanders, MD, is a member of the department of psychiatry at Massachusetts General Hospital.

Helen Schietinger, MS, RN, has developed community-based services for people with AIDS in the United States and Africa.

Maureen Shannon, MS, CNM, FNP, is a nurse-practitioner and certified nurse-midwife in the department of obstetrics, gynecology, and reproductive infectious disease at San Francisco General Hospital/University of San Francisco. She is a clinical nurse researcher for the Bay Area Perinatal AIDS Center.

B. Joyce Simpson, RN, MPH, is pediatric HIV coordinator for the care of children born to HIV-infected mothers at Yale-New Haven Hospital.

Ann Sunderland, MSW, MPH, was the social work supervisor for the perinatal HIV transmission study at SUNY Health Science Center-Brooklyn.

John Tucker, MD, was a perinatologist and assistant clinical professor of obstetrics and gynecology at Harlem Hospital Center. Tucker, an avid and well-loved teacher, died in November 1992.

Sten H. Vermund, MD, PhD, is chief of the epidemiology branch in the Clinical Research Program, Division of AIDS, National Institute of Allergy and Infectious Diseases, National Institutes of Health. He also is associate clinical professor of epidemiology and social medicine at Albert Einstein College of Medicine, New York.

Krystn Wagner, PhD, was formerly with the AIDS Division of USAID. She is currently a student at the Yale University School of Medicine.

Ann Williams, RNC, EdD, FAAN, is associate professor of adult health nursing at Yale School of Nursing and family nurse-practitioner with the AIDS Care Program of Yale-New Haven Hospital.

Sterling B. Williams, MD, is vice-chairman of academic affairs, Columbia-Presbyterian Medical Center, Department of Obstetrics and Gynecology.

Laura J. Wittig is a graduate student in family studies at Purdue University.

Mary Young, MD, is an infectious-disease physician in a research clinic run by the medical center at Georgetown University Hospital.

Michele A. Zavos, JD, is project director of the American Bar Association's AIDS Coordination Project and adjunct professor in Women's Studies at the George Washington University.

Send correspondence to
    Ann Kurth
    Indiana State Department of Health
    Division of Acquired Diseases
    1330 West Michigan Street
    Indianapolis, Indiana 46206–1964

Telephone: (317) 633-0661
Fax: (317) 633-0663

Index

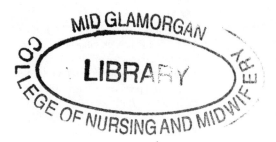